Psychoanalysis and Culture at the Millennium

Psychoanalysis and Culture at the Millennium

Edited by Nancy Ginsburg
and Roy Ginsburg

Yale University Press   New Haven and London

Copyright © 1999 by Yale University.
"The Construction of National Identity" Copyright © 1997
by Peter Loewenberg.
"To the Egyptian Dig: Freud's Exploration in Western Culture"
Copyright © Carl E. Schorske.
All rights reserved.
This book may not be reproduced, in whole
or in part, including illustrations, in any form
(beyond that copying permitted by Sections 107 and 108
of the U.S. Copyright Law and except by reviewers
for the public press), without written permission
from the publishers.

Set in Caslon type by Tseng Information Systems.
Printed in the United States of America.

Library of Congress Cataloging-in-Publication Data
Psychoanalysis and culture at the millennium / edited by Nancy Ginsburg
and Roy Ginsburg
p. cm.
Includes bibliographical references and index.
ISBN 0-300-07190-6 (alk. paper)
1. Psychoanalysis and culture. 2. Popular culture—Psychological aspects.
3. Freud, Sigmund, 1856-1939. I. Ginsburg, Nancy, 1944- .
II. Ginsburg, Roy, 1943-1992.
BF175.4.C84P8 1998
150.40'5—dc21 98-37423
CIP

A catalogue record for this book is
available from the British Library.

The paper in this book meets the guidelines
for permanence and durability of the Committee
on Production Guidelines for Book Longevity of
the Council on Library Resources.

10 9 8 7 6 5 4 3 2 1

CONTENTS

Part IV
Art

Part V
Psychoanalysis and Culture

Part VI
Epilogue

PREFACE

This book is a broad exploration of the relation between twentieth-century thought and psychoanalysis as we approach the millennium. It was inspired by a conference, "Psychoanalysis and Culture: The Contributions of Sigmund Freud," held at Stanford University in January 1991. That interdisciplinary conference was organized by my late husband, Roy Ginsburg, to coincide with the exhibition of Freud's collection of antiquities that Lynn Gamwell had brought to Stanford. Distinguished psychoanalysts and scholars from the United States and Europe gathered to discuss the influence of psychoanalysis on modern thought, and papers on history, art, literature, and philosophy were presented to a large audience.

Roy was the tireless chairman of that conference. He was a man of great energy, enthusiasm, and ideas, and his death in 1992 left many projects undone. This volume was in the early stages of development at that time, and I have completed it with a mixture of sadness and excitement.

Although this volume was stimulated by the conference, Roy and those who attended might not recognize it as an outgrowth of that event. Only four of the fifteen essays here were presented at the conference. Six other contributors to this book participated in the conference but gave different presentations, and five authors were not conference participants but were asked to write for this book. I believe that the result is as lively as is psychoanalysis as we approach the millennium.

I thank all the authors for their invaluable contributions to this book. Not only did they generously allow their ideas and writing to be included, but many were helpful in other specific ways that supported my efforts to get the book published. I want to especially thank Lynn Gamwell, whose exhibition of Freud's antiquities inspired the conference, and whose friendship and enthusiastic support inspired me in the early stages. Richard Almond is gratefully acknowledged for his continued support and for suggesting that I consider Jerome A. Winer as the literature discussant. Peter Loewenberg's support has been greatly appreciated, along with his cheerful willingness to continue to rewrite his essay so that it would be timely. Paul Schwaber gets special thanks because his periodic calls to inquire about the progress of the book kept me from giving up at many discouraging moments. I am grateful to Robert Wallerstein for suggesting that I contact Gladys Topkis at Yale University Press, and I am especially grateful to her for supporting this publication. Special thanks also go to Heidi Downey and Chris Erikson at Yale University Press.

Versions of the following chapters have appeared in other publications.

Richard Almond: *The Therapeutic Narrative: Fictional Relationships and the Process of Psychological Change,* Barbara Almond and Richard Almond. Praeger, 1996. Praeger is an imprint of Greenwood Publishing Group, Inc., Westport, Connecticut. Used with permission.

Lynn Gamwell: *A Century of Silence: Abstraction and Withdrawal in Modern Art.* Exhibition catalogue. Binghamton: Binghamton University Art Museum, State University of New York, 1993.

Ellen Handler Spitz: "Primary Art Objects," in *The Psychoanalytic Study of the Child*. Vol. 44. New Haven: Yale University Press, 1989. Reprinted with permission.

Richard Kuhns: *Contemporary Psychoanalysis* 29, no. 1 (January 1993). Reprinted with permission.

Nancy Ginsburg

Contributors

Richard Almond is a member of the faculty at the San Francisco Psychoanalytic Institute and is clinical professor of psychiatry at the Stanford University School of Medicine. He has a private practice in Palo Alto, California.

Janine Chasseguet-Smirgel is a training analyst at the Paris Psychoanalytic Society and in private practice.

Lynn Gamwell is director of the University Art Museum at the State University of New York at Binghamton, where she is also associate professor of art history.

Charles Hanly is professor of philosophy at the University of Toronto. He is also in private psychoanalytic practice.

Richard Kuhns is professor of philosophy at Columbia University.

Peter Loewenberg is professor of history at the University of California at Los Angeles and a psychoanalyst in private practice.

Paul Robinson is the Richard W. Lyman Professor of the Humanities at Stanford University.

Eli Sagan is professor of sociology at the New School for Social Research.

Carl E. Schorske is professor emeritus of history at Princeton University.

Paul Schwaber is professor of letters at Wesleyan University and a psychoanalyst in private practice.

Ellen Handler Spitz is lecturer, department of art, Stanford University.

Marcelo M. Suárez-Orozco is professor of human development and psychology; member of the executive committee of the David Rockefeller Center for Latin American Studies; and faculty associate, Harvard Center for International Affairs, Harvard University.

John Toews is professor of history at the University of Washington.

Jerome A. Winer is professor of psychiatry at the University of Illinois.

Robert S. Wallerstein is training and supervising analyst, San Francisco Psychoanalytic Institute, and professor emeritus and former chairman of the department of psychiatry, University of California School of Medicine.

Introduction

PSYCHOANALYSIS: FROM MODERNISM
TO POSTMODERNISM?

PAUL ROBINSON

What is the cultural situation of psychoanalysis as we reach the fin de siècle? Historically, psychoanalysis was a product of the last fin de siècle, of the modernist revolt against positivism, Victorianism, and vestigial romanticism. It has been the dominant intellectual presence in Western culture during the intervening century. But as the century ends, and as modernism gives way to postmodernism, we might well expect that Freud's epochal creation would start to show its age.

We can begin with the state of Freud's reputation. As is well known, Freud has come under increasing attack during the past three decades. Feminists like Kate Millett and Germaine Greer have identified him as the chief intellectual force behind modern sexism. Biographical scholars like Frank Sulloway and Jeffrey Masson have questioned his originality and integrity. And philosophical critics like Adolf Grünbaum and Frank Cioffi have raised doubts about his credentials as a scientist. But Freud has not been without his fin-de-siècle apologists. Juliet Mitchell and Nancy Chodorow have vigorously defended him against their fellow feminists. Sulloway and Masson have been countered by, among others, Peter Gay in an authoritative biography. And Freud's philosophical advocates have included such potent hermeneutical voices as Jürgen Habermas and Paul Ricoeur.

The conclusion, I think, must be that Freud's reputation remains embattled. He has not sunk gracefully into the historical woodwork, in the manner, for example, of Charles Darwin, who, save among Christian fundamentalists, enjoys an utterly secure place in our intellectual pantheon. Freud, by contrast, continues to be a subject of fierce contemporary debate. Witness the blasts regularly issued against him by Frederick Crews in the *New York Review of Books*, and the no less impassioned apologias elicited from that journal's correspondents.

The argument will no doubt continue in the twenty-first century. But there are signs that the biographical debate may be entering a new phase, where the matter of Freud's stature will no longer occupy center stage, as scholars begin to explore more subtle questions about the tensions in his intellectual makeup and the trajectory of his career. To such a wished-for genre belongs Carl Schorske's essay introducing the present collection.

Schorske offers a brilliant analysis of the gendered cultural geography of Freud's mind. In Freud's early years, Schorske argues, England stood for masculinity, heterosexuality, discipline, and ethics, while France represented femininity, bisexuality, expressiveness, and aesthetics. Later this dichotomy gave way to a more complex one in which the oppositional poles were taken by Jews and Egyptians. Before the First World War, and above all in the Leonardo essay, Egypt became the locus of Freud's sympathetic interests in the bisexual, the feminine, and the erotically indulgent. But in reaction to the rise of Nazism, ancient Israel, and above all the figure of Moses, emerged as a powerful masculine, heterosexual, and repressive antagonist, transforming even Egypt itself from its prewar libidinal identity into a bastion of the ego. In these shifting allegiances Schorske identifies a fateful choice in Freud's intellectual biography, one that saw him (and the movement he founded) increasingly tied to a hardened "masculinist" and "heterosexist" view of the human situation. The road not taken—the road that led to Freud's first Egyptian dig—might, Schorske implies, have resulted in more accommodating relations with feminism and gay liberation in the latter half of the century. As we shall see, the matter of Freud's views of women and sexual deviation haunts many of the essays in this volume. With characteristic incisiveness, Schorske identifies perhaps the central problematic of psychoanalysis as it enters the fin de siècle.

A second issue is that posed by Freud's universalism, which stands at odds with the more modest intellectual ambitions of postmodernism and its commitment to particularism and difference. This issue is broached above all in the volume's historical and anthropological essays. Peter Loewenberg and Marcelo M. Suárez-Orozco employ the psychoanalytic concepts of splitting and projection (or scapegoating) to interpret the phenomena they examine: nationalism in the case of Loewenberg, aggressive fandom in the case of Suárez-Orozco. Both suggest that the sometimes murderous stigmatization of an "Other" originates in the externalization of personal fears and desires. In his criticism of their papers, John Toews expresses reservation about the unexamined psychic universalism informing both analyses: their comfortable conviction that immutable psychological processes underlie the huge variety of social forms produced by different cultures and different ages. In his moderate way, Toews gives voice to the doubts raised by postmodernism about "metanarratives," like psychoanalysis, that presume to reduce the multiplicity of cultural experience to a single story. He calls for an effort to "historicize" Freud, to understand him, in effect, as a figure of the last fin de siècle, whose ideas were inescapably shaped by the universalist assumptions of modernism, assumptions that have been seriously challenged by our own fin de siècle. Taken together, the three essays of this section document the continuing power of Freud's ideas to illuminate important historical and cultural developments of the late twentieth century (and with every passing day, nationalism and scapegoating of the Other appear to be the most dangerous forces abroad in today's world), but they also suggest an important limitation in the psychoanalytic imagination, one that sets it at odds with the particularizing and multicultural ethos of contemporary thought.

The essays on literature and art reflect what has been perhaps the single most fruitful area of interchange between psychoanalysis and modern culture. The interchange began with Freud himself, who not only was profoundly influenced by literary and artistic figures (from the Greek tragedians, through Shakespeare, to such moderns as Dickens and Dostoevsky) but initiated the work of "applied psychoanalysis"—the effort to bring analytic concepts to bear on the interpretation of individual works of art and literature. Richard Almond's study of *Jane Eyre*, Paul Schwaber's examination of *Ulysses*, and Ellen Handler Spitz's analysis of picture books (especially those of Maurice Sendak) are recognizable heirs to Freud's own essays on Leonardo, Michelangelo's Moses, Shakespeare's *Merchant of Venice*, and Jensen's *Gradiva*. Indeed, one might worry that, for all their valuable insights, they too closely replicate Freud's own interpretative practices (and those of his earlier followers, like Otto Rank, within psychoanalytic literary studies). The modern academic critic will experience a certain unease with their casual assumption that literary characters can be examined as if they were real people—indeed, in the case of Richard Almond's Jane Eyre, as if they were analytic patients with developmental histories and transference relationships. Modern criticism is uniformly hostile to the confusion of art and life; it insists that "characters" be recognized for the artful creations they are.

A more serious issue posed by these essays hearkens back to the questions raised by Carl Schorske's essay: the identification of psychoanalysis with uncritical assumptions about gender and sexual identity. The psychological narrative that

Richard Almond discovers in *Jane Eyre* celebrates the protagonist's discovery of her womanly calling in a mature heterosexual relationship (albeit one with certain maternal overtones): Jane Eyre transcends childish inclinations toward Oedipal revolt (tinged, as always, with incestuous desire), homoerotic object choice, and ascetic withdrawal to find her proper adult role as Rochester's wife. Paul Schwaber tells a similarly upbeat story about Leopold Bloom: tortured by his failed masculinity (which dates from the death of his infant son), Bloom nonetheless triumphs over the emasculating threats and bisexual temptations presented in the "Nighttown" episode to reclaim his identity as father to Stephen Dedalus and, Schwaber speculates, successful lover to Molly. In both cases, the narratives uncovered by psychoanalytic criticism are the "masculinist" and "heterosexist" ones Carl Schorske criticizes as products of Freud's late turn from Egypt to Israel, from the feminine to the masculine, from bisexual indulgence to heterosexual austerity, from aesthetics to ethics. Once again, we sense a tension between the analytic inheritance and our fin-de-siècle preoccupation with difference and heterogeneity.

Psychoanalysis's identification with modernism and its universalizing and masculinist preferences is also on display in the final set of essays treating "psychoanalysis and culture." In his exploration of psychoanalysis and modern philosophy, Charles Hanly links Freud's creation to what Hanly calls the dominant materialism or naturalism of the twentieth century, the conviction that no transcendent reality exists beyond the natural order and that the task of reason is to chart the regularities governing that order and to restrain the dangerous forces of irrationalism. Freud's theory, Hanly asserts, "describes a fundamental truth about the human condition." But, of course, our century has ended with an explosion of doubt about the powers of reason, as well as a categorical rejection of the notion that the human realm is of a piece with the natural realm or amenable to the same modes of inquiry. Indeed, "truth" itself—never mind "fundamental truth"—is now a contested category, as postmodernists prefer to speak of "discourses," no one of which enjoys the privileged status of truth. In the emerging postmodernist canon, psychoanalysis has been reduced to one of several competing systems of knowledge: an admired one, insofar as Freud himself raised doubts about the stability of the self and its power to achieve a disinterested picture of reality, but an arrogant one insofar as psychoanalysis seeks to normalize (or "naturalize") a story about the human situation that "privileges" men over women, straights over gays, sameness over difference.

Janine Chasseguet-Smirgel's examination of perversion and Satanism at once confirms and questions the identification of psychoanalysis with modernism and its preferred narratives. I have suggested that psychoanalysis, like modernism, has come to be associated with ideas of sameness or universality, just as postmodernism champions difference and particularism. But Chasseguet-Smirgel ingeniously argues that, from a psychoanalytic viewpoint, perversions (and their cultural correlates, from the Black Mass to Nazism) aim "to destroy reality, composed of differences, and in its place to establish a reign of anality where all differences have been abolished." Thus she interprets perversion as an attempt to do away with the distinction between male and female (by shifting attention from the genitals, where difference prevails, to the anus, where we are all alike) or the distinction between young and old, as in the Marquis de Sade's imagined incestuous couplings of father and daughter, mother and son. Psychoanalysis condemns these totalizing gestures in the name of a discriminating humanism, which, it might be argued, resembles the postmodernist's critique of totalizing metanarratives. But an ambiguity in Chasseguet-Smirgel's study is her apparent inclusion of homosexuality and bisexuality among the perversions, which leads her, for example, to link the "multiplication of transvestite cabarets in Berlin with the advent of Nazism." Once again the normalizing thrust of psychoanalysis, regretted by Carl Schorske, is on display, and we feel the gulf separating Freudianism from the critical perspectives of postmodernism. Hence, like many of the essays contained in this volume, Chasseguet-Smirgel's study affirms the centrality of psychoanalysis to the intellectual life of our century (as well as its pertinence to understanding the century's political catastrophes) yet hints at the growing dissonance between the intellectual habits of analysis and the emerging zeitgeist of the fin de siècle.

The essays published here grew out of a scholarly conference on the cultural impact of psychoanalysis held at Stanford University between January 11 and 13, 1991. The idea for the conference was planted in 1989 by a group of scholars and therapists, mostly associated with the university. It was nurtured over two years of complex planning that involved a large cast of characters and countless meetings. The immediate inspiration for the conference was the forthcoming visit to Stanford of the collection of Freud's antiquities (whose contents are beautifully displayed and insightfully analyzed in Lynn Gamwell and Richard Wells's volume *Sigmund Freud and Art: His Personal Collection of Antiquities*). From the start the intention was to explore the full range of cross-fertilizations between psychoanalysis and modern cultural and intellectual history.

Although many hands worked to prepare the conference, the main inspiration came from Roy Ginsburg, who as a practicing psychoanalyst and an academic (he held the post of associate professor of clinical psychiatry at Stanford University Medical School) was ideally suited by both training and temperament to the task. Roy Ginsburg died on October 2, 1992, at age forty-eight, just under two years after his brainchild had been realized, and less than a week after he was diagnosed with leukemia. At the time he was president of the San Francisco Psychoanalytic Institute, where he had done his training.

I like to think Roy would have been pleased with the volume that has resulted from the conference. Certainly he would have welcomed its eloquent testimony to the scope and endurance of Freud's legacy. But as a man of irony, modesty, and integrity, he would also have been eager that the volume honestly reflect the ambiguities, the limits, and the unexplored possibilities of the analytic heritage. In my view, the volume successfully balances achievements with ambiguities.

Psychoanalysis was created with the century and has played a more prominent role in the century's intellectual and cultural life than any other movement or tradition. Similarly, Freud has no equal among twentieth-century figures in terms of his influence on modern thought and culture, including popular culture. Indeed, we are now close enough to the end of the century to be able to say with confidence that, for better or for worse, he has been its presiding genius, much as some (such as Frederick Crews) would like to wish him away. But the fin de siècle has ushered in a new intellectual dispensation that may bring an end to Freud's intellectual reign. It remains to be seen whether his heirs can muster the suppleness of imagination needed to meet the postmodernist challenge.

I

FREUD AND CULTURE

To the Egyptian Dig

FREUD'S EXPLORATION IN
WESTERN CULTURES

CARL E. SCHORSKE

In March 1933, a new patient came to Freud. She was an American poet, Hilda Doolittle—better known by her pen name, H. D. The clouds of Nazism hung heavy in the European sky that spring. H. D., severely traumatized by World War I, was frightened. She came to Freud, as she tells us, "in order to fortify and equip myself to face war when it came." In her brilliant *Tribute to Freud,* she writes, "With the death-head swastika chalked on the pavement leading to the professor's door, I must calm as best I could . . . my own personal little dragon of war-terror."[1]

Freud also was possessed by the menace to civilization in Europe. Spurred by the flail of Hitler's rise to power, he was engaged at a new level of intensity with defining the nature of Jewishness, and the place of the Jews in the making of Western culture.

The transaction that ensued between the poet-patient and the professor must have been unique in the annals of psychoanalysis. Because both suffered acutely from the sense of a historical ending in modern Europe, their dialogue—even to the suggestive articulation of their powerful transferences—took the form of cultural discourse about antiquity, its symbols and their meanings. We have but one side of the discussion—H. D.'s—but her report makes us consider anew Freud's lifelong attempt to build, in effect, a meaningful interpretation of Western civilization, and to find his own place in it.

Freud had a large collection of archeological artifacts, in which H. D. evinced an immediate interest. A group of religious figurines stood arrayed on his desk, "like a high altar," she observes, in his study. From the assembled divinities Freud chose a tiny Athena and offered it to his new patient, almost as if it were a flower. " '*This* is my favorite,' he said . . . . 'She is perfect . . . . *only she has lost her spear.*' " H. D. felt the power of the gesture, and allowed it to resonate in her mind. "He knew that I loved Greece. . . . 'She has lost her spear,' " H. D. continues.[2] She does not explore the sexual implication of the loss of the spear for the androgynous goddess, nor its relevance to H. D.'s own bisexual proclivities. Nor did Freud, although he had done some revealing digging into Athena's nature.

Athena and Hellas provided a common ground of culture between the Jewish professor and the Christian poetess. It was a point of departure for a psycho-archeological quest which soon led them to Egypt; first together, in the analysis, later, each individually. In Egypt, Freud and H. D. sought to decipher the origins of human culture in ways that would fortify each in defining his/her own nature amidst the terrors of the modern world. H. D. recorded the yield of her dig in the long poem *Helen in Egypt;* Freud, in the work toward which this essay is directed, *Moses and Monotheism.*

I

That Athena should have been Freud's favorite among his archeological artifacts can come as no surprise. To anyone socialized in Austrian liberal culture in the mid-nineteenth century, as Freud had been, Athena served as a comprehensive symbol of all that that culture held dear. After the Austrian liberals finally achieved a constitutional state in the 1860s, they placed a great statue of Athena before their new Greek-style parliament building. Protectrix of the free polis, she was also goddess of wisdom, a symbol well suited to a liberal elite that believed in the liberating power of science and reason.

What was true of the symbolism of Athena for politics acquired even greater force in the substance of Austrian education. Classical culture was the foundation on which Austria's highly effective reformed, elite education was built. Greek and Roman civilization provided a religiously neutral ground for constructing a secular liberal culture. For no social group did this have more decisive meaning than for the newly emancipated Jews. Jewish children could join their Christian schoolfellows in acquiring a common gentile culture, the religion of which was dead and hence no threat to their own. The classics and ancient history opened for the Jews a road to a deep cultural assimilation into the gentile world without implying either heresy or apostasy.

At home and in separate religious instruction, young Sigmund Freud imbibed Hebrew and Jewish culture. In school, the public realm, he became a Greek. Under Athena's liberal aegis, he could drink deeply of both cultures, finding in the myths and ideas of Greeks and Hebrews the materials to construct his identity, his values, and his stance in a culturally and politically divided modern society.

To use past cultures thus, as reservoirs of human models and symbols, is not the same as exploring cultures as historically specific collective constructions. In his mature work, Freud, despite his enormous historical and cultural erudition, interested himself principally in the exploration of the universal nature and dynamics of the individual psyche, from whatever culture it may have sprung. Only once did he attempt systematically to come to grips with the character and construction of a particular culture, as historians and anthropologists do. This task Freud undertook only at the end of his life, and with considerable hesitation, in *Moses and Monotheism*, where he tried to get at the nature of Judaism. Although deeply attached and indebted to Greece and Rome, he never considered analyzing either as a whole culture. Yet the way he related to them—and especially to Athena/Minerva—sheds light on his deepest personal values and intellectual concerns.

II

Once Freud had defined his scientific mission as the exploration of the buried reaches of the human psyche, he drew an analogy between his work in depth psychology and that of the archeologist in exhuming and decoding buried cultures. It was only natural for this child of nineteenth-century Europe to assign priority to those ancient cultures that were regarded as progenitors of his own: Greek and Roman, Hebrew, and finally, Egyptian. Modern European cultures, by contrast, interested him little in his mature years. Yet as a young man Freud was drawn to two contemporary civilizations that meant much to his intellectual formation: those of England and France. They set a tone of duality that lasted all his life, and deserve a quick look for their prefiguration of the gender dimension in his later approaches to culture.[3]

Like many another Austrian liberal, Freud was a passionate Anglophile. After graduation from *Gymnasium* in 1875, he made a visit to England which, as he later said, "had a decisive influence on my whole life." In 1882, deeply frustrated with his career, he wrote to his fiancée of his longing to escape from Vienna and "that abominable steeple of St. Stefan"—a symbol of Catholic reaction. "The thought of England surges up before me, with its sober industriousness, its generous devotion to the public weal, the stubbornness and sensitive feeling for justice of its inhabitants. . . ."[4]

As a university student, Freud found reinforcement for his admiration for England in two important professors: Franz Brentano and Theodor Gomperz. Both were exponents of English philosophic radicalism, the first in philosophy, the second in classics. On Brentano's recommendation, Gomperz enlisted Freud to translate some of John Stuart Mill's most radical essays, including "The Subjection of Women" and "Socialism." Gomperz also imparted to the young Freud an interpretation of Greek culture consistent with his strongly moralistic Jewish heritage and the English utilitarian rationalism that continued the Puritan religious tradition in a militantly secular form.

Freud wrote to his fiancée of his fidelity to "the works of the men who were my real teachers, all of them English or Scotch; and I am recalling again . . . the most interesting historical period, the reign of the Puritans and Oliver Cromwell, with its lofty monument to that time, *Paradise Lost*."[5] The future intellectual explorer of sexuality was thus an admirer of the Puritans, the exemplars of libidinal repression. For they and their philosophic radical descendants were the builders, stern and rational, of the liberal ego and the England Freud admired: a land of ethical rectitude, manly self-control, public order, and the rule of law—all the characteristics that Matthew Arnold associated with Hebrews, but that Austrian liberals like Freud identified also with Athena and the Greeks.

Three years after Freud considered taking refuge in England's isle of masculine virtue, he fell in love with seductive, feminine Paris, where in 1885 he went to study with Martin Charcot. Paris was for him the absolute antithesis of London: a place of danger, of the questionable, the irrational. Freud encountered the city in a spirit of adventure, thrilling and frightening. He opened himself to the world of forbidden *fleurs du mal* that the

Anglophile and the liberal Jew in him had until then rejected or avoided: the Roman Catholic Church, the bewitching power of the female, and the power of the masses.

Mindful of Freud's hatred of Catholicism, and his longing to escape to England from the shadow of Vienna's "abominable steeple of St. Stefan," one is astonished at his being awed in Paris by Notre Dame. "This is a Church," he wrote. "I have never seen anything so movingly serious and sombre." As for the people of Paris, whom he observed in a year of anti-Semitic unrest, Freud found them frightening, "uncanny." "They are people given to psychical epidemics, historical mass convulsions, and they haven't changed since Victor Hugo wrote *Notre Dame.*"[6]

To the awe of the Church and the fear of the feverish crowd one must include one more element in Freud's simplistic image of Paris: women. Both in the theater—especially that of the bewitching Sarah Bernhardt—and in the salon, Freud responded, as his letters show, with a quite new receptivity, both sensual and intellectual, to the magic of women.[7] One can understand easily the feelings that underlay one of Freud's later jokes: A married couple is discussing the future. The man says to his wife, "If one of us should die, I shall go to Paris."

Paris, and Freud's quasi-stereotypical perception of it, provided the ideal setting for him to receive Charcot's doctrine concerning hysteria, which opened the way to that questionable province of the psyche where Freud would do his pioneering work.

One cannot fail to be struck by the radical antithesis between Freud's characterizations of English and French cultures. The Puritan-rationalist spectacles he wore when he looked at England allowed him to see there nothing of the cathedrals, crowds, or women that so caught his eye in France. By contrast, the image of the feminine so dominated his perception in France that the positivist, rationalist, masculine side of that country's bourgeois culture scarcely entered his field of vision. He made no attempt to establish any relationship between the contrasting values that attracted him in England and France. This polarity was subsequently to trouble both his experience of culture and his thinking about it. He confronted it for the first time in his encounter with Rome, where masculine and feminine, ethics and aesthetics—in short, the ego-world of his England and id-world of his Paris—converged in ambiguous symbiosis.

III

In the years 1895 to 1900, when Freud wrestled toward the intellectual breakthrough embodied in *The Interpretation of Dreams*, Rome, mother of cities, came to occupy a crucial place in his life. When Freud discovered the analogy between depth psychology and archeology, Rome was its focus. In 1896, he began his collection of archaic objects. He also spent passionate evenings with an archeologist friend, Emmanuel Loewy: "He keeps me up until three o'clock in the morning," Freud wrote. "He tells me about Rome." Then a strange problem arose. Freud developed what he called his "Rome neurosis." He, an avid traveler in Italy, could not get to Rome, though the city haunted his dreams. To do so, he had to dig up the Rome in himself, by analyzing his dreams.

I cannot here deal with Freud's Rome neurosis, and the way he resolved it psychoanalytically.[8] What concerns me is rather his cultural perspective. Although it contains classical elements, these are folded into Rome as the Holy City of Christendom. Unlike his approach to either England or Paris, Freud's perspective on Rome is Jewish, that of the outsider; but it is a double perspective. On the one hand, Rome is forbiddingly masculine, the citadel of Catholic power, and his dream-wish, as liberal and as Jew, is to conquer it. On the other hand, other wishes show Rome as feminine, Holy Mother Church, promising gratification, and to be entered in love. His powers were too weak for the project of conquest, his conscience too strong for the opposite possibility: to embrace the Church in conversion. Hence the neurotic impasse. Freud found the roots of these wishes in his psyche: in his childhood relations to his Jewish father and to a beloved Catholic nanny. But Rome had brought into conjunction the affects attached to masculine England and feminine Paris, in a tangled mass. While Freud resolved the problems presented by Rome in his self-analysis by reducing them to family relations, the cultural problems of the Jew in a gentile world troubled him more than ever.

Once more Freud was drawn to the classical era for emotional comfort. This became clear when he overcame his Rome neurosis through his self-analysis, and in 1901 was able to enter the city at last. Medieval and baroque Rome evoked his hatred of Catholicism once more: "I found almost intolerable the lie of salvation which rears its head so proudly to heaven." But beneath Catholic Rome was the city he cherished: classical Rome. His feelings for it as the foundation of European civilization welled up as did Gibbon's when he surveyed the ruined forum from the Capitoline. The focus of Freud's pathos was, not surprisingly, Athena, in her Roman persona, Minerva. He wrote to his friend Wilhelm Fliess, "I could have worshipped the abased and mutilated remnant of the Temple of Minerva."[9]

Was Freud's Roman Athena the same one the liberals of Vienna had chosen as their symbol of rational wisdom and justice? One suspects that she was, for she filled him still with serenity and a sense of intellectual security. But not for long.

Shortly before he described to Fliess his reaction to Rome, Freud had written him to announce his next big psychological study. It would be called "Human Bisexuality."[10] Athena could well symbolize this more ambiguous and ambitious psychoanalytic enterprise, lying beyond her orthodox nineteenth-century signification as goddess of rational order. For Athena, as Freud would soon explain, was an androgynous goddess. In her rational cool and ascetic bisexuality Athena unified the ethical civic spirit that had so attracted him to manly England, and the unsettling feminine beauty and irrational religious power that had so stirred him in seductive Paris. After his conquest of Rome, the pursuit of these related opposites led Freud to new cultural sites, to strata lying deeper both in history and in his psyche than Greece and Rome; namely, to Israel and Egypt.

IV

Before we follow Freud on his explorations in these more remote cultures, let us pause with him in the middle of the journey, on the acropolis of Athens. Freud visited it in 1904. In sharp contrast to his golden moment in the flats of Rome, where he had "worshipped the . . . remnant of Minerva's temple," Freud felt on the heights of Athens an unsettling malaise. He later analyzed that experience in an essay, "A Disturbance of Memory on the Acropolis," concluding that his joy had been undermined by guilt.[11] His whole acquired classical culture, which had served as a solid, secular common ground between Christian and Jew, now appeared to him under the aspect of his own detachment from the Jewish tradition to which his uneducated father had resolutely clung. Thenceforth, the road to Israel beckoned.

A few years later, returning to Rome, Freud felt again a flash of the apostate's guilt. This time it was in confronting Michelangelo's statue of Moses. Freud at first identified himself with the mob of backsliders to the golden calf upon whom the angry prophet's eye is turned, "the mob which had neither faith nor patience, and which rejoices when it has regained its illusory idols." [12] But then Freud detached himself from this guilt as Jew. Michelangelo's Moses, he argues in his famous essay of that name, is not the "historical figure," the angry, tablet-breaking prophet of the Bible. He is rather an exemplar of masculine moral control over the instincts, who governs his rage for the sake of his cause. [13] Most Freud biographers agree in seeing this Moses experience as connected with the tension between Freud and his followers over Freud's effort to make a gentile, C. G. Jung, his successor as head of the psychoanalytic organization so that psychoanalysis might not be a purely Jewish science. Freud found in Moses a model from which to draw strength as the embattled, patriarchal leader of his movement. Far from assaulting the father—that is, Moses—in identification with the backsliding mob of sons, Freud was hardening himself into being a powerful father himself, as he confronted his fractious followers.

The second road that led away from Athens ran in an almost opposite direction, to Egypt. At one level, this would seem a logical counterpart to Freud's renewed preoccupation with his Jewishness. Israel, and especially the two biblical figures that most engaged Freud from childhood on, Joseph and Moses, were fundamentally defined in relation to Egypt. [14] Yet after 1900 Egypt nurtured in Freud interests that were in drastic contradiction to the faith of his fathers and even to the male orientation of psychoanalysis—interests closer to his new project of 1901: "Human Bisexuality." For Egypt was a land of the primal mothers, and of religiously expressed bisexuality. It touched ultimate and even dangerous questions of the psyche to which Freud had devoted scant attention before he fell under Egypt's spell. [15]

Ever since the Renaissance, Egyptomania had periodically

seized the European imagination. That mysterious land promised access to the womb of culture and the tomb of time, to the original and the hidden, the voiceless (*infans*) childhood of humanity. In the fin de siècle it was the finds of archeologists that aroused anew the desire to decipher the culture of the Nile, as the philologists had done a century before. The archeologists' work swept the educated public in its wake.

Freud caught the fever. By 1906 at latest, his intoxication with things Egyptian far exceeded his earlier infatuation with Rome. He began to build a substantial library on Egypt. The most tangible evidence of his passion was in his expanding collection of artifacts, today preserved in the Freud Museum in London. In it Egyptian culture was the most strongly represented. There were no less than six figurines of Egypt's polytheistic holy family: Isis, Osiris, and Horus. Egypt soon dominated Freud's consulting room, in photos and in stone reliefs of Osiris and his family at the doorway to his study. Freud meditated upon—virtually communed with—these ancient images, not only at the desk where H. D. had noticed them and where he worked under their gaze, but even at the dinner table.[16]

Another index of the strength of his addiction is Freud's behavior on a week's visit to his beloved London in 1908, his first since 1875. This time it was not the virtuous character of English culture that captured him. Though he did some sightseeing, his biographer Ernest Jones reports, "What meant most to him [in London] was the collection of antiquities, particularly the Egyptian ones, in the British Museum. He did not go to any theater, because the evenings were given up to reading in preparation for the next day's visit to the museum."[17]

As early as 1907, Freud turned the attention of a prized new disciple, Karl Abraham, toward Egypt. On Abraham's first visit to Vienna, Freud not only gave him his "first Egyptological lessons," but even put two little Egyptian figurines in his guest's briefcase as a surprise farewell gift.[18] The lesson took; five years later, Abraham in turn surprised Freud, presenting him with a brilliant psychoanalytic study of Amenhotep IV, the pharaoh who was later to be the central figure in Freud's *Moses and Monotheism*. Freud wrote his friend in delight and gratitude: "Amenhotep IV in psychoanalytic illumination! That is certainly a big step in 'orientation'" (the pun in German implies also turning toward the East).[19]

In 1910, Freud's interest in Egypt surfaced for the first time in his published work. As his road to Jewish culture had passed through the Renaissance via the art of Michelangelo, so the road to Egypt ran through the art of Leonardo da Vinci. In Moses, the problem Freud addressed was patriarchal control; in Leonardo, it was homosexuality.[20] Freud analyzed a childhood memory of Leonardo's, in which he is visited in his cradle by a vulture that strikes his mouth with its tail. Freud sees Leonardo's homosexuality in this infantile fantasy, in the interpretation of which the vulture represents a new figure on the psychoanalytic scene: the phallic mother. Freud grounds his analysis of Leonardo's fantasy on the vulture-headed Egyptian mother-goddess, Mut. She is one of Egypt's original hermaphroditic divinities who survive alongside later gods who are sexually more differentiated. Freud analogizes the symbolic culture of Egypt, in the childhood of the race, to the infantile fantasy of the pre-oedipal individual. He sees the androgynous gods of Egypt as "expressions of the idea that only a combination of male and female elements can give a worthy representation of divine perfection."[21]

Suddenly, in this connection, Athena reappears in the text on Leonardo. Locating her origins in Egypt, Freud describes her now as a Greek descendant of an Egyptian phallic mother-goddess, Neith of Sais.[22] From this line of inquiry into bipolar unities also stemmed Freud's later interpretations of the Gorgon Medusa, the snakes on whose head are penises threatening castration. It was the Gorgon's fierce face that adorned the breast and shield of Athena to keep her male antagonists at bay.

In 1910, Freud published another fruit of his Egyptian explorations, this time concerning language. The article, "The Antithetical Meaning of Primal Words," took the form of a review of a book published almost three decades earlier. Its author, the philologist Karl Abel, had demonstrated that, in the primal language of Egypt, a single word denoted both an idea and its opposite; that is, both strong and weak, both light and dark. Freud noted that this finding about primal language was the same as his own view of dreams. "Dreams feel themselves at liberty . . . to represent any element by its wishful contrary."[23] Primal words thus have the same character as the primal bisexual divinities of Egypt; they constitute a unity of opposites. Only later are they split into autonomous antithetical, or complementary, terms.

Some of Freud's boldest later inquests into female psychology, bisexuality, and the pre-oedipal mother (for example, "Female Sexuality" [1931]; "Contributions to the Psychology of Love" [1918]) might be traced back to the study of Egyptian culture that so fired his imagination in the prewar years. They yielded new psychoanalytic concepts that pointed beyond the essentially male confines of most of Freud's cultural theory, especially *Totem and Taboo*. But the turn to Moses and the saving of the Jews led Freud away from the new veins he had opened in his first Egyptian dig.

V

Moses and Monotheism, written in the 1930s, explores as history the problem Freud had explored in his own psyche in analyzing his Rome neurosis: the relation of Jew and gentile. The work is both Jewish history and Egyptian history.

As Jewish history the book centers on two sensational, anti-traditional ideas. The first is that Moses was not a foundling Jew but a high-born Egyptian. The second is that, after the Exodus, Moses was killed by the more primitive of the Jews, who could not abide the severity of his law. Both these notions link the Jews, as Freud explicitly aims to show, to the world of the gentiles: the first, culturally, links the Jews to the Egyptians; the second, by analogy with the crucifixion, to the Christians. With these identifications of Jew and gentile through Moses, Freud accomplishes two things. First, he vindicates the Jewish people by defining them as carriers of the highest mark of civilization first achieved by Egypt. Second, in his myth of the killing of Moses, Freud gives the Jews a basis for abandoning their exclusivist self-definition, which in his view prevents them from realizing, as Christians do, their own universality. To achieve this, Freud says, the Jews must recognize as Christians do their own patricidal crime, and assume its guilt as participants in the brotherhood of man.

The particular Egypt that Freud provides as setting for his Moses story in the 1930s is strikingly different from the land of bisexual religion and primal mothers that claimed his attention before World War I. We should see it as a second Egyptian dig. Freud concentrates now on a later phase of Egyptian history, the reign of Amenhotep IV, who renamed himself Akhenaten. That pharaoh of the eighteenth dynasty was the nearest thing Egypt produced to a European enlightened despot of the eighteenth century, like Joseph II of Austria. Akhenaten was a man after Freud's heart, a rebel-reformer. Establishing a monotheistic cult of an abstract sun god, Aton, the pharaoh suppressed the polytheistic religion of Egypt. Akhenaten's monotheistic cult stressed not salvation but truthfulness, ethics, and justice. His was an elitist creed developed "in deliberate hostility to the popular [religion]."[24] But when Akhenaten died, his victory over the superstition and darkness of Egyptian polytheism was swept away by a counterreformation, much as Emperor Joseph II's enlightenment had been by Catholic reaction.

According to Freud, Moses, the Egyptian nobleman, member of Akhenaten's intellectual elite, was caught in the *Götterdämmerung* of Egypt's enlightenment. As Freud put it, Moses was one who, like the enlightened anti-Nazi Gentiles in Freud's time, "lost his fatherland" when the values it stood for under his pharaoh were destroyed.[25] Determined to rescue the pharaoh's cultural achievement from the counterreformation, Moses chose as his vehicle the Jews, a poor alien people settled in a border province, who worshipped a primitive tribal God. In effect, Moses made Egyptians out of the Jews, so that they might preserve the highest culture that his country had achieved. He gave them three Egyptian gifts: monotheism, the ethical code of the Aton cult, and the practice of circumcision. With these three gifts of Egyptian enlightenment, Freud argued, Moses created the most fundamental characteristic of Jewish culture ever after: *Geistigkeit.* That term embraces both spirituality and intellectuality. It is the opposite of *Sinnlichkeit,* the realm of the senses. It is London as opposed to Paris. The eternal task of Geistigkeit is to control Sinnlichkeit and the instincts that drive it. That is what civilization is all about.[26] The Egyptians achieved it first among all peoples in Akhenaten's brief moment in history. Moses imparted its essentials to the Jews, so that they might save it and cultivate it for the future.

It was a man's job. Not for nothing did Freud entitle his book in German, *Der Mann Moses.* He did not say *Der Mensch Moses. Mann* conveys what Freud wanted: manliness, maleness and its attributes: courage, force, principle, uprightness.[27] One recalls his earlier political-cultural heroes, Hannibal and Oliver Cromwell. Freud fantasizes further that Moses, the able, masterful aristocrat, might have aspired to rule Egypt as Akhenaten's successor. In any case, it fit his nature to plan for the Jews: "to found a new empire, to find a new people [ein neues Reich zu grunden, ein neues Volk zu finden. . . .]"[28] Freud associated Moses's imperial manliness of course with his Geistigkeit. Demanding of the Jews instinctual renunciation, Moses liberated them not so much from Egyptian bondage as from their own instinctual drives. A father to the childish people, Moses transformed them into a father-people, exemplifying the victory of male abstraction, the central prerequisite of civilization, over female sensuality and materiality. Thanks to their intellectual and ethical strength, the Jews as *Kulturvolk* par excellence would always be attacked whenever repressed instinct broke loose in civilized society; thanks to the same masculine virtues, they would have the power to endure in adversity.

The ideal historical base for Freud's final exploration in culture in *Moses and Monotheism,* we must by now realize, is no longer Greece, but Egypt. In the Egypt of his second dig, the Jews acquired an honored place in gentile history such as neither Athens nor Rome nor the classicism of the Austrian Gymnasium could provide them. For in Egypt, the Jews became the *Kulturvolk* that rescued the highest gentile civilization from the unholy alliance of priests and ignorant people; just as, in modern times, the Jews and cultured gentiles were, through exodus and exile, saving Europe's enlightenment from Hitler.

VI

Let us look now at the Egyptian side of the equation. What did Freud do with Egyptian history to sustain his image of Moses?

And, in so doing, what did he do to his previous excavations of Egypt for the psychoanalytic understanding of culture?

In the first Egyptian dig, Freud's findings were related to bisexuality, the phallic mother, the union of opposites in religion and even in language. In the second dig, undertaken in search of the origins of the Jews, we find a different Egypt, one wholly oriented toward masculine cultural achievements, with Geistigkeit and instinctual repression at the center.

In pursuit of this difference, I began to look at Freud's sources. The trail led first, of all places, to Chicago. James Henry Breasted, founder of Chicago's Oriental Institute, published in 1905 *The History of Egypt,* a great classic of its time, and Freud's principal source. Breasted had written his doctoral thesis in Berlin on the hymns of Akhenaten's sun god, Aton. There he showed the world's earliest monotheism in birth in poetry. Then, in his comprehensive history, Breasted charted Egyptian culture as it struggled out of chthonic darkness to the achievement of rational enlightenment during the reign of his hero, Akhenaten. In the progressivist spirit of America's New History, which had a principal center in Chicago, Breasted made of Egypt a paradigm for the whole history of Europe, at a time when Greeks and Hebrews were both still in a primitive state.

As Freud was a secularized Jew seeking roots deeper and anterior to those of his faith, Breasted was a secularized Protestant Christian engaged in the same quest: both sought to deny to their respective traditions claims to be the divinely ordained founders of civilization by exalting Egypt as creator of the first enlightenment culture. Even as Freud began work on *Moses and Monotheism,* Breasted was publishing a popular book on Egypt under the title *The Dawn of Conscience* (1933) — what Freud would have called "the origins of the super-ego." Breasted included in its preface an explicit expression of concern about revived anti-Semitism in order to offset the fact that he was undermining the Judeo-Christian claims to primacy in creating our civilization.

Freud's portrait of Akhenaten and his religious revolution is firmly grounded in Breasted's account: monotheism, rationalism, the construction of an ethical code, even circumcision are in it. But Breasted includes another aspect of Akhenaten's culture nowhere mentioned in Freud: a rich, sensual element. No Egyptian nobleman could have escaped it.

If the god Aton was dematerialized, the earthly life and cultural forms of his cult were far from it. Breasted shows how the art of Akhenaten's reign broke the stiff, hieratic geometrical tradition of Egypt in favor of a sensuous, naturalistic plasticity worthy of *art nouveau*. Frescoes depicting Akhenaten and his beautiful queen Nefertiti in tender communion or playing lovingly with their daughters radiate the joy of Sinnlichkeit. "To the sensitive soul of this Egyptian dreamer," Breasted says, "the whole animate world seems alive with the presence of Aton: . . . the lily-grown marshes, where the flowers are 'drunken' in the intoxicating radiance of Aton." The Emersonian Breasted concludes, "The deepest sources of power in this remarkable revolution lay in this appeal to nature, in this admonition to 'consider the lilies of the field.'"[29]

None of the sensual side of the Akhenaten culture described by Breasted appears in Freud's account. Freud selected from Breasted's *History* that which connects the Egyptian enlightenment to the Geistigkeit he sees in the Jews. In his own copy of Breasted's history, Freud marked only those passages that sustained this commonality. The rest—and the richer information on the sensuous culture of Akhenaten in *The Dawn of Conscience*—he ignored.

Another omission in Freud's book is even more astonishing. Neither in text nor footnotes is there any reference to the one major psychoanalytic study of Egyptian culture: Karl Abraham's "Amenhotep IV." This is the long article with which, as I have mentioned, Abraham, the faithful disciple, had surprised the master in 1912.[30] He wrote it under the stimulus of Freud's interest in bisexuality and its presence in the Leonardo analysis and in Egyptian religious culture.

Abraham's psychoanalytic portrait of Akhenaten centers squarely on the pharaoh's androgynous nature. Reared by a powerful mother to whom he remained passionately attached, Akhenaten lived in a permanent state of anger against his strong father. Akhenaten's self-representation in art, no less than his behavior, showed striking androgynous characteristics. It was also marked by allusion to the most primitive styles. Identifying his god Aton with the first sun god, and claiming descent from him, Akhenaten outflanked his father, Amenhotep III, and replaced his cult. His archaism, Abraham argues, betrayed a well-known neurotic symptom: the fantasy of high parentage. Akhenaten made his god a god of love, a completely spiritualized ideal father. "He had sublimated his aggressive instinctual impulses [against his father] to an extraordinary extent," Abraham maintains, "and had transformed them into an overflowing love for all beings, so that he did not use violence even against the enemies of his empire." Though Abraham saw Akhenaten as a predecessor of Moses as monotheist, "[his] conception of god had more in common with the Christian than with the Mosaic conception." A God of love.[31] Finally, Abraham stresses the tremendous influence of women—especially his wife, Nefertiti, and his mother, Tiys—on Akhenaten's court and cult.* If ethical Geistigkeit was one aspect of the

*Not for nothing did glorious Nefertiti, whose elegant portrait head is still a prized object of the Berlin Museum where Abraham worked, enthrall the European fin de siècle as the quintessential femme fatale. "Suave . . . icy . . . an android," writes Camille Paglia in her perceptive

monotheistic god Aton, intense, aestheticized sensuosity was the other. Freud left this dual character out of his account.*

The project of vindicating the Jews as a masculine Kulturvolk led Freud in effect to ignore in his second Egyptian dig the conceptual treasures he had unearthed in his first. He abandoned the shafts he had himself opened into a possible bisexual theory of cultural development. He expurgated or repressed the knowledge of Breasted and Abraham, his best informants, with respect to the integration of Sinnlichkeit with Geistigkeit, female with male, in the culture of Akhenaten. Freud paid a price for his suppression of the truth about the androgynous pharaoh, a price not without its irony: In making of Moses an Egyptian, he ended by making of Akhenaten a Jew.

VII

Our story has been one of a dualism that worked itself out again and again in Freud's explorations in culture. In the 1880s there was puritan, manly England versus fascinating, feminine Paris; in the 1890s, anxiety-provoking Rome, with its menace of masculine papal power conflated with the temptation of the Church as Holy Mother; in the 1910s, virile Michelangelo contrasted with androgynous Leonardo; and finally, Egypt, the

---

analysis of Nefertiti, "she is femaleness made mathematical . . . the triumph of Apollonian image over the lumpiness and horror of mother earth. . . . Head magic." (Camille Paglia, *Sexual Personae* [New Haven: Yale University Press, 1991], 66–69).

*Breasted cites a source (a hymn?) calling Aton "*the father and mother of all he had made*" (*History,* 337; italics mine). This dual character of the god recalls Freud's observation in *Leonardo* that to the Egyptians "only a combination of male and female elements can give a worthy representation of divine perfection."

land of primal bisexual culture confronting the enlightened patriarchal despotism of Akhenaten/Moses.

What, in all this, has become of Athena, who had accompanied Freud throughout his culture odyssey? After the experience on the acropolis in 1904 Freud left her with a sense of guilt about their relationship. In 1910, in the swamplands of the Nile, he found her in a primal form, a phallic mother-goddess. How she would have shocked the good liberals of Vienna, who had chosen her as the virginal symbol of their rational polity! In *Moses and Monotheism,* Athena appeared once more, though only in a footnote. There Freud speculated on the origin of Athena's Greek persona: A great earthquake, such as he thought might account for the tidal wave that swallowed the Egyptians in the Red Sea, had also sealed Athena's destiny as a mother-goddess. Like the matriarchal goddess of Crete, Freud suggested, she had lost all credibility when her womanly powers failed to protect the Greeks against the volcanic eruptions of nature. Then male gods like "earth-shaking Zeus" took over. The mother-goddess Pallas Athena, Freud tells us, "was demoted to a daughter, robbed of her own mother, and through the virginity imposed upon her, permanently excluded from motherhood."[32] Thus denatured by her father Zeus, she had henceforth to serve his patriarchal purposes as intellectual brainchild. We recall Freud's words on Athena to H. D.: "She is perfect . . . only she has lost her spear." In the light of Freud's suppression of bisexuality in his final work of cultural analysis, those words on Athena have a melancholy ring.

In May 1938, Freud fled Vienna for England, the land of civic virtue to which he had thought of emigrating over fifty years before. Taking the Orient Express westward to London, he stopped for a night in the other favored city of his youth, Paris. There he enjoyed the hospitality of a favorite disciple, his "dear Princess," Marie Bonaparte. "An energy devil," Freud had called her; "a quite outstanding, more than half masculine female."[33] As if to justify his characterization, the Princess had smuggled his favorite statuette, Athena, out of Vienna, when he feared his collection of artifacts might be lost.[34] Now she put it into the old man's hands.

Freud carried Athena on to London himself. It was his last voyage with that old androgynous companion from antiquity, whose changes had recorded so faithfully the changes in Freud's understanding of humankind. But as he left for London, it was not to Athena that Freud's thoughts turned to define his situation. "I compare myself," he wrote to his son Ernst, "with the old Jacob, whom in his old age his children brought to Egypt."[35]

For the sake of the Jews in Hitler's Götterdämmerung, Freud banished from his mind the promising insights into sexuality and culture he had found in Egypt, and abandoned them in *Moses and Monotheism*. Now he could go to England to die in freedom with his historical illusions, a Jewish patriarch in the enlightened gentile country of his youthful dreams.

Notes

1. H. D., "Writing on the Wall," in *Tribute to Freud* (New York: Pantheon, 1956), 93, 94.
2. Ibid., 68, 69.
3. For a fuller discussion of Freud's encounters with England, Paris and Rome, see my "Freud: The Psychoarcheology of Civilizations," in *The Cambridge Companion to Freud*, ed. Jerome Neu (Cambridge, Eng.: Cambridge University Press, 1991), 8–24.
4. Quoted in Ernest Jones, *The Life and Work of Sigmund Freud*, 3 vols. (New York: Doubleday, 1953-1957), 1: 178.
5. Ibid., 179.
6. *The Letters of Sigmund Freud*, ed. Ernest L. Freud (New York: McGraw-Hill Paperback, 1964), 183, 187-188.

7. Ibid., 179–181, 196–197.
8. Cf. my *Fin-de-Siècle Vienna* (New York: Knopf, 1979), ch. 4.
9. *The Complete Letters of Sigmund Freud to Wilhelm Fliess*, ed. Jeffrey Moussaieff Masson (Cambridge, Mass.: Harvard University Press, 1985), 449.
10. Ibid., 448.
11. Sigmund Freud, *Works, Standard Edition*, ed. James Strachey et al., 24 vols. (London: Hogarth, 1966–1974), 22: 239–248.
12. Freud, "The Moses of Michelangelo," ibid., 13: 213.
13. Ibid., 13: 233.
14. For the association of Egypt with both sibling rivalry and the death of the mother in Freud's childhood experience and his later dreams, see William McGrath, *Freud's Discovery of Psychoanalysis* (Ithaca: Cornell University Press, 1986), ch. 2.
15. An original and suggestive analysis of Freud's relation to Egyptian mythology and its implications for his theory is provided by Joan Rafael-Leff, "If Oedipus was an Egyptian," *International Review of Psychoanalysis* 17 (1990): 309–335. Leff integrates the perspectives of psychoanalyst, Egyptologist, and feminist.
16. Ellen Handler Spitz, "Psychoanalysis and the Legacy of Antiquity," in *Sigmund Freud and Art*, ed. Lynn Gamwell and Richard Wells (Binghamton, N.Y.: State University of New York, 1989), 154–155.
17. Jones, *Freud*, 2: 52.
18. Sigmund Freud and Karl Abraham, *Briefe, 1907–1926*, ed. Hilda C. Abraham and Ernst L. Freud (Frankfurt: S. Fischer, 1965), 28.
19. Ibid., 115.
20. The Leonardo text also involved a new relationship between mythology and sexuality, bringing Freud closer to Jung but on the basis of misunderstanding. See George B. Hogenson, *Jung's Struggle with Freud* (Notre Dame: University of Notre Dame Press, 1983), 26–40.
21. "Leonardo da Vinci and a Memory of Childhood," Freud, *Standard Edition*, 11: 93–94. Freud conflates Mut with another mother-goddess, Nut, who alone is identified with a vulture. See J. Harnik, "Aegyptologishes zu Leonardos Geierphantasie," *Internationale Zeitschrift fur Psychoanalyse* VI (1920): 362–363.
22. Freud, *Standard Edition*, 11: Freud had initially connected Egypt with Greece in the case of Leonardo's vulture too: "It can be proven that Leonardo was acquainted with the vulture as symbol of motherliness through his reading of Greek authors, who were thoroughly steeped in Egyptian culture." (Presentation in *Minutes of the Vienna Psychoanalytic*

Society, ed. H. Nunberg and E. Federn (New York: International Universities Press, 1967) 2: 342. Freud omitted this claim from the published version.

23. Freud, *S.E.,* 11: 155.

24. Freud, "Moses and Monotheism," *S.E.,* 23: 20–26.

25. Ibid., 28.

26. Ibid., 64; 86 n. 1; 111–123.

27. Bluma Goldstein, *Reinscribing Moses* (Cambridge, Mass.: Harvard University Press, 1992), 102–103.

28. Ibid., 28. I have brought the translation closer to the original German.

29. James H. Breasted, *The Dawn of Conscience* (New York: Charles Scribner's Sons, 1933), 292–298; Breasted, *A History of Egypt* (New York: Charles Scribner's Sons, 1923), 376–378.

30. Karl Abraham, *Selected Papers* 2 vols. (New York: Basic Books, 1955), 2: 262–290; Leonard Shengold, "A Parapraxis of Freud's in Relation to Karl Abraham," *Imago* 92 (1972): 123–159.

31. Abraham, *Selected Papers,* 2: 275, 287.

32. Freud, *S.E.,* 23: 45, n. 2.

33. Quoted by Peter Gay, *Freud: A Life for Our Time* (New York: W. W. Norton, 1988), 541, 542.

34. Jones, *Freud,* 3: 227–28.

35. Ibid., 225.

2

History and Anthropology

The Construction of National Identity

PETER LOEWENBERG

Poets are the unacknowledged legislators of the world.
—Percy Bysshe Shelley

Nationhood is the extension of real or symbolic love felt for the corner of land which belongs to the commune, to an entire valley, an immense plain, the steppe, and the great city such as Paris or Vienna.
—Arnold van Gennep

History . . . is a nightmare from which I am trying to awake.
—James Joyce, *Ulysses*

In the late afternoon of 16 June 1904 a dialogue takes place in Barney Kiernan's saloon on Little Britain Street in which Leopold Bloom is baited by a one-eyed Fenian fanatic known simply as "The Citizen." Bloom's is the voice of humane cosmopolitan reason:

> —Persecution, says he, all the history of the world is full of it. Perpetuating national hatred among nations.
> —But do you know what a nation means? says John Wyse.
> —Yes, says Bloom.
> —What is it? says John Wyse.
> —A nation? says Bloom. A nation is the same people living in the same place.
> —By God, then, says Ned, laughing, if that's so I'm a nation for I'm living in the same place for the past five years.

So of course everyone had a laugh at Bloom and says he, trying to muck out of it:

—Or also living in different places.

—That covers my case, says Joe.

—What is your nation if I may ask, says the citizen.

—Ireland, says Bloom. I was born here. Ireland . . . .

—And I belong to a race too, says Bloom, that is hated and persecuted. Also now. This very moment. This very instant . . . .

—Robbed, says he. Plundered. Insulted. Persecuted. Taking what belongs to us by right. At this very moment, says he, putting up his fist, sold by auction off in Morocco like slaves or cattles.

—Are you talking about the New Jerusalem? says the citizen.

—I'm talking about injustice, says Bloom.

—Right, says John Wyse. Stand up to it then with force like men . . . .

—But it's no use, says he. Force, hatred, history, all that. That's not life for men and women, insult and hatred. And everybody knows that it's the very opposite of that that is really life.

—What? Says Alf.

—Love, says Bloom. I mean the opposite of hatred. . . .

—Ireland my nation says he (hoik! phthook!) never be up to those bloody (there's the last of it) Jerusalem (ah!) cuckoos . . . .

John Wyse saying it was Bloom gave the idea for Sinn Fein to Griffith to put in his paper . . . .

—Isn't that a fact, says John Wyse, what I was telling the citizen about Bloom and the Sinn Fein? . . .

—He's a perverted jew, says Martin, from a place

in Hungary and it was he drew up all the plans according to the Hungarian system. We know that in the castle . . .

—A wolf in sheep's clothing, says the citizen. That's what he is. Virag from Hungary! Ahasuerus I call him. Cursed by God.[1]

Amid the sweet stench of beer in Barney Kiernan's pub, James Joyce dramatizes the emotional valences of exclusion and inclusion, of violence and single vision, which make up the discourses on national identity. He plays with the problematic politico-legal definition of "nation," which may mean whatever one wishes it to mean, and with the complexity of distinguishing "national identity" from "ethnicity," "peoplehood," and "race." Joyce's caricature-in-voice monocular Irish "Citizen" is evocative of Homer's "violent and lawless tribe . . . these Cyclopians have no parliament for debates and no laws."[2] The Cyclopian episode of *Ulysses* displays chauvinism without irony, vision without perspective. Bloom offers us a series of attempts at defining national identity. First is the legal positivist definition: a nation is constituted by those living in the same place. It is expressed in the third person: "He or she belongs . . ." The second definition is cultural: a national identity is composed by those who believe they belong to a nation, and is affirmed in the first person: "I belong . . ." The xenophobic, one-eyed Citizen offers a third definition, which is prescriptive: national identity consists of particular characteristics—racial, religious, ideological, spiritual, physical—that circumscribe belonging and is pronounced in the third person: "You do"; or, as is asserted to Bloom: "You do not belong. . . ."

The dialogue alludes to a complex and neglected Hungarian-Jewish-Bloom-Griffith-Feinian-Irish nationalist relationship with which Joyce played.[3] Bloom was born of a Hungarian-

Jewish father in the year of Hungary's rebirth, 1866, the year of Habsburg Austria's defeat by Bismarck's Prussia in the Seven Weeks War, a war that began on "Bloomsday," 15–16 June 1866. Bloom is rumored in Dublin to be the secret Jewish advisor to Arthur Griffith (1872–1922), founder of the Sinn Fein.[4] The Hungarians had exploited Austria's defeat to negotiate a new constitutional arrangement, the *Ausgleich* of 1867, which gave Hungarians home rule and influence on national policy in a dual monarchy, while accepting the Austrian emperor as the constitutional head of state. In 1904 Griffith advocated the "Hungarian Plan" as a viable blueprint for Ireland's future relationship with Great Britain. He concluded: "None who reflect can doubt that, carried out with the same determination, the policy which resurrected Hungary . . . can end the usurped authority of England to rule our country."[5] The Citizen's curse— "Virag from Hungary!"—speaks of *virago,* a male-like woman. Bloom's character had androgynous qualities, and *virag* in Hungarian means bloom or flower.[6] When Bloom is attacked by the Citizen, he bids farewell to Dublin as *Lipóti Virag,* and the orchestra follows *Come Back to Erin* with *Rakoczy's March.*[7]

Joyce left Dublin for the Continent in 1904—his final line in *Ulysses: "Trieste-Zürich-Paris,* 1914-1921," speaks of cosmopolitan wandering, personal isolation, exclusion, and exile. He articulates in his modern Odysseus the tensions of twentieth-century chauvinist identity politics. Odysseus tricked the Cyclops and made escape possible by telling him, "Noman is my name. Noman is what mother and father call me . . . ."[8] Leopold Bloom is for Joyce "Everyman or Noman."[9] He is the universal hero: Irish, Jewish, Hungarian, Hellenic, the quintessential modern man—a rootless, dispossessed wanderer, "Ahasuerus," without a national home, and not the master in his own house. He is four times exiled, as a Jew, a Hungarian, an Irishman, and displaced at home by Blazes Boylan. Bloom is an ethnic and religious cosmopolite: uncircumcised, multiply baptized, half-Irish half-Jew, born of a gentile Irish mother and a Hungarian father who gave him a Jewish name and visage, married to a half Spanish–half Irish woman, affirming a proud historic Jewish identity. He suffers the torments and the ambiguities of the rise of militant twentieth-century nationalism, which continue to tear asunder both his country and his people. The Fenian "Citizen" and the Protestant Orangeman Crofter, political and religious enemies, can unite in their anti-Semitic hatred of Bloom. "Nothing," said Joyce's friend Frank Budgen, "brings people nearer to one another than community in fearing, loving and hating."[10]

Joyce's central European contemporary, Robert Musil, challenged the concept of "national character" by describing the multiple identities possessed by each person:

> The inhabitant of a country has at least nine characters: a professional one, a national one, a civic one, a class one, a geographical one, a sex one, a conscious, an unconscious and perhaps even a too private one; he combines them all in himself, but they dissolve him, and he is really nothing but a little channel washed out by all these trickling streams, which flow into it and drain out of it again in order to join other little streams filling another channel. Hence every dweller on earth also has a tenth character, which is nothing more or less than the passive illusion of spaces unfilled. . . . This interior space—which is, it must be admitted, difficult to describe—is of a different shade and shape in Italy from what it is in England, because everything that stands out in relief against it is of a dif-

ferent shade and shape; and yet both here and there
it is the same, merely an empty, invisible space with
reality standing in the middle of it like a little toy
brick town, abandoned by the imagination.[11]

Musil deconstructs and subverts the essentialist concept of
identity. Yet, he sees "the national" as not only one of the
nine identity fragments, but ascriptively in the invisible interior space "without qualities" in which the essential spirit
(*Geist*) resides. National identity is culturally, psychologically,
and historically constructed, consisting of a different "shade
and shape" in England or Italy, because relations to the nine
identity fragments which people internalize are essentially different in each nation. Nationality is privileged in defining personal, subjective political and social identifications because it
absorbs into itself all other identity fragments.

II

The three main social science approaches to national identity
are the reflexive sociological model of Pierre Bourdieu, Rogers
Brubaker, and Benedict Anderson; the cognitive socialization
model of Ernst Gellner and Eric Hobsbawm; and the family
communication model of Erik Erikson and Karl Deutsch,
which, I argue, offers the maximum utility and relevance for
research in problems of national identity.

Most sociologists use "identity" ascriptively; as something
which is assigned by others. Bourdieu, undoubtedly with the
history of France in mind, views the state, through its admin-
istrative discourse of symbolic functions, official forms, cer-
tificates, records, credentials, as the institution "which assigns
everyone an identity."[12] Identity, suggests Bourdieu, can be
self-assigned, as when a person intentionally alters language to

adopt the style of a higher social class.[13] Identity is perception which "exists fundamentally through recognition by other people."[14] In seeking to explain the Chinese student protest movement of the night of June 3-4, 1989, in Tiananmen Square, Craig Calhoun tells us that "Identity is a no more than *relatively* stable construction in an ongoing process of social activity. . . . Even at a personal level . . . identity is not altogether internal to an individual but is part of a social process. . . . Identity is not a static, preexisting condition that can be seen as exerting a causal influence on collective action; at both personal and collective levels, it is a changeable product of collective action."[15]

Concordantly, on the national level Rogers Brubaker argues: "We should think about nation not as substance but as institutionalized form, not as collectivity but as practical category, not as entity but as contingent event . . . as something that suddenly crystallizes rather than gradually develops, as a contingent, conjuncturally fluctuating, and precarious frame of vision and basis for individual and collective action, rather than as a relatively stable product of deep developmental trends in economy, polity, or culture."[16] As Brubaker points out, nationality is not quantifiable *precisely* because it is a subjective category: "Nationality is not a fixed, given, indelible, objectively ascertainable property; and even subjective, self-identified nationality is variable across time and context of elicitation, and therefore not measurable as if it were an enduring fact that needed only to be registered."[17]

Benedict Anderson holds that the rich multiplicity of historical, ethnic, and religious roots of national identity require acts of mental invention of a mythic common past, usually glorious but sometimes persecutory, and the suppression of the diversity of sectarian, clan, tribal, dynastic, and polyglot origins of the peoples who constitute the nation. Anderson cogently applies the metaphor of childhood memory amnesia in the creation of a national identity: "All profound changes of consciousness, by their very nature, bring with them characteristic amnesias. Out of such oblivions, in specific historical circumstances, spring narratives. After experiencing the physiological and emotional changes produced by puberty, it is impossible to 'remember' the consciousness of childhood . . . . As with modern persons, so it is with nations. Awareness of being imbedded in secular, serial time, with all its implications of continuity, yet of 'forgetting' the experience of this continuity . . . engenders the need for a narrative of 'identity.'"[18]

Both the power and the feigned quality of nationalism are apparent when we look at such synthetic nations as the United States, Brazil, Indonesia, and Israel. These are invented nations, each with an assertive, self-worshiping, and aggrandizing nationalism, and each worthy of special attention, study, and interest. But the power of "imaginary" nationalism should not be underestimated or deprecated merely because it is "constructed." People are demonstrably willing to die for these national identities, which evoke deeply stirring identifications with family and home, tradition and emotionally freighted symbolism.

Eric Hobsbawm detests nationalism, therefore discounts its power and wishes it would disappear to the trash heap of history with other bourgeois institutions. This wish also determines his analysis. In 1990 he doubted "the strength and dominance of nationalism," holding that it "will decline with the decline of the nation-state . . . the phenomenon is past its peak."[19] Two decades ago Hobsbawm argued for nationalism as "a historic phenomenon, the product of the fairly recent past, and unlikely to persist indefinitely."[20] Bourdieu's critique of Marxist research into the national question reflects that: "it is no coincidence that Stalin is the author of the most dogmatic and most *essentialist* 'definition' of the nation."[21]

Ernest Gellner stresses the role of school transmitted culture, which he terms "exosocialization" or "education proper," as distinguished from family childhood socialization.[22] The historical development which Gellner sees is the nation as a culture/polity based on an educational machine running from grade school to university.[23] Gellner has a distinctively Darwinian view of human nature, and for that reason he points to the superiority of the Freudian model over rational interest models of behavior: "All the assumptions, for instance, contained in the pervasive economist's model, of a *homo economicus* in pursuit of sharply specific aims, simply fail to do justice to the brutality, deviousness, tortuous obscurity of our inner life, to all the things which we know from experience to mask our real driving forces."[24] He therefore believes that: "nationalism does not have any very deep roots in the human psyche. The human psyche can be assumed to have persisted unchanged through the many many millennia of the existence of the human race, and not to have become either better or worse during the relatively brief and very recent age of nationalism."[25] Gellner subscribes to the classical Freudian idea of an unaltered, unconscious instinctual structure in humankind. He legitimately calls for a culture-specific explanation of nationalism, which should place him in the province of modern ego psychology. Our focus must, indeed, be on how political institutions and individual people adapt to the pressures and exigencies of historical forces.

Social scientists currently use the term "identity" widely and artlessly, without reference or acknowledgment to Erik H. Erikson, who first articulated and developed the concept. He drew on "internal" personal and "external" historical experience, calling the integration *psychosocial* identity. A critique of

Erikson's concept of identity for social scientists is that he re-defined it often as he applied it in particular cases.[26] I find this flexibility to be a virtue that enhances the usefulness of psychosocial identity as a concept for comprehending nationalism in its multiplicity of forms. In all of his uses of identity, the sense of *inner* continuity between one's personal, ethnic, social, and politico-national past and one's present interactions with the world remains the important constant factor. Erikson did field work on the Pine Ridge Indian Reservation of the Oglala Sioux in South Dakota in 1937. Children were forced to attend U.S. government boarding schools, where the general affect was slow, apathetic, depressed. A boy who was singled out by his teacher as a problem "radiates . . . a sense of ideal identity" when he can, in the present moment, behave in a way that is in concord with his traditional tribal values of sharing and generosity: "The way you see me now is the way I really am, and it is the way of my forefathers."[27] The Eriksonian model assumes that identity is made up of *identifications*—the internalizations of parents, family, kin, friends, peers, teachers, social and spiritual counsellors, ethnic and religious heritage, transgenerational political and social traditions, geography, and all the elements that make up the growing person's psychosocial surround. But identity is more than the sum of childhood identifications. Ego identity, says Erikson, "is the accrued experience of the ego's ability to integrate all identifications with the vicissitudes of the libido, with the aptitudes developed out of endowment, and with the opportunities offered in social roles. The sense of ego identity then, is the accrued confidence that the inner sameness and continuity prepared in the past are matched by the sameness and continuity of one's meaning for others."[28] People will fight hard to maintain these identities when they are threatened, because the alternative—indentity diffusion—is a painful experience of inner fragmentation.

We need operational definitions of national identity that allow space for the subjective experiences of people, including their sense of continuity and integration with their internalized personal, familial, and ethic past.

Karl Deutsch, in a seminal work which I think deserves renewed attention, emphasizes the intimate family socialization process as the essential building block of nationalism. Deutsch distinguishes between two kinds of communication, bureaucratic and social. Bureaucratic, or what Talcott Parsons termed "instrumental," communication connotes business, professional, and official transactions. Deutsch differentiates "the narrow vocational complementarity which exists among members of the same profession, such as doctors or mathematicians, or members of the same vocational group, such as farmers or intellectuals. Efficient communication among engineers, artists, or stamp collectors is limited to a relatively narrow segment of their total range of activities."

The other field of communication, which Deutsch signifies as "social communication," denotes areas of: "childhood memories, in courtship, marriage, and parenthood, in their standards of beauty, their habits of food and drink, in games and recreation, they are far closer to mutual communication and understanding with their countrymen than with their fellow specialists in other countries."[29] This is what Parsons termed the "affectual" as opposed to the "instrumental" functions, and it corresponds to the distinction Ferdinand Tonnies made between community (*Gemeinschaft*) and society (*Gesellschaft*). For Deutsch there is a fundamental relationship between a people and a community of mutual understanding. "Membership in a people essentially consists in wide complementarity of social communication. It consists in the ability to communicate more effectively, and over a wider range of subjects, with members of one large group than with outsiders."[30]

Deutsch draws on the concept developed by the Austro-Marxist Otto Bauer, that a nation is a community shaped by shared experiences. Bauer specified a common history; "a community of fate" which "tied together" the members of a nation into a "community of character." A "community of culture" remains entirely dependent on a preceding "community of fate" (*Schicksalsgemeinschaft*).[31] Deutsch sees nationalism as grounded in a common social culture, which is a personal, developmental, highly family and home oriented, learned pattern of life: "We found *culture* based on the community of communication, consisting of socially stereotyped patterns of behavior, including habits of language and thought, and carried on through various forms of social learning, particularly through methods of child rearing standardized in this culture."[32] He directly invokes the feeling of comfort and security in knowing that others understand one in the intimate realms of taste, play, family and sexual life, referring to:

> the widespread preferences for things or persons of "one's own kind" (that is, associated with one's particular communication group) in such matters as buying and selling, work, food and recreation, courtship and marriage. . . . At every step we find social communication bound up indissolubly with the ends and means of life, with men's values and the patterns of their teamwork, with employment and promotion, with marriage and inheritance, with the preferences of buyers and sellers, and with economic security or distress — with all the psychological, political, social, and economic relationships that influence the security and happiness of individuals. Nationality, culture, and communi-

cation are not the only factors that affect all these, but they are always present to affect them.[33]

The obvious case to test the family socialization model of Deutsch and Erikson is the history of modern Poland, a naturally poor country with open forest and steppe frontiers, and the geopolitical misfortune of being surrounded by strong, voracious imperial neighbors—Romanov Russia, Hohenzollern Prussia, and Habsburg Austria. As Thucydides said: "Of the gods we believe, and of men we know, that by a necessary law of their natures they rule whenever they can." Poland was four times partitioned and occupied by her hostile neighbors; in 1772, 1793, 1795, and again from 1939 to 1945, between Hitler's Nazi Germany and Stalin's Soviet Russia. In the long nineteenth century (1789–1914) Poles were subjected to Russification and Prussification, their language was banned in schools and offices, their culture deprecated, their church persecuted. The Polish people revolted in 1830–31 and 1863–64, tragic risings which were suppressed with bloody severity. When Poland was re-created in 1919 after the First World War there had been no Polish state for 124 years, or the equivalent of six demographic generations. But the flame of Polish national identity was kept alive and fueled in the Polish family, home, and church.

Erikson and Deutsch provide for the existence and instrumental effectiveness of Musil's reality of an interior space in the person. Their evocation and structuring of the most intimate interpersonal psychodynamic field and their relation of that field to ethnic and national conflict makes their models of nationalism richer, more complex, and superior to Anderson, Bourdieu, and Brubaker's reflexive understanding of nationalism, or Hobsbawm and Gellner's structural models. Deutsch integrates the implications of developmental personality research with social science communication theory to build a dynamic cultural-historical narrative explanation of how nationalism and nation building function in individuals and groups. While Deutsch accurately locates the phenomenology of nationalism in the family and the home, he does not explain the dynamics of how these nationalist messages are communicated, transferred, inculcated, and internalized from caretakers to children in each case in the intimate family ambiance. This is the province of psychoanalytic research on the internalization of trust and fear.

III

Nationalism begins in the family and the home. The decisive questions appear early: "Mama, what are we? What am I? Who are they? Are they good or bad? Can I feel safe with them? Who dominates whom? Who has power, authority, and status?" And, immediately sensed but never articulated, "Why are you anxious?" There is a common folk saying in the Middle East: "I fight my brother, my brother and I are against our cousins, we and our cousins against the other clans, our people versus their people, our nation against the world." This maxim conveys the family socialization process, which begins early and which views outsiders and strangers as a cause for anxiety as well as curiosity and wonderment.[34] The phase-specific distinctions between "us" and "them" that children experience as they grow up can give us a grasp of the roots of national identity.

By the second half of the first year of life the generalized smiling response is reserved for the mother and other special caretaking persons. This preferential smile to the mother is the crucial proof that a bond to another specific person has been established which distinguishes that loved person from all others in the world.[35] Projection, or casting away from the self, and introjection, or taking in, incorporating into the self, are among the most "primitive" defenses. Their roots are in the earliest "oral" phase of life. As Freud put it: "Expressed in the language of the oldest—the oral—instinctual impulses, the judgement is: 'I should like to eat this' or 'I should like to spit it out'; and put more generally: 'I should like to take this into myself and keep that out.' That is to say: 'It shall be inside me' or 'it shall be outside me.' . . . The original pleasure-ego wants to introject into itself everything that is good and to eject from itself everything that is bad. What is bad, what is alien to the ego and what is external are, to begin with, identical."[36]

Melanie Klein and her followers developed the concept of primitive "splitting" in early infancy, which explains the division of people and objects in the world into categories of "good" and "bad."[37] A child who has distinguished between internal and external, between self and nonself, may then use what Anna Freud categorized as the defense mechanisms of projection and introjection: "It is then able to project its prohibited impulses outwards. Its tolerance of other people is prior to its severity towards itself. It learns what is regarded as blameworthy but protects itself by means of this defence-mechanism from unpleasant self-criticism. Vehement indignation at someone else's wrong-doing is the precursor of and substitute for guilty feelings on its own account."[38] The decisive variable is the level of basic trust and confidence based on a consistent, close, warm, and pleasurable interaction with the mother or other primary caretakers. Erikson refers to the conflict of "basic trust versus basic mistrust" as "the nuclear conflict" and "the first task of the ego."[39]

Daniel N. Stern argues that the leap from unpleasurable to "bad" and from pleasurable to "good" is an issue for later cognitive ego development, dependent on verbalization and symbol formation. Stern offers the concept of affectively toned clusters of interactive experiences between infant and mother which constitute "working models" of mother for the child. At a later date these are reintegrated by the older child or adult into higher-order categorization of "good" and "bad."[40] The important point for us is that "splitting" exists in adult attitudes toward conflict in personal, group, and international settings and that the analysis and understanding of this pervasive mechanism is relevant for coming to grips with nationalism, ethnocentrism, and racism.[41]

IV

I wish now to offer a case study of a historic ethnic identity conflict—the island of Cyprus, where I engaged in field work and interviews in the north in the spring of 1997—and apply to it the principles of crisis management, dispute resolution, and tension reduction derived from both clinical practice and political psychology field work.[42] There are three immediate critical strategic issues:

1. The agreement signed 4 January 1997 by the Greek Cypriot Government to purchase from Russia a SA-10 anti-aircraft missile system, and the resulting threats of a military strike by Turkey. President Clinton expressed American vexation: "We have been very concerned about the decision. . . . The United States and its allies tried hard to persuade Cyprus that purchasing these missiles was a step leading away from negotiations, which remain the only way to solve the Cyprus problem. In the context of the already excessive levels of armaments on Cyprus and last summer's intercommunal violence, the government's decision to go forward

with purchases was doubly regrettable."[43] The Republic of Cyprus, under U.S. pressure, agreed to defer the importation of components of the missile system for sixteen months, until April 1998. This Greek Cypriot threat to install missiles remains acute.[44]

2. On January 16, 1997, the Turkish Government accepted a U.S. initiative for a moratorium on flights of Greek and Turkish combat aircraft over Cyprus, provided the Greeks also agree to it. On 17 January Greek Cypriot President Glafcos Clerides said he could not accept a moratorium. President Clerides agreed that no Greek fighter aircraft will be permanently stationed on Cyprus before March 1998. Now there are Greek and Turkish military overflights and landings on Cyprus.[45]

3. The Government of Cyprus' current negotiation for membership in the European Union (E.U.) is a potential opening for Turkish Cypriot participation. President Rauf Denktash expressed the official Turkish Republic of Northern Cyprus (TRNC) position, which is no entry without Turkey. That is not going to happen now or in the near future because the Europeans are not ready to accept an Islamic state. However, Turkish Cypriot entry could be a precursor and prologue for eventual Turkish E.U. entry. Greece threatens to block the E.U. enlargement process if the Cyprus application is held up. Greece has blocked E.U. funds for Turkey and vetoed a renewed E.U. membership overture to Turkey.[46]

Let us now consider the following political, socioeconomic, cultural, and psychological structural problems in the Cypriot situation:

1. Both sides have been severely traumatized. The Turks were rulers of an empire until 1918. As Interior Minister Sukru Kaya Bey put it in 1934, Turks could scarcely be expected to "live as slave where the Turk previously was the master."[47] The Turkish Cypriots were from 1963 to 1974 a beleaguered minority residing in enclaves encompassing 3 percent of the territory. The Greeks were most recently traumatized by the Turkish amphibious military intervention of 20 July 1974, which expelled them from the northern one-third of the island. This, of course, only compounded the traumas of five hundred years of Ottoman rule and the history of prolonged Greco-Turkish wars and massacres (War of Independence, 1821–31; Cretan Revolts, 1866–68, 1896–97, 1905–13; Thessaly, 1878–81; Anatolian campaign, 1919–22).

2. Once traumatized, people will desperately avoid returning to a position of vulnerability where the trauma could be repeated. The demographic situation on the island is substantially different now than it was before 1974. What amounts to a massive population exchange took place after 1974, with all of the island's Turks seeking refuge in the north and all Greeks fleeing south. With a contiguous band of settlement in the north, are the Turks in fact today as exposed to annihilation as they fear?

3. With 18 percent of the population, the Turkish side now controls the northern 37 percent of the island. What percentage of the land they hold are they willing to negotiate in order to achieve recognition and a stable peace? This is the Camp David formula for exploiting an asymmetry in vital interests: land for political recognition.

4. President Denktash professes commitment to a Federal Republic of Cyprus, "a bi-national, bi-lingual, bi-cultural partnership state."[48] How is the sovereignty of a binational state compatible with a Turkish right of military intervention, which the Turkish Cypriots demand for their security? Do Denktash and the other TRNC leaders see that it is not possible for Greek Cypriots to agree to a constitutional arrangement under which the Turkish army comes in whenever the Turks ask for them?

5. How real is the security of waiting on the Turkish motherland for intervention? Sometimes she chooses to come when asked, at other times she will not or cannot. The U.S. has blocked past interventions and could do so again. It took eleven years last time. The question is: What constitutes reliable security under which Greek and Turkish Cypriots feel safe? The most reliable security is a political solution.

6. Are the Greek Cypriots as monolithic in their opinions as the Turkish Cypriots believe? There are fissures and there have been coups (1974), assassination attempts, and civil wars on the Greek side.

7. Is the E.U., which is mistrusted, a homogenous, pro-Greek force as is believed? The E.U. has a record of sensitivity to ethnic minority rights (the German right to own land in Danish Schleswig; Åland [*Ahvenam-maa*] Island's autonomy between Finnish sovereignty and a Swedish population).

8. The advantages of E.U. membership for all of Cyprus are multiple, and recognized by the TRNC. E.U. membership brought booming economies and modernization to Spain, Portugal, and Ireland. As things stand the advantages will accrue only to the Greek

side: no tariffs for exports to Europe, such as now hurt the TRNC; massive loans, investment, and credits (the E.U. poured $3 billion into Ireland); increased tourism resulting from direct flights from northern and western European cities to the TRNC, which are not now possible. The Greek side now has two million tourists per year, and an annual per capita income of $12,000, compared to $4,000 for the TRNC. What is not taken into account is the dynamic impact of economic development and infrastructural integration in creating conditions of stability. A Franco-German war is today unthinkable for structural reasons.

9. What useful contemporary models of interethnic, intercommunal comity exist? TRNC President Denktash invokes Swiss cantonal federalism. The Swiss "magic formula" (*Zauberformel*), which assures minorities (Franco-Italians, Catholics, Peasants, Socialists) representation on a national level, may be relevant. The Italo-Austrian accommodation on the South Tirol (*Alto Adige*) should be of special relevance because Austria, the non-sovereign power, is guaranteed an international protective function (*internationalen Schutzfunktion*) for the German-speaking population under international law.

10. A distinct civic culture has developed in Cyprus which distinguishes the island population from the Greek and Turkish motherlands. One ambivalent identification they share is a historic background of British rule, from 1878 to 1960. There are still two British bases on the Greek side. Cypriots drive on the left side of the road. The TRNC, unlike Greek Cyprus, where the church is powerful and controls education, is a secular polity where the Welfare Party, Turkey's recent ruling

party, has *no* representation. At President Denktash's annual Bayram Reception, celebrating the end of the Mohammedan Feast of Ramadan on 18 April 1997, among the military, police, civic, and commercial dignitaries there was not a single Imam or Moslem cleric in evidence. President Denktash threatens closer integration with Turkey if the Republic of Cyprus enters the E.U. What would this mean for the now secularized, partially Anglophone northern Cyprus?

11. Differences of opinion exist in the TRNC. Two of the four parties in the Legislative Assembly are willing to consider entering the E.U. without Turkey after a settlement of the Cyprus issue.

12. The 1974 populations were 641,000 Greeks and 116,000 Turks. What is the effect on the civic culture of the TRNC, whose 1996 population was 198,215, of the immigration of Anatolian peasants from Turkey? No one knows the figures. President Denktash asserts that it is 15,000; it may be as high as 100,000 according to the *New York Times*.[49] Both the Ottomans and the Turkish Republic encouraged internal and foreign immigration, believing "that a large population was the pre-condition for economic development as well as for a strong defense against outside enemies."[50] How long will it take until there is an Islamic political movement because of this internal immigration? What is the potential effect of this influx on a final settlement?

13. Militarization of the island is an issue. There are between 30,000 and 40,000 Turkish troops and additional TRNC conscripts stationed in the north. There are 11,500 Greek Cypriot national guard conscripts in the south. A 1,200-strong U.N. force patrols a 111-mile buffer zone between them.

14. The threat of castration by the enemy is invoked in language, material symbolism, folklore, and oral tradition. The Nicosia International Airport is now closed. On arrival at the new TRNC Erçan Airport, I inquired what the name meant. I was told Erçan was the only Turkish jet pilot shot down in the 1974 war. He parachuted to Earth, was captured and taken to Nicosia, tortured, and his penis was cut off. Various minarets, the slender lofty towers attached to mosques from which the faithful are summoned to prayer, were deliberately toppled by the Greeks. This is understood as symbolic castration. The implicit message is: *If we again fall under Greek control, we will be castrated.* Nicoletta Gullace recently wrote of British propaganda in World War One as eliciting "public outrage through accounts of rape, mutilation, and barbarism . . . . Images of sexual violation retain an extraordinary potency in the arsenal of symbols deployed against a common enemy."[51]

To return in a Joycean mode to where we began, with *Ulysses;* Joyce knew and portrayed the nightmarish side of Irish, Hungarian, and Jewish identity. An important personal and political meaning of his novel is that national identity may haunt us, but it is also essentially who we are—internalized identifications with loved and hated persons and places, dreams and disasters, wounds and triumphs, grievances and entitlements, rituals and symbols, that constitute meanings for life. Nations as polities can, at least in theory, exist with only an "imaginary past." The imaginary, however, carries great demonstrable power to move individuals to action. On the other hand, persons and nations who believe they are reborn anew each day are living a fantasy of denial that will exact a cost in pain and destruction. I have undertaken to demonstrate that humanistic and psycho-analytic understandings of national identity incorporate inner subjective dimensions of experience that are needed for understanding politics and history, inasmuch as they make us conscious that we are *not* born anew daily—we carry internalized pasts within us. Persons and groups have histories that interact with current crises and opportunities. Perspectives that include a place for the continuity of history and cultural discourse in the personality are a prerequisite for a satisfying contemporary social science understanding of national identity.

Notes

I thank the Hon. Gündüz Aktan, deputy undersecretary for Europe, Turkish Foreign Ministry, Ankara, for candid exposures to Turkish foreign policy problems in May 1996; H. E. Rauf Denktaş, president of the Turkish Republic of Northern Cyprus, for consultations in April 1997; and Hon. Kostas Karistinos, press attache, Embassy of Cyprus, Washington, D.C., for consultation and research materials. I acknowledge with gratitude the hospitality and good offices of Vamik and Betty Volkan, both for making possible hands-on field work in Cyprus and for his psychodynamic conceptualization of the interplay of enemy images. I am indebted to the thoughtful analysis of James J. Sheehan in "National History and National Identity in the New Germany," *German Studies Review,* Special Issue: "German Identity" (Winter 1992): 163–174. I benefited from the discerning discussion of this topic at the fifth annual meeting of the University of California Interdisciplinary Psychoanalytic Consortium at Lake Arrowhead on 10 May 1997. I thank Lynn D. Lampert for her resourceful research assistance.

1. James Joyce, *Ulysses* (1992; reprint, New York: Random House, 1961), pp. 331–338, *passim.*

2. Homer, *The Odyssey: The Story of Odysseus,* trans. W. H. D. Rouse (New York: Penguin, 1937), p. 102.

3. Little scholarly attention has been paid to the Hungarian identity theme in *Ulysses.* A rare exception is Roger Tracy, "Leopold Bloom Fourfold: A Hungarian-Hebraic-Hellenic-Hibernian Hero," *Massachusetts Review* 6 (Spring–Summer 1965): 523–538.

4. Hugh Kenner, *Ulysses* (London: George Allen & Unwin, 1980), p. 133; Vincent Sherry, *Ulysses* (Cambridge: Cambridge University Press, 1994), p. 12.

5. Arthur Griffith, *The Resurrection of Hungary: A Parallel for Ireland; with appendices on Pitt's Policy and Sinn Fein*, 3rd ed. (1904) (Dublin: Whelan and Son, 1918), p. 95.

6. I thank Professor Gyula Gazdag for aid in translation from the Hungarian.

7. Joyce, *Ulysses*, pp. 342–343.

8. Homer, *The Odyssey*, p. 107.

9. Joyce, *Ulysses*, p. 727.

10. Frank Budgen, *James Joyce and the Making of Ulysses* (Bloomington: Indiana University Press, 1960), p. 274.

11. Robert Musil, *The Man Without Qualities*, vol. 1, *A Sort of Introduction: The Like of it Now Happens (I)*, trans. Eithne Wilkins and Ernst Kaiser (New York: Perigee, 1953), p. 34. Musil disliked Joyce's work and the comparison with *Ulysses* annoyed him.

12. Pierre Bourdieu, *In Other Words: Essays Towards a Reflexive Sociology*, trans. Matthew Adamson (Stanford, Calif.: Stanford University Press, 1990), p. 136.

13. Pierre Bourdieu, *Language and Symbolic Power*, ed. John B. Thompson, trans. Gino Raymond and Matthew Adamson (Cambridge, Mass.: Harvard University Press, 1991), p. 88.

14. Ibid., p. 224.

15. Craig Calhoun, "The Problem of Identity in Collective Action," in Joan Huber, ed., *Macro-Micro Linkages in Sociology* (Newbury Park, Calif.: Sage Publications, 1991), pp. 52, 59.

16. Rogers Brubaker, *Nationalism Reframed: Nationhood and the National Question in the New Europe* (Cambridge: Cambridge University Press, 1996), pp. 18–19.

17. Ibid., p. 56, n. 1.

18. Benedict Anderson, *Imagined Communities Reflections on the Origins and Spread of Nationalism*, revised ed. (London: Verso, 1991), pp. 204–205.

19. E. J. Hobsbawm, *Nations and Nationalism Since 1780: Programme, Myth, Reality* (Cambridge: Cambridge University Press, 1990), pp. 182–183, and n. 22. This analysis prompted the *New York Times* to comment that Hobsbawm's "survey, conducted with the traditional Marxist loathing for anything so backward-looking, merely reveals nationalism's faults rather than proves that its emotions have lost their pulling power" (28 July 1990).

20. E. J. Hobsbawm, "Some Reflections on Nationalism," in T. J. Nossiter,

A. H. Hanson, and Stein Rokkan, eds., *Imagination and Precision in the Social Sciences* (London: Faber and Faber, 1972), p. 406.

21. Bourdieu, *Language and Symbolic Power,* p. 288, n. 11.

22. Ernest Gellner, *Nations and Nationalism* (Oxford: Basil Blackwell, 1983), pp. 36–38.

23. Ibid., p. 57.

24. Gellner, "Psychoanalysis as a Social Institution: An Anthropological Perspective," in Edward Timms and Naomi Segal, eds., *Freud in Exile: Psychoanalysis and Its Vicissitudes* (New Haven: Yale University Press, 1988), pp. 223–229. The quotation is from p. 226.

25. Gellner, *Nations and Nationalism,* pp. 34–35.

26. John J. Fitzpatrick, "Erik H. Erikson and Psychohistory," *Bulletin of the Menninger Clinic* 40 (1976): 295–314; Howard I. Kushner, "Pathology and Adjustment in Psychohistory: A Critique of the Erikson Model," *Psychocultural Review* 1 (1977): 493–506; Paul Roazen, *Erik H. Erikson: The Power and Limits of a Vision* (New York: Free Press, 1976). For an appreciation, see Robert Coles, *Erik H. Erikson: The Growth of His Work* (Boston: Little, Brown, 1970).

27. Erik H. Erikson, *Childhood and Society* (New York: Norton, 1963), 2d ed. p. 129.

28. Ibid., p. 261.

29. Karl W. Deutsch, *Nationalism and Social Communication: An Inquiry into the Foundations of Nationality,* 2nd ed. (Cambridge, Mass.: MIT Press, 1966), p. 98.

30. Ibid., p. 97.

31. Ibid., pp. 19–20. Otto Bauer, *Die Nationalitätenfrage und die Sozial-demokratie* (1907), *Werkausgabe* (Vienna: Europaverlag, 1975), 1: 172, 192. Cf. Peter Loewenberg, "Austro-Marxism and Revolution: Otto Bauer, Freud's 'Dora' Case, and the Crisis of the First Austrian Republic," in *Decoding the Past: The Psychohistorical Approach* (New Brunswick, N.J.: Transaction Publishers, 1996), pp. 161–204.

32. Deutsch, *Nationalism* p. 37.

33. Ibid., pp. 101, 106.

34. Margaret S. Mahler, Fred Pine, and Anni Bergman, *The Psychological Birth of the Human Infant* (New York: Basic Books, 1975), p. 209. Mahler et al. stress the variety of reactions to strangers, of which anxiety is only one. They regard "stranger anxiety" as a "one-sided" and "incomplete" description (p. 56), preferring the term "stranger reactions": "In addition to anxiety, the stranger evokes mild or even compellingly strong curiosity. That is why we have emphasized throughout this book that *curiosity*

and *interest* in the new and the unfamiliar are as much a part of stranger reactions as are anxiety and wariness."

35. John Bowlby, "The Nature of the Child's Tie to His Mother," *International Journal of Psychoanalysis* 39 (1958): 350–73.

36. Sigmund Freud, *"Die Verneimung"* (1925), *Studienausgabe*, Hrsg. Alexander Mitscherlich et al., (Frankfurt am Main: S. Fischer Verlag, 1975), vol. 3, p. 374; "Negation," Sigmund Freud, *Standard Edition of the Complete Psychological Works*, ed. James Strachey et al. (London: Hogarth, 1961), vol. 19, p. 237.

37. Melanie Klein, *The Psycho-Analysis of Children* (London: Hogarth Press, 1932); *Contributions to Psycho-Analysis, 1921–1945* (London: Hogarth Press, 1948); *Envy and Gratitude and Other Works, 1946–1963* (London: Hogarth Press, 1975). See also Otto Kernberg, *Borderline Conditions and Pathological Narcissism* (New York: Jason Aronson, 1975).

38. Anna Freud, *The Ego and the Mechanisms of Defence* (1936) trans. Cecil Baines (New York: International Universities Press, 1946), p. 128.

39. Erikson, *Childhood and Society*, p. 249.

40. Daniel N. Stern, *The Interpersonal World of the Infant: A View from Psychoanalysis and Developmental Psychology* (New York: Basic Books, 1985), pp. 252–253.

41. Vamik D. Volkan, *The Need to Have Enemies and Allies: From Clinical Practice to International Relationships* (Northvale, N.J.: Jason Aronson, 1988), pp. 28–29. See also Kurt R. and Kati Spillmann, *Feindbilder: Entstehung, Funktion und Möglichkeiten ihres Abbaus, Zürcher Beiträge zur Sicherheitspolitik und Konfliktforschung,* Nr. 12 (Zurich: ETH, 1989); and Group for the Advancement of Psychiatry, *Us and Them: The Psychology of Ethnocentrism* (New York: Brunner-Mazel, 1987).

42. Peter Loewenberg, "Crisis Management: From Therapy to Government and from the Oval Office to the Couch," in *Fantasy and Reality in History* (New York: Oxford University Press, 1995), 217–224; see particularly the work of Alexander George, ed., *inter alia, Managing U.S.-Soviet Rivalry: Problems of Crisis Prevention* (Boulder, Colo.: Westview Press, 1983); *Avoiding War: Problems of Crisis Management* (Boulder, Colo.: Westview Press, 1991).

43. President William J. Clinton to Speaker of the House of Representatives and the Chairman of the Senate Foreign Relations Committee, 25 April 1997. Office of the Press Secretary, The White House.

44. Stephen Kinzer, "Greek and Turkish Jets Lead New Round of Cyprus Tension," *New York Times,* 20 June 1998.

45. "Cyprus Talks for U.S. Envoy on Athens Stop," *New York Times,* 22 June 1998.

46. "Controversy Over European Union Talks With Cyprus," *Time International,* vol. 150, no. 33 (April 13, 1998), p. 16.

47. Brubaker, *Nationalism Reframed,* p. 156, quoting Joseph B. Schechtman, *European Population Transfers, 1939–1945* (New York: Oxford University Press, 1946), p. 490.

48. President Rauf Denktash, "Talking Points" with Malcolm Rifkin, secretary of foreign affairs, United Kingdom, 16 December 1996, p. 3.

49. Celestine Bohlen, "Greek and Turk Cypriots Dispute Who is Living in Island's North," *New York Times,* 23 January 1997.

50. Kemal H. Karpat, *Ottoman Population, 1830–1914: Demographic and Social Characteristics* (Madison: University of Wisconsin Press, 1985), p. 62.

51. Nicoletta F. Gullace, "Sexual Violence and Sexual Honor: British Propaganda and International Law During the First World War," *American Historical Review* 102, no. 3 (June 1997): 714–747. The quotation is from pp. 746–747.

A Psychoanalytic Study of
Argentine Soccer

MARCELO M. SUÁREZ-OROZCO

If one were to make a list of major social events in which millions of men in most corners of Earth invest curiously large
amounts of affective energy, the soccer spectacle would most
likely occupy a comfortable place among the top ten (see Bayer
1990; Scher 1988; Romero 1985). Despite this, a glance at the
scholarly works on the psychosocial nature of the soccer spectacle shows an alarming lack of coherent documentation of and
insight into the dynamics of the cathexis the soccer fan so intensely invests in the soccer show.

As a child growing up in Argentina, I became a captive of
the addicting webs of the soccer spectacle. It is perhaps this
early involvement with the game that led me to search for the
tools in anthropology, folklore, and psychology needed to unravel the meaning of this show, which had such a narcotizing
effect on me as a child.

The first inkling of the questions I raise here was perhaps
formulated when, as a child, I was taken most weekends to
the soccer stadiums by neighbors to join others in passionately
rooting for our home team. Although I had no clear idea of
what was really going on, in my frantic shouting and mimick-
ing of the older fans I must have had the first real feeling of
social belonging. My soccer fixation continued. When I was a
bit older, I and was allowed (not without frowns from my parents) to go to the stadiums, no longer with a guardian, but with
my adolescent friends. Soon we recognized the real dangers in
going to a stadium, where up to twenty thousand fans for each

of two rival teams gathered to root for their teams, and thus (at least in theory) help them win. However, the emotional involvement, the delirious and unrestrained shouting, the ritualized exchange of insults between fans of the same and opposite teams, their vicious throwing of bottles and stones, and the general state of dissociation bring to attention (even to the eye of an untrained adolescent) the fact that much more than mere rooting for the victory of one's team is occurring in soccer stadiums throughout Argentina (and probably in other places of the world, where the soccer phenomenon has reached equivalent dimensions). My parents' frowns were thus not without reason.

The questions this paper explores include: Why are hundreds of thousands of men attracted to soccer stadiums every weekend all over Argentina? What force is there in the soccer spectacle that addicts men, possessing them during the ninety minutes in which twenty-two players, eleven for each team, try to kick a ball—in its ancient form a pig's bladder (Mafud 1967: 34), sometimes stuffed with hair (Pickford 1940: 82)— into the rival team's goal more times than that team kicks it into their goal?

Sufficient Reasons

Scholarly works on the psychosocial nature of the soccer spectacle have for the most part been conducted by either European (both British and Continental) or Latin American researchers.[1] These writers have proposed a wide array of reasons to explain why every weekend soccer attracts millions of fans to stadiums all over the globe. In this section of the paper I review these proposed explanations and briefly evaluate their strengths and weaknesses in explaining the unusual behavior of fans at the stadiums.

Buytendijk, in his *Le Football, une Etude Psychologique* (1952), argues that spectators seek sensationalism in the soccer stadium. This after-the-fact statement is inherently circular and does not satisfactorily explain what underlies the fans' desire for sensationalism in the first place. Buytendijk also argues that fans seek diversion from the pressures of everyday life. At first glance, no one would disagree with this line of argument; however, it does not address why it is that fans overwhelmingly seek soccer games, and not, for example, polo matches or other diverting shows. Further, no one who has seen a considerable number of soccer spectacles would agree with his proposition that soccer is pressure free. A quick glance at the statistics of tragic violence at the stadiums (Taylor 1969, 1971a, 1971b; Romero 1985, 1986) would convince even those who have never seen a professional soccer game that the opposite is true.

Buytendijk further argues that the game offers fans a sense of belonging with their fellow fans and their beloved players. Regrettably, he does not document the specifics of the soccer fan's structural scapegoating of the "other" as a means of defining one's group. As I shall later document, this scapegoating, or, more precisely, projecting, is of central importance in the Argentinian soccer stadium, as a means for defining not just one's group, but also one's masculinity. Interestingly, and in accordance with Foster's image of "limited good and machismo" (1979: 130), the fan must define his manliness at the expense of that of other fans. And as we shall see, this is only the tip of the psychodynamic iceberg. Lastly, Buytendijk views soccer as offering fans an opportunity to be experts, due to the well known and rather simple rules that govern the game. Although this view of the "cerebral fan" does have some validity, the affective and irrational involvement of the fan in the game is, in my opinion, a far more fundamental underlying factor, which must be accounted for if we are to understand the basic dynamics of the fan's behavior.

Da Silva views spectators as inherently voluble and emotional, and he argues that any frustration will automatically lead to aggression, "the most frequent being verbal aggression directed toward the athlete, who becomes an easy and readily available scapegoat" (1970: 307). Since he fails to document specific instances of verbal aggression toward athletes,[2] and as my data indicates that the most frequent form of verbal aggression is not directed at the players but at the rival team's fans, at least in the Argentinian case, we must question the validity of his statement.[3] Further, I must note that the frustration-aggression hypothesis of Dollard, Doob, Miller, Mower, and Sears (1939), inherent in da Silva's argument, can be seriously questioned in its ability to explain aggression in the soccer stadium. Consider Hopcraft's discussion of the problem of violence in and around British soccer stadiums: "Initially it seemed possible to align the vandalism directly with the disappointment of supporters who had travelled far to see their side go down. Later on it became clear that the result of the game had no causative effect on this kind of behavior at all: win, lose, or draw, there could be trouble or there could be none" (1968: 183). Again, dissociative, irrational behavior with no apparent causes appears to be a recurring theme of the behavior of both British and Argentinian fans, and I have no reason to believe that Brazilian fans are much different.

For da Silva, aggression in the stadium provides fans "a catharsis and an outlet not only for the spectator's sportive frustrations, but also for his economic and even existential anxieties" (da Silva 1970: 307). Again, he regrettably fails to outline and illustrate the dynamics of the catharsis. Further, his implied understanding that it is the violent nature of the spectacle that attracts fans is an oversimplification of the complex dynamics of the event. I shall briefly evaluate more critically this hypothesis.

Freud's student Helene Deutsch brilliantly explored the relationship between castration fears, associated in their genesis with oedipal rivalry, and the attraction males have for soccer. Briefly, she viewed soccer as a mechanism used, even by non-markedly neurotic individuals, for the "projection of a source of anxiety into the outside world and discharge of the anxiety" (1926: 226). Later I shall more thoroughly explore Deutsch's thesis in the context of the symbolism of the game itself. Suffice it to say here that from her argument it logically follows that one reason, among many others, that millions of males are attracted to stadiums every weekend is the opportunity the game offers them to "project" themselves into their idols, and with them to vicariously master "the ball," and by extension their own masculinity. We shall return to this point.

Dunning and Elias have done more than any other English speaking scholars to document the history and sociology of soccer.[4] Dunning views soccer as an institutionalized means of channeling aggression: "Many of the more brutal practices of earlier times were rooted out, but the chances for participation in a physical struggle were not eliminated entirely" (1967: 884). By extending his logic we can infer that the pleasure of watching the "physical struggle" between the teams is, at least in part, what attracts fans to the show. The idea of fans taking sadistic pleasure in watching the violence on the field and around them is shared by Hopcraft, who sees soccer as being an essentially conflictual sport: "People enjoy watching violence, and they are fed it in children's comics, in pop music and by cinema and television. When it occurs on the football terraces there is relish as well as condemnation in the way the seated ranks and the newspapers respond to it" (1968: 185). Although this is partially true, it does not explain why fans are addicted to soccer and not to other more violent games.

Later, Elias and Dunning (1970) argue that the spectacle and color of professional soccer function as a relief from the constraint and control of civilization. Fans are perceived as searching for excitement in "unexciting societies." No one would really question this argument, but the question still remains, why soccer and not other "colorful" spectacles?

Frankenberg views soccer as a symbol of village prestige and unity in the face of the outside world, in the community he studied in North Wales (1957). Soccer is viewed as a functional, cohesive bond which provides the community a sense of common destiny and belonging, especially when relating to the outside. This may be true for the rather remote village he studied, but in my opinion it would be a mistake to extend this rather romantic view of the game to the rest of world soccer. The inherent conflictual nature of the game (Hopcraft 1968; Taylor 1969, 1971a, 1971b) makes untenable the extension of Frankenberg's observations in North Wales to soccer generically.[5]

Lever, in her theoretical works on soccer in Brazil, describes the game as "the opium" (1969) of the Brazilian people, and more generally as "a Brazilian way of life" (1972). However, "to make such a statement is not to give an explanation of why some seek opiates and others do not," as DeVos (1978: 7) insightfully commented on Marxists' views on religion. And the same applies to our research problem: Why do fans seek soccer and not other "opiates"?

Mafud, in his *Sociologia del Futbol* (1967) views the game, following Buytendijk (1952), as a basic regression from culture to nature. The game attracts crowds, in the eyes of this Argentine sociologist, for a variety of reasons. First, borrowing from Buytendijk, soccer is pictured as a diversion, allowing both players and fans to escape everyday reality. Secondly, by pitting groups against each other the game offers fans and players alike an opportunity to discharge aggression. And third, in Mafud's reasoning, the game attracts crowds by offering them a "chivo emisario" or "scapegoat" into which to project "la propia culpa, el propio miedo, la propia agresividad sobre el otro o sobre los otros" ("one's own guilt, one's own fear, one's own aggression into the other or the others") (1967: 111).[6] Although he briefly discusses the mechanics of scapegoating, his examples are few, and clearly need further elaboration to prove the usefulness of his hypothesis.

Others, for example Patrick (1903), an adherent of nine-teenth-century unilinear evolution theorizing, see games such as soccer as offering a de-evolutionary return to savagery, thus allowing the "higher centers" of the brain to momentarily rest. Medner (1956) views games such as soccer as intensifying hu-man vitality. Dundes (1978) reports the following views of an-cient soccer: "The ancestral form of football, a game more like rugby or soccer, was interpreted as a solar ritual—with a disc-shaped rock or object supposedly representing the sun,"[7] and also "as a fertility ritual intended to ensure agricultural abun-dance" (1978: 76). Pickford (1940, 1941), in his rather romantic historical studies of the origin and development of the game, sees it again as a constructive use of aggression. In her doc-toral thesis, Reaney (1916) relates the popularity of soccer to the fact that the game brings into play the primitive instinct of propelling a missile toward an aim (the goal). Schwartz (1973) reviews what he considers to be the most important determi-nants of spectator sports. For him, the pleasure-of-observing-excellence hypothesis, the need-for-excitement hypothesis, and the release-of-tension hypothesis are probably the most im-portant in determining fans' attendance. However, Schwartz grimly concludes, these hypotheses remain to be tested.

The problem with all of the above views, which reflect a belief that soccer's popularity is primarily due to its acting as an outlet for aggression, has been correctly outlined by Dundes in his psychoanalytic study of American football: "It is insufficient to state that football offers an appropriate outlet for the expression of aggression" (1978: 76). Dundes goes on to quote Arens, who argues that it would be an oversimplification "to single out violence as the sole or even primary reason for the game's popularity." As far more violent sports do exist in Argentina (boxing, wrestling, and so forth), and are far less popular than soccer, Dundes' objection applies also in our case.

Stokes's ingenious study points, in my opinion, to a more fruitful area of research by looking at the symbolism inherent in the game itself (1956). His psychoanalytic study of ball games views soccer specifically as a stage in which oedipal fantasies are acted out in a disguised, ego syntonic way. Each team is perceived as defending the symbolic maternal vagina (the goal) from the aggressive father (the rival team). At the same time, the teams are seen as trying to conquer new lands (women), thus developmentally moving from infancy to adulthood. In his own words: "When football teams canter out of the natal tunnel beneath a stand, the crowds applaud, surrender to them the field of play. Then, each team defends the goal at his back; in front is the new land, the new woman, whom they strive to possess in the interest of preserving the mother inviolate, in order, as it were, to progress from infancy to adulthood: at the same time, the defensive role is the father's; he opposes the forward of youth of the opposition" (1956: 187). Stokes's theoretical bias made him, in my view, arbitrarily perceive the goals as either the symbolic maternal vagina or the symbolic vagina of the "new woman." This view is contrary to my data, which in fact show that the goal, which each team defends at its back, is symbolic of the players' masculinity. However, Stokes's symbolic interpretation opens new avenues to arrive at the possible psychosocial meanings of the game.

Two other important works on soccer must be evaluated before we move on to our own analysis. Veccia, in his "Sunday Orgasm" (1976), states ex cathedra that soccer can be viewed as dramatizing collective unconscious impulses of a sexual and aggressive nature. This is easily detected, Veccia argues, in the game's symbols and in the spectators' emotions. The conduct of the athletes, officials, and spectators is interpreted as having sexual content, with specific sexual meaning. The author further argues that voyeurism, de-individuation, and interaction are the three most important factors which induce spectators to attend soccer stadiums. His failure to illustrate his imaginative points with even a single datum makes his propositions mere speculations.

In what remains the best researched monograph on the soccer phenomenon in Europe, Vinnai (1973) reviews the most salient features of the spectacle, emphasizing its relation to the larger society. Vinnai views the soccer game as providing a stage for the fans to observe the inherent nature of their working hours. "Here, twenty-two sportsmen provide the thousands on the terraces with routinized performances paralleling those of working hours" (1973: 39).

Thus, for Vinnai the soccer spectacle appears to fulfill the same function myths serve in the view of Lévi-Strauss (1958): It is a stage upon which the inherent contradictions of life are enacted in a disguised form. This view is in direct contradiction to most of the scholars discussed above, who view the game as offering both players and fans an escape from reality. Furthermore, for Vinnai the spectacle has become a mere capitalistic plot, preventing the working classes from directing their energies toward their true enemy, the bourgeoisie. "The same holds for the struggle for a better life, but the pseudoactivity

of football canalizes the energies which could shatter the exist-
ing power structures" (1973: 90). He concludes: "Sport, which
has long belonged to the realm of unfree activity, is also a part
of the system of capitalist mass culture, designed to keep the
victims of the alienated industrial apparatus under close control" (1973: 14). This Marxist view of soccer, which reduces the
game to a mere mirror of the struggle of the classes, fails to address the issues of meaning and value which both players and
fans attach to the game. Further, Vinnai's etic construct does
not address the obvious problem of why fans should get such
orgasmic pleasure, as they in fact do, from observing their own
tragic struggle being enacted.

The Spectacle and the Unconscious

In this section, I describe and interpret soccer stadium ethos as
revealed by both its folklore and game symbolism. An emphasis
will be placed on the former, with the intention of explaining
why it is that fans are so emotionally involved with the soccer
spectacle. Further, insight into the meaning of the symbols inherent in the game itself will help us understand why the game
triggers such peculiar fantasies and behavior from the fans.

I have chosen to discuss fans' folklore following the proposition endorsed and elegantly documented by Dundes that folklore is unconscious and that "among its functions, folklore provides a socially sanctioned outlet for the expression of what
cannot be articulated in the usual direct way" (1976: 1503).
Dundes goes on to argue, "It is precisely in jokes, folk tales, folk
songs, proverbs, children's games, gestures, etc., that anxieties
can be vented." The Argentinian fan, as will be documented,
has plenty of anxieties to vent, especially about his masculinity.

Thus, borrowing from Geertz (1973), a "thick description"
of the "deep" aspects of the Argentinian soccer spectacle, in-

cluding fans' folk songs and verbal duels, may help us uncover the underlying dynamics that motivate men to go to stadiums and tell us more generally about Argentinian male psychology.

A typical journey to the soccer stadium starts after the big Sunday lunch, when the average working class fan is picked up by *la barra,* the "gang," who are of course all fans for the same team.[8] The soccer show is, for all practical purposes, an all-male spectacle; only males play it professionally,[9] and the overwhelming majority of the fans are male.[10] With this point in mind, I turn to a description of a typical day at the soccer stadium. As la barra[11] meet, they will immediately begin a passionate discussion of how their team should line up; guess which of their beloved stars will first score a goal; and perhaps anticipate in paranoid fashion that the referee for that day's match has probably been "bought" by the rival team.[12] The integrity of the referee will surely be a topic of discussion on the way back home from the game if one's team lost in a close match.

By now, as they get closer to the stadium, they will begin to be increasingly excited, especially as they join other barras of their team and, waving the team's precious flag, chant lines such as:

| Soy de Boca, | soy de Boca, | de Boca yo soy. |
| (I) am of Boca, | (I) am of Boca, | for Boca I am. |

"Boca" is the name of their team. As they eventually meet barras from the opposing team, the chanting will get louder. Cursing and ritualized insulting will automatically start. The more elaborate songs and insults will not start until the fans for both teams are inside the stadium and the game has begun.

Once inside the stadium the more verbal and fanatic rooters[13] will lead their barras to the terraces in back of one of the two goals, facing directly the barras of the other team, who traditionally will be in back of the opposite goal. Facing each other from opposite sides of the soccer field, thousands of fans will loyally join their fellows in insulting and humiliating the rival team's fans, players, coach, and owner, the game's referee, and, when felt necessary, the players of their own team. The neutral spectator will avoid the heated polar ends of the stadium and will most likely either buy a more expensive ticket for the safer *platea* (covered grandstand) along the lateral side of the stadium, or find a seat in the uncovered portion along the opposite lateral side, thus having to his right hand and to his left hand the fans of each of the two teams. Although this type of more neutral, less fanatic observer does have a role in the soccer spectacle, for reasons of space I will discuss only the folklore of the more active fans, who due to their larger numbers form a group more relevant to this study.

The Macho Ethos

With this more or less typical background setting in mind, we can now begin to document soccer stadium folklore. The fans' dissociation will reach its pregame peak as the players of both teams emerge from an underground tunnel. At this point the fans will compulsively shake their team's flag and throw clouds of confetti, and sooner or later the fans for one of the teams (let us call them team A) may chant this song, which is commonly heard at the beginning of games:

> Vamos a ganar,   vamos a ganar
> We will win,   we will win
>
> Porque sino   los vamos a vejar
> Because if not   we will rape them

This song is particularly common at decisive games that one's team has to win at all costs. Fans use the song to warn the opposing team and its fans that if their team does not win this critical game they will rape the members of the rival team. Such homosexual rapes, of course, almost never actually occur. Nevertheless, the chant is an important datum, as it represents a vehicle for threatening to put one's rivals in the shameful position of a passive recipient of a homosexual encounter. It thus indicates that if they cannot attain power (victory) on one level, by winning the game, they will have to ascertain their superiority on another level: by overpowering their rivals with rape. This need to ascertain one's masculinity by victimizing the other appears to be a recurring pattern in soccer stadium folklore. But before further speculating on this theme, let us search the data further for more convincing evidence.

To the above threat the enraged fans of the other team (let us call them team B) may respond with the following statement about the nature of their team:

No tenemos a Maradona,	no tenemos a Filliol
We have not Maradona,	we have not Filliol
Pero si tenemos huevos,	huevos para salir cam-
	peon.
But yes we have eggs,	eggs to come out
	champion.

The meaning of this is that even though they do not have Mr. Maradona — the once loved and respected star of Argentine soccer (nicknamed "the white Pelé"), recently disgraced in a drug-related scandal — or the almost equally famous goalkeeper Mr. Filliol, they do have the hyperphallusness (*los huevos*, that is, "balls") that is, in their estimation, required to win the championship.

A concern with the power inherent in possessing a hyper-phallic sexual organ is also evident in other aspects of Argentinian folklore. For example, as this song indicates, a big compliment payed to Juan Domingo Peron (nicknamed "El Macho") by his loyal *Peronistas* was that he had an oversized sexual organ:

> La poronga de Peron
> The prick of Peron
>
> Es mas grande que un jamon
> Is bigger than a ham.

In their view Peron, the true macho, was a great man in part because he had a great phallus. Both songs, thus, mirror the belief held among many Argentine men that a "real macho" must be endowed with a large penis, which in turn is a metaphoric source of power. In the soccer stadium we can see this occurring: Although the fans admit to lacking great players, they boast that they and their team have *huevos*, the ultimate symbol of masculinity, superiority, and courage. The inherent power derived from their phalluses will enable them to subjugate all rival teams and thus eventually win the championship.

If the two hypothetical teams playing our typical game were really mismatched, a song such as the following might be heard:

> Señor Armando, Señor Armando
> Mr. Armando, Mr. Armando (the club's owner)
>
> A su cuadrito lo cogemos caminando
> Your little team we fuck walking

Freely translated this means, "Señor Armando, we screw your little team effortlessly." I heard this song at the Banfield Club stadium some years back, when the home team, a rather small and second-rate club, was facing the most-feared of the nation's teams, the Boca Juniors, owned by Mr. Armando. The Banfield fans began nervously to sing to Armando how their team was "screwing his little team," not even playing hard but just casually "walking" the field.

This song illuminates several theoretical issues. First, it shows how in the unconscious mind of the fan, the game symbolizes a homosexual encounter. So, "Mr. Armando, we play better soccer than your little team" becomes "We screw your little team."[14] This point is important in refuting Stokes's proposition that the goals in the soccer stadium symbolize the "maternal" and "new woman" vaginas. In fact, in Argentina at least, the folk, in their projective symbolic systems, associate the goals with their masculinity, more specifically their *culos* (backside). We shall briefly return to this critical point.

A second critical process that appears to recur in the Argentine data, which the above song beautifully illustrates, is the process of "projective inversion" as described by Dundes. For Dundes, projection in the psychoanalytic sense occurs in two distinct ways. Direct projections, in folklore, are "more or less direct translations of reality into fantasy." But projective inversion occurs with those "human problems which evidently require more elaborate disguise" (1976: 1521). In the last song we have a clear example of projective inversion. The fans for the lesser team—who undoubtedly fear, like all other Argentine fans, the powerful Boca Juniors team and their fans—project, in an inverted disguise, their own very founded fears of being "screwed" in the stadium by their rivals.[15] Thus, the unconscious fear "you are going to screw us" becomes the pseudo-aggressive, ego syntonic "we will screw you effortlessly."

Back to our stadium. At this point of the heated verbal exchange, Boca's fans might likely want to remind Banfield's fans who they are, and warn them not to step over the line:

Hinchada, hinchada, hinchada hay una sola
Fans, fans, fans, exist one only

Hinchada es la de Boca que le rompe el culo a todas
[Fans is the of Boca that it] breaks the ass of all

This freely translates, "Real fans are Boca's, who fuck and tear open the anuses of all other fans." This song, in its manifest content, indicates that the fans, and obviously by extension, real men, real machos, are Boca's, who, as noted previously, have a reputation for being hypermanly machos, because they are superphallic (that is, they have "balls"). They are superphallic because they not only force other teams' fans to submit to homosexual encounters, but they also "tear their anuses open" (*romper:* to tear open or to break). Another song articulating this fantasy was chanted in Argentina during the 1978 Jules Rimet soccer World Cup. In order to make it to the final rounds the home team of Argentina had to score a decisive victory (victory by *goleada,* that is, by scoring many goals) over the Peruvian national team. As they approached the stadium, Argentinian fans deliriously chanted:

Salta, salta, salta, pequeño canguro
Jump, jump, jump, little kangaroo

Hoy a los Peruanos les rompemos el culo
Today to the Peruvians we break the ass

This freely translates into "Today we will tear open the anuses of the Peruvians."

Beneath such sadistic fantasies an interesting picture develops, which will enable us to explore a dimension of machismo which has largely been ignored by social scientists who have studied the macho syndrome. Machos, as illustrated in their collective fantasies, are sadists who tear open the anuses of other men. Chapman notes: "Moreover, in many instances the sexual sadist has profound doubts about his sexual adequacy and masculinity, and he attempts to assuage these doubts by exaggerated aggressiveness in his sexual activities" (1967: 206). Although in our folklore data we are dealing, of course, with sadistic *fantasies,* and Chapman is describing the psychiatric profile of practicing sadists, his point nevertheless offers us a tool to explore the possible meanings of this aspect of macho behavior.

The important point is that in fact the macho, as documented by his unconscious fantasies, has "profound doubts about his sexual adequacy and masculinity," and these doubts are evident in his paranoid fear of being anally penetrated by other machos. This important point on the psychology of the hypermanly macho, which has emerged from my data, escaped the eyes of social scientists working on the macho syndrome in other parts of the world (Bolton 1979; Gilmore and Gilmore 1979; Chinas 1976; Fromm and Maccoby 1970; Foster 1979). Bolton, for example, describes the macho "ethos" as a set of beliefs, values, attitudes, emotions, and behavioral patterns found most commonly in Latin America (1979: 318). I would add that machismo in Latin America was inherited from Spain. Brandes's superb documentation of masculine metaphors in southern Spain (1980), and Gilmore and Gilmore's more shallow interpretation of the ontogenesis of machismo in an Andalusian town (1979), corroborate my argument.

According to Bolton, for a male to qualify as a true macho he must "be assertive, powerful, aggressive and independent" (1979: 319)—a rather similar profile to our Argentine macho fans.[16] Bolton further argues that a macho competes with other machos, as for example in trying to outdrink them. He also discusses the well known fact that a true macho must dominate his women. However, he fails to discuss the salient feature of machismo, inherent in the Argentine data; that the hypermanly macho is *afraid of being homosexually attacked by other machos.* Evidence of the macho fear of being anally penetrated is not limited to my data. As Brandes reports, "The threat of anal penetration" is an important male concern in southern Spain (1980: 95) and in fact is part of a larger Mediterranean preoccupation, which has been naturally inherited in Latin America (Dundes and Falassi 1975: 189; Dundes et al. 1970; Miner and DeVos 1960).

Fromm and Maccoby (1970), in their study of a Mexican village, also appear to have overlooked the homosexual dimension of the macho syndrome. For them "machismo indicates an attitude of male superiority, a wish to control women and keep them in an inferior position" (1970: 16). The point to be made is that the macho, who spends so much psychic energy keeping his women in an "inferior position," with all the status anxiety this brings along, must at all times guard his own "mas culus (male anus)" (Dundes 1978: 87) or "masculinity" from the perceived phallic threat of other males.

Foster also fails to discuss the possible homosexual aspects of machismo, although he does discuss his idea of the image of "limited good and machismo" in the Mexican village he studied (1979: 130). We must not assume that because these eminent social scientists fail to report the possible homosexual dimensions of the hypermanly behaviors of machos, the syndrome must therefore not exist in Mexico. It is interesting to note that the Mexican poet and essayist Octavio Paz, in his now classic humanistic portrait of Mexican national character, *The Labyrinth of Solitude,* briefly discusses the possible homosexual components of the Mexican macho. Paz notes: "It would not be difficult to perceive certain homosexual inclinations also, such as the use and abuse of the pistol, a phallic symbol which discharges death rather than life, and the fondness for exclusively masculine guilds" (1961: 82). Of course it is not "difficult to perceive" such homosexual inclinations. What *is* difficult is to understand how and why these inclinations arose in the first place—a topic beyond the scope of this paper—or to document and interpret how and *why* these tendencies, which seem to be in direct contradiction to all other aspects of the macho ethos, surface in their expressive life.[17]

With this understanding in mind, let us return to the soccer spectacle to further document how these homosexual preoccupations surface. A most common song, only heard after a goal is scored, will help us elucidate how the fans, in their unconscious, view the game in symbolic terms. This one-liner goes:

> Oh, oh, oh, por el horto
> Oh, oh, oh, through the asshole

Thus, after their team has scored a goal, the fans in orgasmic joy chant how their team has just put the ball "through the asshole" of the rival team, meaning, of course, the goal. Here we have further unequivocal evidence that, in the fans' folkloristic free associations, the goals do not in fact symbolize vaginas, as Stokes asserted, but that in the Argentine case they symbolize the *horto* (asshole) of the opposite team. The game, thus, can be viewed not so much as a stage on which oedipal fantasies are acted out, as Stokes suggested, but rather as a stage on which macho homosexual fantasies and the macho's need to put down other males, very specifically by depicting them as the shameful recipients of a forced homosexual encounter (perhaps due to an exaggerated fear of being penetrated), are acted out.

Let's examine a more elaborate song to illustrate this basic process.

> Ya todos saben que Brasil esta de luto
> Now all know that Brazil is mourning
>
> Son todos negros, son todos putos
> Are all niggers, are all faggots

This freely translates, "By now all know Brazil is mourning, they are all a bunch of niggers, they are all a bunch of faggots." An acquaintance of mine heard this song during the 1978 Jules Rimet soccer World Cup semifinals played in Argentina. As the Brazilian team, then the natural rivals of the Argentine national team, was eliminated, joyous Argentinian fans all over the city of Buenos Aires took to the streets singing this song. Again, as in other cases, more than one function and meaning can be extracted from the chant. On the surface the song mirrors the eternal national rivalry between Argentina and Brazil.[18] At a deeper level of analysis the song nicely illustrates the Freudian process of projecting onto the outside thoughts and affects of a taboo nature that originate within the self. So, again on the surface, the chant functions to put down the Brazilians by calling them *putos* (faggots) and thus assigning to them the passive, recipient role in a homosexual encounter. At the deeper level of meaning we see how these machos' "unresolved bisexuality" (Gilmore and Gilmore 1979: 283) and potential recipient homosexuality is projected onto the rivals.

An important culturally constituted issue in the construction of (homo)sexuality in the Spanish-speaking world surfaces in these songs and the phenomena they relate to. According to Latin American folk definitions, male homosexual behavior is only the behavior of a passive recipient in a homosexual encounter (that is, he who is anally penetrated). According to this folk view, the penetrator may not be considered, or indeed consider himself a homosexual as long as he remains the active partner in the sexual act. Note the monumental significance of this folk belief and practice in the context of the AIDS epidemic and its specific impact on the Hispanic population. Many Hispanic males, thinking that AIDS is a problem affecting mainly homosexuals, may think that as long as they are the penetrators and not the penetrated in a homosexual act, they need not worry about the disease!

Many soccer chants relate to homosexual themes. An interesting psychodynamic process is at work in this next song:

> Soy de Boca, soy de Boca . . . que puto yo soy.
> (I) am of Boca, (I) am of Boca . . . what (a) faggot
> I am

I myself heard this song at the Boca Juniors Club stadium during a national soccer championship season. This game was an important one, as the mighty Boca Juniors team, then leading all teams, was facing the second most respected team that season, the San Lorenzo de Almagro Club. The San Lorenzo de Almagro fans began singing, "I am for Boca, I am for Boca," thus puzzling the whole stadium, especially Boca's fans, who began wondering why the San Lorenzo fans were rooting for their rivals. Then the second part of the song was chanted and everything became clear. "I'm for Boca, I'm for Boca . . . . what a faggot I am." This song was perceived by all as being so creative that even the most loyal of Boca's fans nervously laughed and even applauded its ingenuity.

The song clearly shows how machos' fears of turning into passive homosexuals surface in their folkloric fantasies.[19] The song is in fact saying that Boca's fans are a bunch of passive homosexuals, unlike us San Lorenzo fans, who are straight *but could possibly turn into passive homosexuals if we were to become fans of the wrong team (Boca).* At the surface the song serves to put down Boca's fans; at a deeper level the internal taboo and anxiety-producing thought of being a passive homosexual is projected to "the other," in this case, interestingly, one within the self (of every macho)—a potential homosexual that might emerge were one to become a fan of the wrong team. It is precisely a paranoid fear that other machos might see this potentiality for passive homosexuality that determines, of course unconsciously, much of the macho's well-known hypermasculine behavior.

To the above song, Boca's fans may eventually reply:

> La copa, la copa, se mira y no se toca
> The cup, the cup, is seen and not touched

This can be seen as reflecting the pride the Boca Juniors fans take in the fact that their team has won, and thus possesses, the last national championship cup. However, it is also immediately clear that the cup is a symbol which stands for other things. First and foremost, the cup symbolizes victory and superiority, which in the Argentine cultural context equals power, which equals virility or masculinity. So the song now reflects—through the symbolic equation, the cup = victory = macho—an exhibitionist wish to expose one's masculinity, which can "be seen" but "never touched" or penetrated in any way. The fear of being homosexually penetrated, as reflected by our data, is the basic psychodynamic process at work, a process which is surprisingly similar (although cultural differences do exist) to the syndromes described by Miner and DeVos (1960) in their study of Algerian males, and by Dundes et al. (1970) in their study of Turkish boys.

This next song gives us a good summary of the macho's views on homosexuality:

> Sol y luna, sol y luna
> Sun and moon, sun and moon

> Sol y luna, sol y luna
> Sun and moon, sun and moon

> La poronga de Armando
> The prick of Armando (name of Boca's owner)

> En el culo de Labruna
> In the ass of Labruna (name of rival team's owner)

What are some twenty thousand of Boca's hypermanly fans meaning to say with this song? Obviously they think that the sexual organ of the owner of their team, Mr. Armando, belongs up the anal orifice of the coach of the rival team (Mr. Labruna), thus mirroring how true machos, like Mr. Armando, beloved by the fans of his team and even nicknamed "the Peron of soccer," with his powerful organ or, *poronga*, penetrates Mr. Labruna. I must repeat that in macho world view it is fine to engage in homosexual acts as long as one's role is the active, penetrating aggressor and not the passive, female-like recipient. This song, of course, is consciously aimed at debasing the rivals to the lowest, most humiliating level. This is also evident in the manifest content of this next song:

> Ahora, ahora, nos chupan bien las boles
> Now, now, suck well our balls

> los de Lomas de Zamora
> they of Lomas de Zamora

By inviting the Lomas de Zamora fans and players to engage in oral sex with them, they automatically (in their own eyes) put them in the lowest role imaginable to a macho, performing fellatio on another man.

Another common strategy found in the Argentinian soccer stadium verbal duels is to put the rivals down by calling them animals. This animal is almost always a chicken, which in the

Argentinian cultural context is loaded with specific symbolism. This is found in the next song:

> Mandarina, Mandarina, Mandarina, Mandarina
> Mandarin, Mandarin, Mandarin, Mandarin
>
> Me parece que los de River
> It appears that they of River
>
> Son todos unas gallinas.
> Are all chickens.

The song, in its manifest content, dehumanizes River's fans and symbolically makes them into animals—interestingly enough, female animals.[20]

In Argentina, *gallina* is not used to refer to women, but very specifically to cowards, who in theory stand in binary opposition to the machos (see Paz 1961). Furthermore, in Argentine humor, another genre of folklore, the gallina is typically the ideal prey for the sex-hungry macho. Indeed, the gallina is the object of countless jokes, because it is the preferred sexual partner of the lonesome gaucho, an archetypical macho. According to folklore, lack of contact with females for extended periods drives the gaucho to bestiality, preferably with a gallina. The following joke confirms how the "gallina"—which never directly refers to women but to passive cowards—is in fact a recipient of macho sexual penetration: A gaucho, after having been in the deserted pampas for an extended period of time, returns to the city and goes directly to a house of prostitution. There the owner tells him: "Go to room number one, open the door, put your prick next to the red light, and have sex." The young, desiring gaucho religiously follows the instructions; he goes into the dark room and puts his phallus in the hole next to the red light. After having an orgasm, the gaucho cries, "Tell me you loved it!" The reply is ki-ki-ki, the supposedly onomatopoeic voice of a gallina, or chicken.

As with homosexual intercourse, a real macho sees nothing wrong in engaging in bestial intercourse so long as he "gives" but does not "receive."[21] The gallina motif forms a whole cycle of folksongs in Argentinian soccer stadiums.[22]

CONCLUSIONS

I have attempted to document the thesis that machos in Argentina are attracted to the soccer field in order to find a collective therapeutic outlet for their taboo thoughts regarding their fear of being debased into a passive, emasculated role. This is most evident in the fans' fantasies of penetrating or being anally penetrated by other males. It is the very symbolism of the game that, in my view, triggers these homosexual fantasies, which surface in the folkloristic free associations common to stadium crowds. In the game, eleven men from each team protect the goal at their back from the penetration of the aggressive rivals. As my data have shown, the goals are highly symbolic of the players', and by extension the fans', anuses. Each time the ball penetrates one's goal, the fans' and players' masculinity is at stake.

In soccer, as opposed to rugby or to American football, we can infer that the ball is unconsciously experienced as an inherently dangerous and dirty object. The players must never touch the ball with their hands during the game, under penalty for foul play (except for the goalkeeper—in his restricted area—and by any of the players when the ball leaves the field of play). Pickford noted this symbolism when he wrote, "In 'soccer,' the player seems afraid that he will dirty or endanger himself by touching the ball with his hand" (1941: 283). Then he goes on to argue how naturally persons with unconscious desires to "spurn them [soccer balls] with his feet or to use them as weapons of attack . . . may fall in love with 'soccer'" (ibid.). Regrettably, the author fails to make the critical connection between the player's own fears of his "balls," more specifically his underlying *fear of castration,* and the player's pseudoaggressive use of a phallic symbol, the soccer ball, to penetrate the rival's goal, at the rival's back.

We may now return to Deutsch's (1926) psychoanalytic views of the game, to show how in fact the above connection that Pickford failed to make is of critical importance for understanding how the symbolism inherent in the game directly affects the surfacing of the fans' homosexual aggression. Deutsch bases her thesis on the analysis of a patient suffering from impotence, anxiety, and depression. The patient could only feel "full of power" by playing ball games such as soccer. Clearly the patient felt better turning from being passive to having active control of the "ball." Deutsch concludes that soccer must offer a mechanism for "the projection of a source of anxiety into the outside world and discharge of the anxiety" (1926: 226).

From Deutsch's case study we can see how, in the game, a fear of castration is projected onto the ball, and is symbolically mastered by the player—and by extension, by the cathected fan. This fear of castration is evident in the symbolism of the game, and is also present in the *"no me rompas las bolas"* ("do not break my balls") cycle in Argentine folklore. This latter body of male folklore is rich with metaphors articulating and venting castration fears—yet documenting this cycle is beyond the scope of this paper.

This castration threat appears to be at the root of machos' obsessive fears of being anally penetrated by other males. Miner and DeVos (1960), in their study of Algerian males, endorse this psychodynamic point: "The fear of retreating into passive homosexuality is one of the dangers besetting an individual who retreats from genital masculinity in the face of subconscious castration threat" (1960: 141).

The macho's excessive fear of being penetrated represents an unconscious and forbidden wish, which is at times disguised in the form of ego syntonic projective inversions. Further, this form of pseudoaggression has been shown to be connected to an underlying fear of homosexuality (Chapman 1967: 266). The other side of the coin of such an obsessive fear is, of course, a taboo wish.

These intrapsychic conflicts are enacted in disguised forms within the soccer spectacle. This is found in the game symbolism and in its structural equivalents—in the fans' folk songs and verbal duels.[23] The game symbolism evokes the fantasies so eloquently articulated in the songs and verbal duels reviewed here—in the game, as in the songs, you use your ball to get into the other team's backside. Understanding this anxiety venting nature of the spectacle is critical for understanding the addictive effect the soccer show has for hypermanly machos, at least in the Argentine case.

Notes

An earlier and shorter version of this essay appeared in *The Journal of Psychoanalytic Anthropology* 5 (1): 7–28. It is dedicated to Alan Dundes. I am indebted to Professor Stanley Brandes and Professor Howard Stein for their insightful comments and suggestions.

1. With, of course, exceptions, among them Yale sociologist Janet Lever (1969, 1972).
2. da Silva does, however, present the case of a soccer player who was referred to him with "a serious psychological problem" due mainly to his being sensitive to "the shouting of the rooters" (1970: 309). However, the author fails to include a description of what it was that the rooters shouted that had such an impact on the player's psychological functioning.

3. Note that I am not arguing that verbal aggression toward the athletes is not common in Argentina; what I am arguing is that it may not be the *most frequent* form of verbal aggression found in the stadiums.

4. See Dunning (1971), a selection of readings on the sociology of sport, which provides the student of theoretical works on soccer the best single source of articles dealing with the historical development and sociology of British soccer. See also Dunning and Elias (1971) for a well documented historical account of the development of the game in England from the early Middle Ages to the end of the nineteenth century. A careful description of the most significant structural changes in the developing game is the central feature of this sociological survey.

5. It would be naive not to recognize that intragroup conflict and violence are active aspects of the soccer spectacle. I have witnessed countless times fans rooting for the same team exchanging insults and fists over who the real star of their team was, how the team should be aligned, or who the captain should be.

6. All translations are mine.

7. Dundes refers to Johnson (1929).

8. In Argentina first division games are played Sundays and the less important, but also spectacular, second division games are played Saturdays— see Muñiz 1995, Bayer 1990.

9. I must note that very early in the game's history the English Football Association excluded women from playing. In 1946 the association exhorted its members to "take steps to prevent clubs letting their grounds or otherwise creating opportunities for female players to participate in irregular football matches" (quoted in Vinnai 1973: 75).

10. In the smaller, less known stadiums, I would argue, soccer is essentially a male affair, with all male fans. Women are sporadically seen in the bigger, more modern stadiums, but almost always accompanied by men, and typically in the expensive *plateas*, or covered seats under a roof, the best section of the stadium. This rather small section, reserved for officials and members of the upper classes, who occasionally find amusement in the spectacle, is separated from the larger terraces by wire fences. Note that for all practical purposes women are not "real" fans, and go to the stadiums by and large to find exotic amusement.

11. *La barra* (the gang) are usually neighbors who have most likely grown up together. Their beloved team has been a source of group cohesion at times (usually of victory), but when disaster strikes and their team loses, in-group conflict is sure to occur. Fights over team issues may break lifelong friendships, especially among the most emotional fans.

12. I myself have countless times observed and participated in all three of these hypothetical topics of conversation among fans.
13. Sometimes called the "owners" of the barra rooting for a given team.
14. Please notice that no a priori theoretical categories are being imposed on the data, they just emerge.
15. Boca Juniors Club fans are feared perhaps more than any others, due to their reputation, most likely deserved, for being more violent, destructive, and in general more aggressive than most other fans.
16. My data do not tell us how "independent" Argentine macho fans are.
17. See Gilmore and Gilmore for an attempt to describe the ontogenesis of machismo in southern Spain as a "reaction formation against unresolved bisexuality" (1979: 283). Amazingly, they fail to report the macho's fear of being anally penetrated, which Brandes (1980: 95) reports in the same region of southern Spain.
18. Of course, this song also reflects Argentine racial prejudice.
19. There is an important difference between these two roles (passive vs. active), at least for Latin men. Professor Alessandro Falassi in a personal communication pointed out to me how the homosexual film director Pier Paolo Passolini was murdered by a male prostitute he picked up. Apparently the "active" male prostitute was enraged when, after he had been the aggressive "giver," Passolini demanded that he now be the passive "recipient." At that point the male prostitute, apparently disgusted with the idea, is said to have killed Passolini. *"Puto"* ("faggot") implies passivity.
20. In Spanish, the article in front of the noun determines the gender of the noun, so "la" gallina is feminine.
21. Please note that I do not imply that homosexual and bestial intercourse are equivalents.
22. For example: "Aunque sean campeones, aunque sean campeones, siguen siendo una gallinas, la puta que los pario." ("Even though they may be champions, they are still a bunch of chickens, the sons of bitches.") Or: "Cuide señora su gallinero, porque esta noche vamos a afanar una gallina para el puchero." ("Madam, take care of your chicken coop, because tonight we will steal a gallina for the stew.") There are many others.
23. I again concur with Dundes when he argues convincingly that in both American football and in male verbal duelings, the object is "to put one's opponent down; to 'screw' him while avoiding being screwed by him" (1978: 81). The same applies to my data.

References

Arens, William. 1975. The great American football ritual. *Natural History* 84: 72–80.

Bayer, Osvaldo. 1990. *Futbol argentino: Pasion y gloria de nuestro deporte mas popular.* Buenos Aires: Editorial Sudamericana.

Bolton, Ralph. 1979. Machismo in motion: The ethos of Peruvian truckers. *Ethos* 7(4): 312–342.

Brandes, Stanley. 1980. *Metaphors of Masculinity.* Philadelphia: University of Pennsylvania Press.

Buytendijk, F. J. J. 1952. *Le Football: Une Etude Psychologique.* Paris: Desclee de Brouwer.

Chapman, A. H. 1967. *A Handbook of Clinical Psychiatry: An Interpersonal Approach.* Philadelphia: J. B. Lippincott.

Chinas, Beverly. 1973. *The Isthmus Zapotecs: Women's Roles in Cultural Contexts.* New York: Holt Rinehart and Winston.

da Silva, A. R. 1970. The role of the spectator in the soccer player's dynamics. In *Contemporary Psychology of Sport: Proceedings of the Second International Congress of Sport Psychology.* Chicago: Athletic Institute. pp. 307–310.

Deutsch, Helene. 1926. A contribution to the psychology of sport. *International Journal of Psychoanalysis* 7: 221–227.

DeVos, George. 1978. Selective permeability and reference group sanctioning: Psychocultural continuities in role degradation. J. Milton Yinger and Stephen J. Cutler, eds. *Major Social Issues: A Multidisciplinary View.* New York: Free Press.

Dollard, I., L. W. Doob, N. E. Miller, O. H. Mower, and R. R. Sears. 1939. *Frustration and Aggression.* New Haven: Yale University Press.

Dundes, Alan. 1976. Projection in folklore: A plea for psychoanalytic semiotics. *Modern Language Notes* 91:1–133.

———. 1978. Into the end zone for a touchdown: A psychoanalytic consideration of American football. *Western Folklore* 37: 75–78.

Dundes, Alan, and Alessandro Falassi. 1975. La Terra in Piazza: *An Interpretation of the Palio of Siena.* Berkeley: University of California Press.

Dundes, Alan, Jerry Leach, and Born Ozkok. 1970. The strategy of Turkish boys' verbal dueling rhymes. *Journal of American Folklore* 83 (329): 325–349.

Dunning, Eric. 1967. The concept of development: Two illustrated case studies. In P. I. Rose, ed., *The Study of Society: An Integrated Anthology.* New York: Random House, pp. 879–893.

———, ed. 1971. *The Sociology of Sport: A Selection of Readings.* London: Frank Cass.

Dunning, Eric, and Norbert Elias. 1971. *The Making of Football.* London: Frank Cass.

———. 1970. The quest for excitement in unexciting societies. In G. Luschen, ed., *The Cross-Cultural Analysis of Sport and Games.* Champaign, Ill.: Stipes.

Foster, George. 1979. *Tzintzuntzan: Mexican Peasants in a Changing World* (rev. ed.) New York: Elsevier North Holland.

Frankenberg, Ronald. 1957. *Village on the Border: A Social Study of Religion, Politics and Football in a North Wales Community.* London: Cohen of West London.

Fromm, Erich, and Michael Maccoby. 1970. *Social Character in a Mexican Village: A Sociopsychoanalytic Study.* Englewood Cliffs, N.J.: Prentice-Hall.

Geertz, Clifford. 1973. *The Interpretation of Cultures.* New York: Basic Books.

Gilmore, Margaret, and David Gilmore. 1979. "Machismo": A psychodynamic approach (Spain). *The Journal of Psychological Anthropology* 2 (3): 281–299.

Hopcraft, Arthur. 1968. *The Football Man: People and Passions in Soccer.* London: Collings.

Johnson, Branch W. 1929. Football: A survival of magic? *Contemporary Review* 135: 228.

Lever, Janet. 1969. Soccer: Opium of the Brazilian people. *Transaction* 7 (2): 3.

———. 1972. Soccer as a Brazilian way of life. In Gregory P. Stone, ed., *Games, Sport, and Power.* New Brunswick, N.J.: E. P. Dutton.

Lévi-Strauss, Claude. 1973. The structural study of myth. In P. Bohannan and M. Glazer, eds. *High Points in Anthropology.* New York: Alfred A. Knopf, pp. 409–428.

Mafud, Julio. 1976. *Sociologia del Futbol.* Buenos Aires: Editorial Americalee.

Medner, Siegfried. 1956. *Das Ballspiel im Leben der Volker.* N.p., Aschendorff.

Miner, Horace, and George DeVos. 1960. *Oasis and Casbah: Algerian Culture and Personality in Change.* Ann Arbor: University of Michigan.

Muñiz, Juan Carlos. 1995. *El picado: Una pasion argentina*. Buenos Aires: Ediciones Urraca.

Patrick, G. T. W. 1963. The psychology of football. *American Journal of Psychology* 14: 368–381.

Paz, Octavio. 1961. *The Labyrinth of Solitude*. New York: Grove.

Pickford, R. W. 1940. The psychology of the history and organization of association football. *British Journal of Psychology* 31: 80–93.

———. 1941. Aspects of the psychology of games and sports. *British Journal of Psychology* 4: 279–293.

Reaney, Mabel Jane. 1916. The psychology of the organized group game. *British Journal of Psychology, Monograph Supplements* 4.

Romero, Amilcar. 1985. *Deporte, violencia y politica: Cronica negra, 1958–1983*. Buenos Aires: Centro Editor de America Latina.

———. 1986. *Muerte en la cancha*. Buenos Aires: Editorial Nueva America.

Scher, Ariel. 1988. *Futbol, pasion de multitudes y de elites: Un estudio institucional de la Asociasion de Futbol Argentino*. Buenos Aires: Centro de Investigaciones Sociales sobre Estado y Administracion.

Schwartz, J. Michael. 1973. Causes and effects of spectator sports. *International Review of Sport Sociology* 3–4 (8): 25–45.

Stokes, Adrian. 1956. Psychoanalytical reflections on the development of ball games, particularly cricket. *International Journal of Psychoanalysis* 37: 185–192.

Taylor, Ian R. 1969. Hooligans: Soccer's resistance movement. *New Society* 7 (2): 4–206.

———. 1971a. Football mad: A speculative sociology of football hooliganism. In Eric Dunning, ed. *The Sociology of Sport: A Selection of Readings*. London: Frank Cass, pp. 352–374.

———. 1971b. Soccer consciousness and soccer hooliganism. In Stanley Cohen, ed., *Images of Deviancy*. Harmondsworth, Middlesex: Penguin, pp. 134–164.

Veccia, Sergio. 1976. Sunday orgasm. *International Journal of Sport Psychology* 7 (1): 3–39.

Vinnai, Gerhard. 1973. *Football Mania: The Players and the Fans. The Mass Psychology of Football*. London: Ocean.

Historicizing the Psyche of Psychohistory

COMMENT ON LOEWENBERG
AND SUÁREZ-OROZCO

JOHN TOEWS

The practice of "applying" psychoanalytic perspectives to the documentary materials studied by historians and anthropologists, the use of psychoanalysis as a hermeneutic method for unveiling the psychological dynamics which make possible, and the hidden meanings which make comprehensible, the phenomenal evidence of past and foreign cultures, has been around almost as long as psychoanalysis itself. The papers by Suárez-Orozco and Loewenberg are thus written within the history of a discourse, and, we might also say, within a certain psychoanalytic disciplinary "culture" in which interdisciplinary relations are defined by the primacy of the psychoanalytic method as the assumed ground or foundation from which the materials of other disciplines can be comprehended. Neither of the papers directly addresses Freudian theory as a specific historical/cultural discourse; rather, both use it as a window onto an otherwise obscured world of unconscious subjective reality. Implicit in the papers, however, are critical tendencies and tensions that place the traditional modes of practicing "applied psychoanalysis" in the areas of historical and anthropological studies in question, and, in an inversion of the conventional patterns of relations in psychoanalytical anthropology or psychohistory, make psychoanalytic theory the object as well as the "subject" of investigation; that is, they raise questions about the cultural and historical determinants of Freudian theory.

Instead of engaging in particular criticism of arguments and claims within areas in which my professional expertise is at the very least severely limited, I will define my own task as the articulation of some of the implicit assumptions and implications of the Suárez-Orozco and Loewenberg papers, and will return the discussion, at the conclusion, to the work of Freud. In my view the most interesting and problematic issues raised by the two papers are centered around questions relating to the construction (historical and cultural) of self-identity, especially as it relates to the ways in which personal identity is defined as gendered and communal.

Professor Suárez-Orozco indicates that the frame within which he would like to situate the anthropological dimensions of his psychoanalytic anthropological study is derived from Clifford Geertz's view of ethnography as a "thick" or contextualizing description of cultural events that aims at the reconstruction of the conditions of the meaning of those events within the webs or networks of signifying actions which constitute a culture. The Argentinean soccer game would thus be analogous to the Balinese cockfight, that "deep" play or spectacle in which the Balinese, or at least certain groups of Balinese males, provide a self-interpretation of their experience through an acted text, "a story they tell themselves about themselves."[1] The acted text or "play" or cultural "spectacle" of the soccer game in Suárez-Orozco's work also seems to provide its own interpretation, or at least clues to its meaning from the "native's point of view," in the songs, chants, and verbal duels of the spectators and/or participants. In Geertz's ethnographic practice, however, a "thick description" of the spectators' relation to the spectacle is the starting point for reconstructing the general semiotic codes which define the distinctive identity of Balinese culture, the acted patterns of meaning regarding fundamental ordering categories like nature/culture, masculinity/femininity, and especially the hierarchical classification of individuals into stratified social groups, within which the Balinese define and recognize themselves. Suárez-Orozco, however, seems uninterested in expanding his analysis beyond the soccer stadium. His object seems in fact to be something we might call "soccer culture," which can be disassociated to a large extent from the webs of significance that define cultures in ethnic, national, civic, or linguistic senses. Although the title and much of the data imply Argentina (or perhaps even the Boca Junior Club) as the relevant cultural context, the text itself moves from "most corners of the earth" to the Mediterranean world (specifically including Algerians and Turks), to the Spanish-speaking world, to the "natural inheritance" of Latin America (including the Portuguese-speaking Brazilians), in a bewildering pluralism that strongly suggests universality, or at least potential universality. Similarly, little significance is given to historical contexts, to changes over time. As long as the game remains the same, the implication is, so will its meanings. Finally and most surprisingly, there is little attempt to move beyond "soccer culture" to other institutions of a male subculture, or institutions of gender formation, that might provide some cultural framework for the conflicts regarding male identity implied in the sung and acted texts of fans and players.

The explanation for what might seem striking and even cavalier "omissions" within the framework and apparent logic of the Geertzian perspective, is of course quite obvious. For Suárez-Orozco, the relevant context for explaining the meaning of the phenomena of soccer culture is not a Geertzian conception of semiotic cultural worlds at all, but the psychological dynamics of male desire as (very generally) modeled in psychoanalytic theory. The soccer stadium is a theater in which unconscious male fantasies are acted out in a disguised fashion. The strong implication is that unconscious wishes and fantasies are not constructed within particular cultural worlds, but are universal, a common ground of meaning that articulates or "expresses" itself with some limited variations within different historical and cultural contexts.

There thus emerges what seems to be a radical disjuncture between the anthropological (at least in the culturalist version of Geertz) and psychoanalytic projects. The self-defined logic of Geertz's position leads to a conception of the psyche as culturally constructed. There are no universal dynamics of psychic life that can be used to explain cultural phenomena. Rather the structures of psychic life can only be explained within the context of the semiotic cultural relations from which they emerge into existence. One of the most striking assumptions of contemporary forms of ethnographic description and cultural analysis is that subjective experience at its most fundamental levels, the experience of selfhood and its boundaries and of emotional or affective states, is a historical/cultural construct; that is, subjective experience, the contents and forms of selfhood, are "produced," not merely "shaped," within the codes of meaning available in particular historical cultures. Gender identities, experiences and self-conceptions of masculinity and femininity, as well as sexual identities, conceptions of selfhood as oriented by homosexual or heterosexual desire, would, of course, be primary components of such constructions.[2]

The logical path of a psychoanalytic analysis, however, seems to move in exactly the opposite direction—toward an assertion of universal psychic structures and processes of male psychology as the hidden origins of the meanings of cultural phenomena. Ultimately, the words and actions of fans, as well as the rules and purposes of the game, can be traced to unconscious fantasies of homosexual rape, anal penetration, and castration, which emerge from the conflictual relations of the oedipal complex. Fears of feminization or victimization by stronger males, of being condemned to the passive, powerless, exposed position of the passive homosexual, fuel fantasies of phallic prowess and mastery over humiliated, victimized others. These wishes and conflicts are "expressed" in the empirical phenomena of soccer culture. From this angle, one might say, psychic processes seem to construct cultural relations.

Such a dichotomy is much too simplistic, however, for the conflict between expressive and constructive notions of masculinity also (implicitly) characterizes the psychoanalytic project itself, at least as it is pursued by Suárez-Orozco. In its most obvious aspects the psychoanalytic sections of the paper are focused on the processes of identification, on the dynamics of "narcissistic" libidinal relations in which the other appears as the other "self."[3] The unconscious desire appears as the desire to be like or even actually be another subject—the triumphant player, the owner of the triumphant players who penetrate the opponents' anuses, the master who screws the victim—and to repudiate the self in the other which represents the position of the victim, the possessed, the mastered, the penetrated. The desire here is "subject-related," to be somebody, rather than "object-related," to enjoy or possess something; it is more tied to identification than to consumption. The goal of the game is not to possess the anus of the other as a love object, but to take up the position of the master who expresses his superiority, affirms his independence and power, by screwing the victim. But this line of analysis soon comes very close to the cultural constructivist position, in which the desiring self is constructed through its identifications, actually created in historical, cultural acts of identification. The implication is that there is no center of desire on which the process of self-formation is grounded, but only an endless series of displacements and identifications in which subjectivity is constructed in the relations and exchanges of the symbolic world of cultural meanings.

There is, however, also a countercurrent of object-related, oedi-pally defined wish-fulfillment analysis in the paper, in which fantasies of sadistic and masochistic pleasure, and thus of li-bidinal fulfillment in relation to the object, are highlighted. This latter perspective also sustains a view of the primacy of a genital masculine subjectivity that is distorted through threats of victimization, rather than the view that machismo is not so much a "distortion" of "normal" masculine desire as a pattern of cultural identification in which masculinity is constructed as a radical repudiation of "feminine" passivity in certain histori-cal contexts.

One aspect of the psychoanalytical "identification" argument in Suárez-Orozco's paper is that the processes of masculine identification as mastery of potential passivity, of the "femi-nine" within, are tied to group identification. As he notes in an autobiographical comment, his experiences within the soccer *barra* provided him with a feeling of "belonging" as well as of masculine identity. In Freud's own theorizing, of course, from the Schreber case to *Group Psychology and the Analysis of the Ego*, homosexuality as a form of masculine self-identification and the construction of group identity in the "mass" or band of brothers were often very closely related.

The more theoretically oriented part of Professor Loewen-berg's presentation might be interpreted as bringing to ex-plicit articulation some of the underlying assumptions inform-ing Suárez-Orozco's analysis of the human core of emotional dispositions (a fundamental ambivalence of aggressive/erotic feelings) and of the psychological processes involved in the complex intertwined construction of personal and group iden-tity (splitting, projection, and introjection). The scapegoating and repudiation themes in Suárez-Orozco's account certainly seem to imply or assume a defensive displacement of intrapsy-chic conflict onto the relation between self and other. In both cases the perspective is critical. The projection of intrapsychic conflicts into the realm of interpsychic relations and group behavior and consciousness introduces a divisiveness and destructive violence into human social relations that might be resolved or at least moderated through a self-conscious therapeutic mastery of inner psychic conflicts.

In Loewenberg's paper the contextual, constructionist dimension in the formation of subjective identity or character is represented by a survey of social scientific communications and socialization theory as it relates to the processes of nation formation and nation building. Two dimensions of these processes (as exemplified by the works of Deutsch and Gellner) are separated out for analysis.

The first is the apparently infinitely expanding network of relations which bind individuals together in webs of social relations and social communication, the contexts of meaning that make up the experience of cultural belonging in everyday life. This process of acculturation or assimilation into a world which provides the contextual frame of meaningful activity on various levels is obviously an immensely complex, multidimensional and dynamically transformative process which includes subcultural systems of meaning that inform identification in terms of, gender, race, familial relations, kinship, ethnicity, class, language, profession, etc. Within the webs of these associational processes one would have to imagine every individual as living an array of communal or social identities of varying intensity and extension, as a kind of dynamic coalition of "subject positions" rather than a single coherent subject. One of Freud's Austrian contemporaries, the novelist Robert Musil, provided in his novel *The Man Without Qualities* what has since become a "classical" account of the multiplicity and confusion of identities, and thus ultimately the subversion or disintegration of the concept of identity in an essentialist sense, in modern or modernizing European societies like turn-of-the-century Austria:

> It is always wrong to explain the phenomena of a country simply by the character of its inhabitants. For the inhabitant of a country has at least nine characters: a professional one, a national one, a civic one, a class one, a geographical one, a sex one, a conscious, an unconscious, and perhaps even a private one; he combines them all in himself, but they dissolve him, and he is really nothing but a little channel washed out by all these trickling streams, which flow into it and drain out of it again in order to join other little streams filling another channel. Hence every dweller on earth also has a tenth character, which is nothing more or less than the passive illusion of spaces unfilled. . . . This interior space—which is, it must be admitted, difficult to describe—is a different shade and shape in Italy from what it is in England, because everything that stands out in relief against it is a different shade and shape."[4]

It is noteworthy, of course, that Musil uses nationality not only as one of the nine subject positions but also as a way of designating the peculiar differentiating contours of the "interior space," in which we assume the essential subject or soul somehow resides. The implications of his position are that this "essential" self is itself historical, culturally constructed, a product of a series of relations to the various subject positions with which individuals identify in a modern culture. Yet Musil also captures the point made by Loewenberg that in the modern world, or at least those worlds increasingly absorbed into the political and economic networks of Eurocentric "westernization," nationality has gained hegemony, or at least relative superiority, in defining societal or cultural identification, superceding or absorbing into itself most other shapes of the communal bond.

The artificially constructed regulation of the proliferating associative networks (represented by Musil's first nine characters) through the boundary setting and hierarchically ordering structures of political power and its consciously articulated strategies of coercive disciplinary socialization and more indirect patterns of acculturation, is the second aspect of national formation (represented by Gellner) in Loewenberg's account. This perspective implies that national community, and the creation of a national self-identity, cannot be comprehended as a kind of synthesis of associational networks in the cultural sphere, but that it involves a forceful imposition of a specific order and meaning on the heterogeneity of cultural identities, that it is a historical product of political action. Nationality is thus seen as the artificial, imaginary creation of a unitary community, as the historical successor to the formerly "sacred" bonds of kinship, religious faith, and dynastic loyalty as the representative of an ideal collective subject with which the individual self can identify.[5]

The psychology of nationalism, of belief in an underlying or all-encompassing, totalizing identity somehow expressing a collective essential subject informing and shaping the dynamic diversity of cultural association seems to involve the mental transformation of open-ended dynamic relational webs into a bounded, unified essence. It remakes the plurality of intertwining genealogical narratives into a single historical narrative, and interprets the artfully constructed closure of a particular part of the web of human association as the revelation of a hidden reality, a "nature" to which in most countries one can be "naturalized," mysteriously informing the activity of each of its members. Nationalism as an ideology transforms Musil's enigmatic "interior space" into the essential self that finds expression in all "secondary" subject positions.

What are the psychological motives and psychological processes which produce this denial of the reality of difference and heterogeneity and open-endedness, and fuel the insistent desire to believe in a particular imaginary community, an illusion of identity, homogeneity, and closure? Loewenberg provides two examples of alternative conceptions in which national identity is defined in terms of a shared recognition of difference, but no account of the psychological conditions within which this might be possible. In fact in his essay Loewenberg has a tendency to merge the construction of a national identity with the processes of group formation, socialization, or acculturation per se, thus reproducing the conception of the nation as the "natural" social bond. Such a maneuver, of course, also allows the easy "application" of universalistically construed psychological categories as an explanation for a particular historical formation. Psychohistory in this instance as well apparently has great difficulty connecting psychic processes to the specificity of a major historical phenomenon. But perhaps this is because Loewenberg, like Suárez-Orozco, ultimately remains loyal to a Freudian theory of universal unconscious desire in its oedipal object-related dimension, a desire hidden as the essential meaning within the deceptive, distorted articulations of the phenomena of clinical analysis and cultural description, and ultimately does not pursue the implication of Freud's theory of the narcissistic desire for identity, and its historicist, constructivist implications.

In both papers, and in the tradition from which they speak, it seems to me, there is a significant gap in the argument about the displacement of intrapsychic conflict into the social and political relations of group formation. How does the process of identification of the individual self with the essentialized representation of gendered selfhood or social association (the ideal fiction of masculinity or the imagined community of the nation) actually occur? Neither Suárez-Orozco nor Loewenberg seems to think that Freud's own analysis of group formation through processes of both identification and displaced oedipal desire in *Group Psychology and the Analysis of the Ego* is adequate or even relevant to his current project. Is this because a close reading of that text would reveal the contingent, historical foundations of the categories in which Freud grasped and analyzed processes of social or gender identification? Has going back to the Freudian texts become more of a threat than a foundation for the continuation of a belief in the universality of the Freudian categories? Are the psychodynamics of socialization or acculturation processes universal? Does it matter whether the group is a traditional tribe or kinship group, a religiously centered culture, a gendered association, a social class or social status group, or a politically organized nationality? Are all forms of group identification, of cultural integration, in some sense pathological? Is homogeneity always also hegemony that marginalizes difference, and does unity always involve repudiation and denial of otherness? Do homogeneity and unity always represent a regression to "primitive" modes of splitting and projection as ways of resolving psychic conflict? In the heterogeneous cultural multiplicity of modern societies and the complex overlapping associational involvements of their members, must there be a primary or totalizing group identification that somehow defines who the individuals "essentially" are? (Must Musil's tenth character be transformed from an absence into a thing?) Is the psychological identification with imagined communities so powerful because integration into "real" communities is collapsing or has already collapsed? Or were all historical forms of human social identity as imaginary and constructed as nationalism? There is a clear moral and moralistic tone in both papers. Does this tone emerge from moral assumptions inherent in the psychoanalytic perspective? Is the norm of a mature, centered individual, recognizing and managing his or her unconscious conflicts, rationally and pragmatically choosing forms of association without relinquishing autonomy and the ultimate particular "thisness" of his or her existence, the basis on which cultures and subcultures of the past and present are to be judged? Is a psychoanalytically informed cultural history which is not at the same time a diagnosis of personal pathology a contradiction in terms?

Some of these questions concerning the historical determination of Freudian assumptions and categories may seem less pertinent on this particular occasion than they might be if the subjects of the essays were somehow more "alien," more foreign or ancient. The phenomena analyzed are, at least in part, culturally synchronous and contemporaneous with the theory used to analyze them. One doesn't have to know a great deal about Freud's own personal/cultural formation as Austrian and Jew in the period before World War I to recognize the extent to which his theoretical and moral positions were influenced by the emergence of the homogenizing and exclusionary politics of German nationalism and Jewish responses to it, and how much of his work was focused on the task of reconstructing the psychological foundations of a secular, cosmopolitan, humanist association of rational and autonomous individuals. Questions of ethnic, national, and religious identity, especially as they pertained to culturally assimilated Jews in German culture, were a critical component of the cultural malaise psychoanalysis was constructed to address and resolve. Similarly, it is becoming increasingly obvious that the issues of gender difference and asymmetry in the Freudian conception of subject-construction or self-identification are inextricably bound up with Freud's participation in a cultural crisis of what we might call gender identity in turn-of-the-century Europe. As a specialist in nervous diseases treating female hysterics Freud was on the front line of the struggle to redefine gender definitions in European bourgeois culture.[6] And this should not be seen simply in terms of the defense of traditional patriarchal values against the new claims of organized feminism. The reordering of the meaning of femininity was involved from the beginning in a questioning and subversion of masculinity, and Freud's self-analysis and self-cure, the resolution of his own "hysteria" in the late 1890s, was intimately connected to the problematic of defining his own masculinity through a repudiation of a "femininity" he defined in terms of the assumption of a passive, subordinate "homosexual" relationship to representatives of autonomy, control, and authority.[7] For a contemporary historian of bourgeois and male liberal culture in central Europe at the turn of the century, Freud's writings are obviously a primary document in the genre of self-interpretation, a critical report of the culture's workings from an alienated "native" assimilated to its ideals, or at least some of its most powerful ideals, and dissimulated from its reality.

The question of the extent to which both Freud and the culture within which he operated and which formed his identity have become historical and foreign is a question that has been persistently raised in the past twenty-five years in the growing body of literature engaged in historicizing Freud, in situating Freud's writings in cultural contexts of various kinds. The question of the application of Freudian concepts to the phenomena of history and anthropology cannot be separated from the question of the historical and anthropological or cultural contexts of the formation of those categories. Do Freud's writings present us with a particular construction, a critical theoretical vision and narrative "fictional" account of human experience and possibility, that is ultimately contained, and only makes "sense" within the cultural context in which it was created? Rather than formulating this question in terms of the conventional contrast between a universally valid theory of human nature and a historically and culturally confined expression of local knowledge, I would like to reformulate it in terms of the problem of the extent to which the cultural patterns and conditions within which Freud wrote are still a part of the cultural experience of some, perhaps most, of us, and inform our assumptions about human cultures and their historical dynamics.

Conceptions of the world of inner experience and the identity of the individual subject as culturally constructed, heterogeneous, and dynamically changing artifacts clearly place some of the conventional modes of psychohistory in a critical perspective, at least insofar as these methods assume not only a uniform biological foundation of the psyche, but also a set of "natural" emotions, feelings, and desires whose temporal and spatial variation is determined by their "external" relations with the forming, disciplining institutions of society, politics, and culture. But this does not necessarily mean that psychohistory requires a new, post-Freudian theoretical foundation. There is already a substantial body of Freudian commentary and interpretation which construes the central focus of psychoanalytic theory as a critical analysis of the ways in which somatic forces are transformed into, or constructed as, meaningful subjective experience, and define personal identity in the processes of cultural formation or acculturation (a commentary that within American culture goes back at least to the writings of Philip Rieff in the late 1950s). In recent years this tradition has received a powerful infusion of creative energy from the feminist appropriation of Freudian theory on the cultural production of asymmetrical gender identities, the incorporation of semiotic and linguistic conceptions of culture into psychoanalytic discourse about the nature of psychic reality (Lacan and co.), and the "post-colonial" analysis of the processes of group formation and cultural homogenization. In other words, the investigation of the "Freud and Culture" problematic has not only produced a consciousness of Freud's writings as embedded in various cultural contexts, but also highlighted the ways in which Freud's theories self-consciously illuminate this process of the cultural construction of subjectivity. Freud's writings have not been abandoned or ignored, but are present everywhere in recent debates concerning both gender and sexual identity and the processes of group formation and marginalization.

The interpretation of Freudian theory as an account of the cultural construction of individual subjectivity in general, and subjectively lived sexuality in particular, contains its own ambiguities and conflicts. First, it has had to come to terms with the apparently contrasting assumptions underlying Freudian psychological analysis and therapeutic practice. As a critical diagnostician of the unconscious dynamics of psychic formation, Freud created a conception of a porous, decentered, tentatively structured and restructured psychic life in which the individual subject or ego was determined and often overwhelmed by forces emanating from the body, the archaic personal and collective pasts, and determining restraints of sociocultural order, and personal identities were constructed in an apparently interminable process of proliferating identifications. As a metapsychological theorist and therapist, however, his goal was the conceptualization and construction of an autonomous, centered, and integrated subject in which the ego was the rational, self-conscious manager of its psychic household. (To cite again one of Freud's most famous lines: "Where it [Es] was, there the subject [Ich] must come into being: this is a work of cultivation [education]"—"Wo Es war soll Ich werden, es ist ein Werk der Kultur.")[8] Second, in both of these dimensions of his work Freud assumed a universality apparently incompatible with contemporary notions of cultural otherness, difference, heterogeneity, and pluralism. With the theory of the oedipus complex (however variable and flexible, it might work itself out in individual cases) Freud affirmed the ultimately homologous character of the processes of acculturation in all human cultural formations across space and time; the production of the human was presented as a single plot with variations. His conception of the cultural construction of subjectivity assumed, in the final analysis, a definition of culture as singular (having one origin in the dynamics of unconscious desire) rather than plural. Moreover, Freud's therapeutic ideal projected a view of a centered, autonomous subject which transcended the determination of all particular cultural meanings, and appeared to emerge as the teleological goal of the history of unconscious desire: the ultimate form and transformation of unconscious wish was the wish to be free and thus in conscious control of one's self as the center of wishing. In this sense Freud constructed as universal a norm tied to his own cultural formation in time and space (as liberal, bourgeois, European, patriarchal, and male).

The problem of integrating a psychoanalytic perspective into the historical project of recreating the subjective dimension of the individual and collective pasts of human populations thus seems to have two dimensions. First, it entails a recognition of the extent to which psychoanalysis can be interpreted as providing a theoretical foundation for grasping the subjective dimension of human historical existence as a cultural construction. Second, it requires a critical revision of Freud's universalist assumptions in terms of our contemporary understanding of cultural pluralism or multiculturalism, both in terms of the otherness of the past and the foreign (what Loewenberg's paper describes so well in terms of the Swiss notion that all human communities are equal before the bar of history), and in terms of the porous, conflict-ridden, eclectic nature of the organizations of heterogeneity into meaningfully unities within our own temporal and cultural contexts. This would involve, as has in fact been evident for some time, a relativizing critique of the Freudian oedipal story as the story of acculturation per se, as well as of the assumed universality of the therapeutic norm of the autonomous, culturally "deconverted," self-contained subject.

The problem with using Freudian theory in the tasks of reconstructing the past is certainly *not* that psychoanalysis is a narrowly conceived individual psychology. As an investigation of the cultural construction of subjectivity, psychoanalysis is a sociocultural theory not only in its peripheral applications but in its conceptual foundations, as Freud himself insisted.[9] The nodal point of a psychoanalytically conceived individual history, the unconscious dynamics of the oedipus complex, is also the moment of entry into the collective, public, historical world of cultural signification and social relations. It is true that the investigation of this process, of the subjective dimension of social and cultural history, of the modes through which we come to live our bodies as historically encultured human beings—if it is to move beyond the general reconstruction of conventional, publicly articulated standards and deal with the actual processes through which inner experience is formed and defined— must focus on the individual case study, moving outward from individual experience through the thick contextual networks of linguistic and social action which define that experience as real and meaningful within specific cultural worlds. But this procedure is in conformity with the investigative methods and practices of the most innovative and influential contemporary cultural historians. In this instance as well, Freud's practice in the writing of his case histories can still provide stimulating, positive models for the contemporary psychohistorian. Although the time will surely come when Freud will appear as a messenger from an alien, foreign culture, articulating a conception of subjective identity and emotional experience that will be perceived as a self-interpretation of another world, that time has not yet arrived. He remains, especially in his role as the analyst of the cultural construction of subjective identity and experience, a viable, present interlocuter in ongoing attempts to construct our own heterogeneous web of associated but not identical narratives of emancipation and integration within the cultural cacaphony of the present, and thus also of current attempts to engage in a meaningful encounter and genuine dialogue with the past.

Notes

1. The two essays to which Suárez-Orozco indirectly refers through phrases cited in his text are "Thick Description: Toward an Interpretive Theory of Culture" and "Deep Play: Notes on the Balinese Cockfight." Both are printed in Clifford Geertz, *The Interpretation of Cultures* (New York, 1973). The connections to the article on the Balinese cockfight seem particularly close. Geertz describes this event in analogy to athletic events in America and emphasizes its exclusively male aspect. The citation in the text is from p. 448.

2. For a classic statement of the cultural construction of self-identity see Clifford Geertz, *Local Knowledge* (New York, 1983), p. 59. The constructionist position on gender and sexual identity is presented persuasively in Joan Wallach Scott, *Gender and the Politics of History* (New York, 1988); Judith Butler, *Gender Trouble: Feminism and the Subversion of Identity;* and David M. Halperin, *One Hundred Years of Homosexuality and Other Essays on Greek Love* (London, 1990).

3. There is a detailed textual analysis of the conflict in Freud between a theory of mimetic desire or identification and object-related desire or wish-fulfillment in Mikkel Borch-Jacobsen, *The Freudian Subject,* translated from the French by Catherine Porter (Stanford, 1988).

4. Robert Musil, *A Sort of Introduction: The Like of It Now Happens,* vol. 1 of *The Man Without Qualities,* translated from the German by Eithne Wilkens and Ernst Kaiser (New York, 1965), p. 34.

5. The proliferation and intensification of nationalisms in the post-colonial and then post-cold-war eras has produced a new wave of scholarship on nationalism that focuses on its constructive, imaginary aspect as it makes new subjects out of old and becomes the matrix of subjectivation in the wake of the collapse of traditional communal bonds. See especially the path-breaking study by Benedict Anderson, *Imagined Communities: Reflections on the Origin and Spread of Nationalism,* revised edition (London, 1991), and the essays by a group of post-colonial post-modernists in Homi Bhabha, ed., *Nation and Narration* (London, 1990).

6. On the significance of the diagnosis and treatment of hysteria for gender reconstruction in late nineteenth-century western cultures see Lisa Appignanesi and John Forrester, *Freud's Women* (New York, 1992), pp. 63–70, and the literature cited there.

7. See Shirley Nelson Garner, "Freud and Fliess: Homophobia and Seduction," in Dianne Hunter, ed., *Seduction and Theory: Readings of Gender, Representation, and Rhetoric* (Urbana, Ill., 1989), pp. 86–109, and Madelon Sprengnether, *The Spectral Mother: Freud, Feminism and Psychoanalysis (Ithaca, N.Y., 1990).*

8. "Neue Folge der Vorlesungen zur Einfuehrung in die Psychoanalyse," in Sigmund Freud, *Gesammelte Werke,* 19 vols. (London, 1940–87), 15: 86.

9. In the opening paragraph of *Group Psychology and the Analysis of the Ego* (1921).

3
LITERATURE

Psychoanalytic Process and Literary Narrative

TRANSFERENCE AND

COUNTERTRANSFERENCE IN *JANE EYRE*

RICHARD ALMOND

The relationship between psychoanalysis and literature has a long history. Freud's application of psychoanalytic ideas to the understanding of creative works and to the personalities of artists is well known (S. Freud, 1908). Freud's writing is replete with literary references introduced to lend weight to his clinically derived ideas. The best known example is his use of the story of Oedipus to epitomize the universality of incestuous wishes and their psychological consequences: "This discovery is confirmed by a legend that has come down to us from classical antiquity: *a legend whose profound and universal power to move can only be understood if the hypothesis I have put forward in regard to the psychology of children has an equally universal validity*" (S. Freud, 1900, p. 261; italics added). Freud's argument is intuitively convincing. If major artistic and mythic themes correspond to our clinical, psychoanalytic understanding, then we can assume that our insights are not peculiar to the psychoanalytic situation or to the neurotic personality. The clinical discovery of themes that are found in literature in turn suggests that artistic expression may be moved by universal as well as individual psychological experience.

In a series of studies of nineteenth- and twentieth-century novels, Barbara Almond and I have observed how frequently two characters struggle with each other psychologically, often with a positive effect on at least one of the participants (B. and R. Almond, 1996). It is our assumption that certain authors have tapped into what might be termed the universal capacity for therapeutic involvement (Bird, 1972). These fictional relationships are not representations of psychotherapy itself, but rather a reflection of the writers' understanding that one person can help another to open up psychological development and to reverse pathological patterns of thought and behavior. Most of our literary "cases," in fact, come from a time before psychoanalysis existed as such. In other words, we suggest that change as we understand it in psychoanalytic therapies may partake of more universal processes, ones that have been recorded in literary narratives.

I will argue that we can learn about the change process by examining *Jane Eyre* and the way in which crucial relationships affect its protagonist as she struggles with developmental tasks and neurotic conflict. I will look at the process of change in the light of both normal development and analytic treatment. In recent years psychoanalysis has increasingly sought to understand process from direct observations from the consulting room and the nursery. Here, the data are fictional interactions that come from the perceptions and imaginations of an author.

While I do not wish to pursue a psychobiographic discussion of Charlotte Brontë herself, it is likely that she was addressing, through her protagonist, her own psychological situation — that of a strong personality in an era when the role of women required submission and indirectness (Fraser 1988). There are, of course, many fascinating parallels between Brontë's life and Jane Eyre's. Since my interest is *not* in psychobiography, but in the question of how Brontë depicts psychological change, I shall not introduce biographic data, nor pursue the many issues in women's psychology and social position that the novel addresses.

In an earlier work (R. Almond, 1989; B. and R. Almond, 1996) I proposed a framework for discussing positive intrapsychic change. I suggested three major aspects of the change process: (1) The parties have intrinsically, or develop, an *engagement* that makes them highly significant to one another. (2) A powerful pattern of *mutual influence* develops in their relationship. In this pattern the influence of one party leads to alterations in the behavior of the other in reciprocal fashion. (3) This pattern of action-reaction, or influence, has a positive *directionality* to it—a pull toward resolution of conflict, growth, and widened adaptiveness.

The parallel to analytic process is compelling: *Engagement* is implied in the development of transference, the investment of the specially structured analytic situation with intense personal significance. *Mutual influence* summarizes our understanding that the enacted interplay of transference and countertransference contributes to change (Renik, 1995). *Directionality* corresponds to the clinical principle that a special attitude is required to ensure that the treatment process is constructive (Almond, 1995).

In examining a work of fiction, of course, we do not expect to find these elements elaborated in just the same form in which we find them in therapy. *Engagement, influence, directionality*— each will appear in a form that fits the narrative structure the author has chosen. Thus, for example, where we expect the analytic attitude of the analyst to make a large contribution to the positive impetus for change, in certain sections of *Jane Eyre* change is impelled by the love and sexual attraction of one or both participants.

Jane Eyre (1847) is a rich literary text for exploring the mutative qualities of relationships depicted in fiction. The novel spans Jane's life from age ten to nineteen, describing a number of developmental stages, tasks, and problems. I shall concentrate specifically on psychological issues embedded in the five phases of Jane's life the novel describes: her home life with the Reed family; her school years; her months as a governess; her life with her second family, the Riverses; and her reunion with Rochester. The central action of the novel—most memorable especially to the early adolescent girls for whom the novel is a perennial favorite—is the romance between Jane and Mr. Rochester. This relationship is both a stimulus for Jane's emergent sexuality and a source of conflict. Issues of development and character intersect with those of intimacy, a combination that frequently brings patients to analytic treatment. Brontë presents relationships as crucial both to development and to the internal conflict resolution that allows a young adult to form a successful sexual-affectional bond. My focus will be on the elements and patterns of interaction that Brontë depicts as effecting these transformations in each phase of Jane's development.

The novel begins when Jane Eyre is ten years old, not long past the age when coherent memory generally begins. *Jane Eyre* encompasses issues of childhood, latency, puberty, adolescence, and young adulthood. It is the story of a woman of strong will, one who accepts deprivation, hard work, and adversity but does not accept submission to persons or standards that are at odds with her internal self-concept and values. In addition to the interplay of character with life events, the novel explores Jane's defenses at each developmental level, and how they shift. *Jane*

Eyre is written in five major episodes, each in a different geographic locale, and each delineating psychological issues of a different developmental stage. Each episode addresses internal developmental changes brought about by interactions with one or several persons she is close to.

Gateshead

Orphaned early in life, Jane is the Cinderella of her Aunt Reed's household, Gateshead, where she is abused by her stepbrother and slighted by her stepsisters and stepmother. In a dramatic opening scene Jane is provoked by her stepbrother, John Reed, who taunts and demeans her. When Jane calls him "wicked and cruel," he runs at her, and she defends herself by hitting and biting in return. *She* is held responsible—"Did anybody ever see such a picture of passion?" says Mrs. Reed, ignoring her son's provocation and putting all blame on Jane. The apothecary is summoned, and he suggests that Jane be sent away to a cheap boarding school.

Mr. Brocklehurst, the director of Lowood School, comes to meet Jane. He admits her to the school following an interview in which Mrs. Reed conveys to the piously sadistic Brocklehurst her view of Jane's wicked character. Afterward Jane for the first time confronts her stepmother about how she has been treated:

> Shaking from head to foot, thrilled with ungovernable excitement, I continued—
>
> "I am glad you are no relation of mine. I will never call you aunt again as long as I live. I will never come to see you when I am grown up; and if any one asks me how I liked you, and how you

treated me, I will say the very thought of you makes me sick, and that you treated me with miserable cruelty."

"How dare you affirm that, Jane Eyre?"

"How dare I, Mrs. Reed? How dare I? Because it is the *truth*. You think I have no feelings, and that I can do without one bit of love or kindness; but I cannot live so: and you have no pity." (p. 30)

Here we have a description of a psychologically abused child who reaches her limit and finally speaks her mind. The poor-relation orphan has endured the family's slights because she has no choice, she rebels only when driven to the extreme. From a developmental point of view, this episode represents certain issues a child experiences in early latency. During the normal genital phase (about age four to six) children face some painful realities. They realize that possessing a parent's love and attention in the way they would like is impossible. This situation is addressed in the Cinderella story, which according to Bettelheim (1975) is children's most popular fairy tale. In that story the wrongs of childhood are magically righted, but only after suffering and a lesson in the delay of gratification.

Mrs. Reed is greedy and self-indulgent; she accuses Jane of these very faults. From a child's point of view, parents do just this—they prevent the child from gratifying wishes but gratify themselves. Jane knows the "truth" of this and rebels against frustration; the plot gives a justification to this outburst that speaks to the frustrated child in all of us. Mrs. Reed, depicted in a child's-eye caricature, is the foil for an outburst that is true to the internal conflict of the child between wishes for oedipal gratification and dominance over the same-gender parent, and powerful, early superego pressures. Rebellion and its consequence—Jane's being sent away to boarding school—symbolize the harsh transition into latency and the potential regression to pre-oedipal defenses under stress (Bornstein, 1951). Mother, once the source of all love and protection, becomes all bad, heartlessly sending the child out into the world. The stage is also set for the transfer of the child's oedipal desire to homo-erotic peer-love, while sexual curiosity is sublimated into learning (Sarnoff, 1976; Shapiro and Perry, 1976).

This series of events is hardly a "therapeutic" interaction in Jane's life, but it does depict the inner experience of an important developmental transition. Mrs. Reed, in her negative way, is a catalyst for Jane's psychic movement. She essentially forbids the satisfaction of Jane's wishes — embodied in her indulged stepsibs — and drives her into the solution of latency defenses. By being such an obviously bad parent, Mrs. Reed stimulates Jane's outburst, which in turn helps Jane crystallize important elements of her character structure — her strong will and her dedication to psychological and moral truthfulness. Intrapsychically, the rudiments of more advanced superego functioning are represented in the combination of Jane's self-righteousness, her steadfast holding to what is fair and right, and her idealization of her self-concept.

Lowood

In the second phase of *Jane Eyre,* the heroine is a pupil at Lowood School for ten years. Here, too, there is a bad parent: Mr. Brocklehurst, who is greedy, punitive, and withholding. In contrast is Miss Temple, who does what little she can for the girls. A second positive female figure is Helen Burns, a starry-eyed classmate whom Jane comes to love and admire. Helen eventually dies of consumption, submitting to her untimely death with masochistic Christian resignation.

The school years are ones of deprivation and sublimation in learning. The first episodes of Jane's school life have the same quality as the events occurring at the end of her time at Gateshead—the powerful adults, the "bad parents," are cruel and arbitrary. But now at Lowood there is also a "good parent" and a sib—a substitute mother and sister—with whom to commiserate and identify. Miss Temple supports Jane against Brocklehurst's attempt to make her a social outcast, a "servant of the Evil One." Jane excels in her studies and quickly becomes a leader and a favorite. At the end of eight years Jane graduates and becomes herself a teacher at Lowood, education has now put her in an adult role, albeit an unworldly, celibate one. Jane has learned to restrain her frustration at limitations on her power. The rule of Mrs. Reed and Mr. Brocklehurst is replaced by the increasingly benign authority structure of the school. Jane has developed a capacity for sublimation into education and art. Like a child at the brink of puberty, she now has adult capacities though still many of the wishes of childhood.

Appropriate to the object relations typical of latency, during the Lowood period Jane's love is directed toward the two important female figures in her life. She also learns from them. Miss Temple is a reassurance to Jane that she can return to the love of a mother figure after her alienation from Mrs. Reed; Helen Burns is an important alter ego—far less willful than Jane, and more submissive and masochistic. Helen tolerates her punishments and deprivation through a defensive withdrawal from reality to an internal fantasy world. From Helen, Jane learns to turn aggression inward; a move to higher-level defenses, but also the source of the internal conflict between assertiveness and masochism that runs through the next two phases of Jane's life.

To summarize: in the Lowood phase the anger and resentment previously focused on Mrs. Reed are directed toward the bad father, Mr. Brocklehurst, just as the latency girl may focus resentment on father or boys, and turn love toward mothers and female peers. Through her love for these female figures Jane is stimulated to turn outwards, towards real love objects; a forward step from the end of Gateshead, when she had only herself to rely on. She also learns to subdue her strident independence and assertiveness (perhaps not as positive a change, according to twentieth-century values). The psychological alterations at Lowood are those of latency: movement from angry competition to idealization and identification; replacement of the oedipal love object (completely implicit in *Jane Eyre*) with a homoerotic peer-love object.

When Jane is eighteen, Miss Temple marries and leaves Lowood. Jane becomes restless; this loss generates old feelings of loneliness and unhappiness. She advertises for a position as a governess and is hired to tutor a young girl at a large estate in another part of England.

Thornfield

The romance of Jane Eyre, governess, and Edward Rochester, tormented master, is one of the best known in English literature. Jane has left Lowood for Thornfield in search of love. She is not aware that it is heterosexual love she is now seeking, but if she had wished only to replace the loss of her homoerotic school attachments she might well have done so by staying at Lowood and loving her pupils. Or, at Thornfield she could have continued a sublimated, teacher's love by focusing on her charge, Adele. It is her master who soon becomes the object of her desire. Rochester has the gothic qualities that inspire girls' preadolescent fantasies. He is erratic, powerful, dangerous, dark, impulsive, sexual—attractive, despite being "not handsome." But it is not a simple gothic plot that emerges in their interaction.

The relationship that develops is one that reflects Jane's defenses and character as much as it reflects her emerging sexual feeling and interest. At first, Rochester deals with Jane in a circumspect, indirect manner. Like a therapist, he encourages her to voice *her* thoughts and feelings, and does not reveal his own. The roles of master and governess allow a great deal of contact without the social constraints of the courtship situation (Poovey, 1988). These protective conditions, along with Rochester's evasiveness, allow Jane to grow into her awareness of adolescent feelings gradually, giving her time to confront a number of conflicts these feelings arouse.

The first meeting contains an element that will be emblematic—Jane assists Rochester. His horse slips and falls on an icy path. He is slightly hurt, and Jane, who is standing nearby, helps him remount. In every other respect—his powerful, spirited horse and his dog—the scene emphasizes Jane's experience of Rochester's dangerous maleness. A pubescent girl can cope with the images suggested by adult sexuality if she can maternalize the situation: the *man* is vulnerable, not *she; she* will care for *him.* Dangerous sexual-aggressive ideas are displaced onto the man and his animal companions. From the first, the relationship with Rochester is imbued with an aura of specialness and animal intensity.

In their next encounter Rochester is the master, in charge, interviewing Jane about her training and abilities. He pursues her artwork in particular, and notes three striking drawings in her portfolio. Rochester says they come from "an artist's dreamland." The author's description of the drawings is hazy, as is Jane's explanation of them; she complains that she has not captured on paper the vision in her mind. From the psychoanalytic point of view we could hardly have a better description of the experience of a dream after waking.

In psychoanalysis we would understand the "dreams" through the patient's associations—the preceding and following thoughts. While we do not have Jane's direct "free" associations to the striking images in the drawings, there is no doubt they suggest loss and yearning. Without conscious intention, Jane exposes powerful internal imagery to Rochester. He comments that "the drawings are, for a schoolgirl, peculiar. As to the thoughts, they are elfish." He notes some striking technical features of the work and of the locations, saying that the landscape of one "must be Latmos," presumably one of the places Rochester has traveled in his search for love and peace. The idea that she has imagined where he has been suggests an incipient intimacy and identity between them—that her inner landscape relates to his outer one. The images are complex and confusing, but powerful. It is significant that this confusion is exposed to Rochester at an early point in their relationship. Like a patient early in therapy, caught between eagerness and defense, Jane reveals much, but keeps meanings obscure.

A few days later Rochester initiates a conversation with Jane that establishes what will become the pattern of their interaction. He asks her direct, penetrating, and highly personal questions. She answers with a proportionate directness, evoking half-revelations from him. The conversation begins on a note of such directness:

> "You examine me, Miss Eyre," said he: "do you find me handsome?"
>
> I should, if I had deliberated, have replied to this question by something conventionally vague and polite; but the answer somehow slipped from my tongue before I was aware, "No, sir." (p. 122)

Rochester notes her bluntness, contrasting it with her nun-like posture and quietness. He prefers honesty over flattery and servility. A few minutes later, to learn more of her, he "orders" Jane to talk; she refuses, pointing out that, though she is a governess to his ward, she is under no obligation to converse with *him* on command. They banter over this; Rochester accepts her position and restates his request as a desire for talk between conversational equals. Now that he has such a peer he can speak, though with disguise, about his dilemma of wishing for love but being prohibited from it. While she advises morality, he confronts her with herself:

> "You are afraid of me, because I talk like a sphinx."
> "Your language is enigmatical, sir; but though I am bewildered, I am certainly not afraid."
> "You *are* afraid—your self-love dreads a blunder."
> "In that sense I do feel apprehensive—I have no wish to talk nonsense."
> "If you did, it would be in such a grave, quiet manner, I should mistake it for sense. Do you ever laugh, Miss Eyre? . . . believe me, you are not naturally austere, any more than I am naturally vicious. The Lowood constraint still clings to you somewhat; controlling your features, muffling your voice, and restricting your limbs; and you fear in the presence of a man . . . to smile too gaily, speak too freely, or move too quickly; but in time I think you will be natural with me." (p. 129)

And, indeed, further conversations and revelations by Rochester *do* alter Jane's response. He has addressed her defensive pride and restraint, and then the vulnerability that the acknowledgement of these repressed feelings would create:

> The ease of his manner freed me from painful restraint; the friendly frankness, as correct as cordial, with which he treated me, drew me to him. *I felt at times as if he were my relation rather than my master:* yet he was imperious sometimes still; but I did not mind that; I saw it was his way. So happy, so gratified did I become with this new interest added to life, that I ceased to pine after kindred: my thin-crescent destiny seemed to enlarge; the blanks of existence were filled up; my bodily health improved; I gathered flesh and strength. (p. 137, italics added)

Jane's emergence, her bodily development, are followed by a disturbing sequel: Rochester's bed is set on fire (unknown to Jane, by Bertha Mason, the mad wife secretly kept in an attic room). Jane saves him by dumping the contents of his wash basin on him. Afterward, having thanked her for saving his life, Rochester wants Jane to remain with him longer. When she insists on returning to her room, he says, "At least shake hands" (p. 141). Back in her bed, Jane is "tossed on a buoyant, but unquiet sea, where billows of trouble rolled under surges of joy" (p. 142). The sexual arousal that their growing intimacy and mutual need has stimulated is dangerous; its fire must be "put out" by Jane. She can fend Rochester off, but her own desire has become partially conscious.

When Rochester invites the local gentry for a stay of several weeks, he appears to be enamored of Blanche Ingram, an eligible, attractive, but mercenary local beauty. Jealousy awakens Jane's consciousness of loving and desiring him. During this visit competitive issues are primary—Rochester insists Jane attend the social gatherings, where she is treated as a domestic in the household, inferior to the company. She has become accustomed to interacting with Rochester as an equal. Her humiliation and jealousy make it clear to her that she loves Rochester, and not as servant to master. He tries to get her to acknowledge this to him. He points out her loneliness, her "coldness," and her refusal to "stir one step to meet it [love; sexuality] where it waits for you" (p. 185). Jane stands firm; she will not be maneuvered into being the first to act on desire. Rochester acknowledges her independence, self-sufficiency, reason, and judgment—and her conscience.

Jane maintains a confused belief about who is responsible for the fire and later mysterious and ominous acts, attributing them to Grace Poole, a servant. Bertha Mason remains unknown to her, despite many hints that might have alerted her that something is not right at Thornfield. She does not want to admit the existence of another woman who has a rightful claim on Rochester. The young adolescent would like to carry forward the dreamy Prince Charming (father) fantasy of latency into the era of adult sexuality; in this fantasy she has no mother, especially not a sexual one.

What Jane particularly wants to avoid thinking about is dramatized when George Mason, Bertha's brother, is attacked and stabbed during an attempt to talk with his sister. Jane is made a conspirator in helping Rochester deal with the incident, helping hide it from a house full of guests. She remains unaware of the attacker's identity, and she accepts Rochester's request that she not ask more. The pubescent girl's fantasies about sexuality are heavily tinged with aggression as she comes closer to thinking about a sexual mother and the primal scene. Jane's confusion about the other woman remains in place so that she can continue to desire Rochester. He confides further about his past and his dangerous present situation and even his peace in having come to know her—but all in allusive form. Again, Jane counsels propriety; she denies the parental bedroom and her own associated fantasies and wishes. When she hears Rochester's description of his dilemma of living a life without love due to a youthful mistake, she rejects the implicit invitation to advise him to ignore morality in the service of love.

Jane is called to the deathbed of Mrs. Reed, where she learns that in retaliation for her childhood rebelliousness, her aunt has deceitfully hidden from Jane an inheritance from an uncle. This episode bolsters the movement away from the (bad) mother and towards the father/Rochester. Returning to Thornfield Jane tells Rochester that she feels "strangely glad to get back again to you; and wherever you are is my home—my only home" (p. 233). Now the pendulum swings toward her attraction to Rochester.

In the most romantic scene of the novel Jane and Rochester meet on Midsummer Eve in the Thornfield orchard. He teases her about her belief that he intends to marry Blanche Ingram and then admits his own attachment to Jane. She expresses her happiness living at Thornfield and her dread of having to leave him. Recognizing that she will not be lured by love *or* jealousy into an illicit affair, but freed momentarily from a sense of complete responsibility for his action by Jane's admission of love, Rochester asks her to marry. Jane, ignorant of the truth, happily accepts.

On their wedding day the ceremony is disrupted dramatically by the sudden arrival of George Mason, who declares "the existence of an impediment"—a living wife. Rochester, crushed and angry, takes the wedding party to see the deranged Bertha Mason, and explains the facts of his situation to Jane and the others. When they are alone he pleads with her to understand, to live with him away from England as his wife, to respond with her love and understanding to his dreadful dilemma. Rochester's plea is scandalous in a mid-Victorian context. Jane refuses, however, for reasons other than those of propriety. Her *internal standards,* her superego, will not allow her to be happy or make Rochester happy. "Conscience, turned tyrant, held Passion by the throat" (p. 282).

The incestuous quality of her situation could hardly be clearer, and Jane's scruples make the most sense seen in this light. Certainly her next actions support such an interpretation; she flees Thornfield during the night, taking almost nothing with her, and exhausting what money she has on coach fare to travel as far as she can. Developmentally, the recognition of mature sexual desire at puberty reawakens oedipal meanings and requires drastic defensive action—dramatic renunciation. Though Jane is chronologically a young adult, her experience and defensive reactions are those of the post-pubertal adolescent. She reacts to the emergence of (incestuously tinged) sexuality with a self-destructive flight into asceticism (A. Freud, 1936).

Morton

The next phase of Jane Eyre's life concerns her psychological reaction to this adolescent brush with incestuous temptation. All impulse, almost life itself, must be foresworn in an effort to disavow, deny, and distance herself from the temptation just narrowly averted. "Tyrant Conscience" takes Jane close to death from cold and starvation, far from the Thornfield she has fled. The imagery of the landscape into which she escapes has strong maternal overtones; it is Nature, the good mother, who keeps her alive during her flight from incestuous danger (Rich, 1982; Williams, 1989). Jane stops just short of starvation; she begs at a strange home for food, work, and shelter. She is taken in by a young minister, St. John Rivers, and, as she recovers, is given a place in his household.

This new home combines the elements Jane now needs—family, and an atmosphere of high-mindedness. The Riverses, St. John and his two governess sisters, provide a peer group united by their morality, culture, and dedication to good works. This atmosphere is an external confirmation of Jane's motives for fleeing Thornfield. There can be love without impulsive loss of control; one can love "sisters" and a "brother" rather than the dangerous Rochester. Jane is set up by St. John as the local schoolteacher, a return to the earlier latency solution disguised in an adult role. But issues aroused earlier cannot be avoided.

St. John emerges as the voice of passion in this episode—inverted passion. He asks Jane to marry him and go with him as a fellow missionary to India. St. John makes clear that he is not drawn to her out of his needs or by love for her but by her potential for submission to him in the form of religious dedication. His proposal offers a masochistic, conscience-satisfying resolution to Jane's guilt and anxiety. She now struggles with a new form of conflict—that between her defensive asceticism and her wish for loving attachment (Williams 1989). Just as she cannot submit in sin to Rochester, she finds herself unable to submit in self-denial to St. John. When he makes his proposal, and presses her for a reply she must face this conflict.

> "Once more, why this refusal?" he asked.
>
> "Formerly," I answered, "because you did not love me; now, I reply, because you almost hate me. If I were to marry you, you would kill me. You are killing me now."
>
> His lips and cheeks turned white—quite white.

> "*I should kill you—I am killing you?* Your words
> are such as ought not to be used: violent, unfemi-
> nine, and untrue." (p. 394)

Jane has detected the hostile component of asceticism, the invitation to join St. John in turning "Tyrant Conscience" upon love. The encounter makes Jane aware of the aggressiveness of her own superego pressure as she experiences St. John's insistence that she give up love for his life of idealistic self sacrifice. Her vigorous negative reaction to St. John shows her how guilt has been dominating her, and implicitly allows Jane to reinterpret her love for Rochester.

One night soon after her confrontation with St. John, she hears the "voice" of Rochester calling to her: "'Jane! Jane! Jane!' . . . it was the voice of a human being—a known, loved, well-remembered voice—that of Edward Fairfax Rochester; and it spoke in pain and woe, wildly, eerily, urgently" (p. 401).

In turning from St. John to Rochester Jane takes an important maturational step. The renunciation of sexuality, which had seemed necessary earlier, now gives way to the acceptance of intimacy. With difficulty Jane recognizes that the appeal of St. John's proposal is masochistic and narcissistic. Rochester's call to her is a plea from an other, one truly in need, and one who will offer her love in return. It is not St. John's invitation to a fundamentally aggressive solution—sexual denial joined with turning of frustrated desire against oneself—but an appeal based on human need for companionship and mutuality of positive feeling and desire. Jane has experienced both incestuous danger and superego danger, and is now in a position to deal with herself and Rochester in a more realistic way.

Ferndean

Jane returns to learn that Thornfield has been destroyed in a fire set by Bertha Mason. Rochester has been injured trying unsuccessfully to save Bertha; he is left blind and with a maimed hand, living in a small house, Ferndean, a few miles away from Thornfield. Jane goes to him and, in a scene that reverses earlier ones, she teases him about her affections and his jealousy, but finally admits her continued love and wish to marry him. The final chapter begins in an active, authorial voice: "Reader, I married him," and continues with descriptions of the worldly and happy direction of Jane's life, as well as those of Rochester and her female Rivers cousins. The book ends with St. John's "successful" martyred death in missionary service. The tempting self-punitive idealism (or masochism) of adolescence is part of the past for Jane; the more tangible and less fantasy-based satisfactions of love and responsibility with a flesh-and-blood partner are now desirable and acceptable. Sexual intimacy is now possible, freed from anxiety about incestuous fantasies. Jane can now enter an adult, sexual relationship safely as the result of a number of factors: the "working through" she has done with St. John; the death of the dangerous mother (Bertha Mason); the injury to Rochester that symbolizes that he is now mortal, no longer the dangerous oedipal figure of the past; the inheritance that allows Jane to enter marriage with a sense of equality rather than dependence.

Discussion

The schema for the change process outlined earlier—*engagement, mutual influence,* and *directionality*—can be applied to the developmental sequence in diagram 1.

Diagram 1

Phase of Jane's Development	Foil (and Jane's reaction)
1. Oedipal	Mrs. Reed's punitiveness and self-indulgence propel Jane into latency.
2. Latency	Mr. Brocklehurst is now the "bad" parent, a cruel father. Jane turns to a love of women; Miss Temple and Helen Burns facilitate feelings of homoerotic love, idealization, and masochistic defense.
3. Puberty	Rochester is the stimulus for weakening of latency defenses and emergence of desire. He is, however, still an oedipal love object; his prior marriage has incestuous meaning for her; positive feelings emerging in Jane arouse conflict.
4. Adolescence	The Rivers family restores equilibrium and love, but with a return to latency defenses. St. John's proposal makes Jane aware of her ascetic solution to the problems of genitality.
5. Adulthood	Rochester as a vulnerable figure is now less the feared and desired oedipal parent, and is safe for genital love. Sexual and emotional intimacy are now possible.

Engagement

In each phase Jane first becomes intensely involved with an agent of change, whom I have designated as the "foil." This engagement may take time to develop, as with Helen Burns, her schoolmate, or it may occur almost instantaneously, because Jane is primed for a certain sort of relationship, as with

Rochester or Miss Temple. Engagement establishes the opportunity for interaction that will have a significant psychological impact; the "foil" is not simply a character, but a potential influence.

Mutual Influence

Once involved, the dyad interact in a way that brings certain issues to the foreground for Jane. The quality and complexity of these interactions increase as the heroine matures. In phases 1 and 2, influence is a relatively straightforward process of loving and emulating those who treat her well and love her, and angrily confronting those who are unfair or cruel, rejecting them as models. During phases 3 through 5 Jane encounters more complex foils, and the interplay with them is more complex. When Jane first encounters Rochester, she is, as he puts it, "under the Lowood constraint." Her prolonged latency as student and teacher have suppressed her natural spirit, and repressed her sexuality. Defenses of self-denial and a quietly proud self-sufficiency enable her to tolerate a position of financial dependence and social inferiority, and keep instinctual pressures far from awareness.

I have already commented on Jane's readiness for engagement with Rochester when they first meet. But Rochester must help her to overcome her defensive tendency to deny attraction to a man, especially one who is socially superior to her. Rochester takes an interest in Jane, not just as a governess, whom he might quiz her about her "accomplishments," but as someone he wishes to understand. Asking her appraisal of his appearance goes beyond role limitations to the personal, and stimulates an involvement with him that is more intimate than her station would dictate. The way Rochester banters with her also hints at his attraction. Jane recognizes this, and is not put off; she feels steadily more recognized as a person. The fire episode can be viewed both as an evolution of the interplay between them and as a representation of a heightened level of intensity of engagement.

Diagram 2

Jane	Rochester
Problem	*Response*
1. Mistrust of others' values and purposes, based on early experience.	1. His basic good-heartedness, his underlying humanness and need for another gradually win her trust.
2. Masochistic, submissive style as a solution to frustration over limitations on her power.	2. He treats her with the respect due an emotional equal, despite her inferior social status.
3. Proud self-sufficiency dominating over object-relatedness.	3. He sees through her defensive pride and points it out. His love for Jane draws her into a relationship.
4. Inhibition of impulses; defenses against all expressiveness.	4. He values expressiveness; he detects her underlying emotionality.
5. Repression of sexuality, denial of her body.	5. He is sensual and physically expressive; he is comfortable with his own body and sexually experienced.

Diagram 2 presents the process of mutual influence in detail during the Thornfield phase. While my focus is on Jane, it is important that Rochester is reciprocally involved in his responses. Jane's personality, her qualities, bring out in Rochester responses that confront, and allow her to modify, her behavior and its underlying psychological structure. The engagement aspect of the relationship puts both Jane's latent wishes and her defenses into active play. Now these are amenable to influence. Each "problem" listed in the diagram also has an "outcome" (not shown), part of which is the opening of a new issue.

Directionality

Psychological movement in the Thornfield phase is fueled by libido. Rochester's need for an empathic companion fuses with his intense sexuality to provide a powerful pull on Jane. This is highlighted in problem 5, but in fact supplies orientation to all the mutual influences of this phase. That is, the eventual result of the changes in Jane's various defenses (problems 1–4) is that she is able to recognize desire in herself and accept it in Rochester. In this phase each outcome is in the direction of softening the repressive and inhibiting effect of defenses, leading toward a release of impulse and the experience of affect. When Jane notes her physical flowering living at Thornfield, it attests to the powerful impact of her physical attraction to Rochester.

Not contained in diagram 2 is the fact that a problem results from the interactions of this phase—the release of libido when it still has a largely incestuous significance. In the same paragraph in which Jane notes her physical improvement she thinks, "I felt at times as if he were my relation rather than my master."

Engagement, Mutual Influence, and Directionality
in the Morton Phase

While at Morton Jane must deal with a whole new set of issues
that follow from her experience at Thornfield. Appropriately,
from the point of view I am taking here that each phase is
a maturational step, the slate of relationships is wiped clean;
Jane begins a new set of connections with the Rivers family.
Once she is engaged psychologically with them, the disturbing reactions to Thornfield can be approached. I shall not outline fully the process of this phase; it is the most complex of
the novel, integrating prior personality development with the
developmental crisis of adolescence: the explosion of puberty
and its disorganizing, regressive impact. Jane's response to this
crisis begins, as I have indicated, with a flight into asceticism. Though the urgency of this defensive reaction quickly
eases, Jane returns to an earlier style of self-containment, self-
sacrifice, and submissiveness.

The unfolding and resolution of these issues occurs in relation to St. John and his two sisters, who have, respectively,
resonances with Brocklehurst and Miss Temple. Though there
is a pull toward self-denial that echoes the Lowood phase,
now Jane is familiar with intimacy, desire, and mutuality. Her
inheritance of a large legacy while living at Morton provides
her with independence; it also symbolizes her psychological
coming-into-her-own. In other words, Jane brings to her important relationships a richer, more complex capacity for *engagement,* one that enables her to deal with defensive reactions
to powerful conflicts.

During this phase *mutual influence* is a blend of the positive feminine identifications that are stirred in relating to the
Rivers sisters and the inverted desire of St. John. The problems
being processed concern higher-level versions of those in earlier

phases—self interest versus relatedness; autonomy versus submission; repression versus desire. These problems are worked out through interactions with St. John and his sisters, in a sort of counterpoint. The sisters love Jane, and she loves them in an object-related, mutual way. For example, when Jane inherits, she insists on dividing her fortune with the Riverses in four equal shares. She makes it clear she is not motivated by guilt, but by a wish not to be separated from her newfound family by wealth (the Riverses, she eventually learns, are actually her cousins), and by a desire to give them the same independence she now has.

At the end of the Morton phase Jane is able to articulate to St. John the destructive quality of his offer, in the face of the intensity of his demand on her. While he is a "negative foil," like Mrs. Reed, it is their powerful interaction that helps Jane clarify her internal conflict over intimacy.

Directionality is now provided in part by Jane's increasingly integrated character, so that the motives that have operated more monolithically in earlier phases now blend—her sense of the "truth" of her own needs; her uprightness; her recognition of the legitimate claims of intimacy. These qualities are reinforced by the Rivers sisters, who also see things clearly and quietly stand their own ground. In an ultimately negative way, St. John also contributes to the directional pull in this phase, by contaminating the appeal of service and self-sacrifice with his blatantly stated grandiose ambitions. His ultimate selfishness makes Jane more aware of, and comfortable with, her wish for gratification and intimacy.

Change Processes in Fiction and Psychoanalysis

I have shown that *Jane Eyre* can be compared to a developmental sequence, and to an analytic treatment, through the vehicle of a general schema proposed for the study of intrapsychic change. Now I shall turn to a more specific comparison between fictional change, as represented by Charlotte Brontë in this novel, and psychoanalytic change. The points of similarity and difference will help us identify those aspects of analytic technique and process that partake of universal themes, and those that are more unique.

The descriptions and changes that go on early in *Jane Eyre* can be viewed as a prologue to the central action of the novel that I have referred to as the Thornfield and Morton phases. As depicted by Charlotte Brontë, Rochester acts in many ways like a psychoanalyst. He is interested, but often silent; he is inquiring, but enigmatic. This facilitates Jane's use of Rochester as a transference figure. Jane becomes deeply involved, but—like many psychoanalytic patients—resists awareness of her feelings. Rochester encourages Jane to admit these feelings; she resists. If we view the "events" of the plot that occur between Jane's talks with Rochester as the equivalent of dreams or extratherapeutic enactments, then the parallel with analytic process is more obvious. The powerful sexual feelings stirred by the episode of the fire; Jane's jealousy and feeling of exclusion during Blanche Ingram's visit; her uneasiness and confusion about Bertha Mason—each can be compared to a manifestation of transference neurosis. In the clinical psychoanalytic situation we recognize the presence of the transference neurosis—the presence in the here-and-now relationship of the patient's central conflicts—by the patient's emotional intensity, preoccupation with the analysis, confusion, and intensified struggle between impulse and defense.

Amid this, Rochester serves a dual function as the object of Jane's feelings and as an observer who draws her out. The issues Jane deals with are not just *enacted*, they are also *discussed*— in highly charged moments. Brontë includes the self-awareness we associate with insight in her depiction of change. For example, Rochester reflects to Jane the defensive function of certain qualities—her pride, self-containment, her need to be right—and ultimately he makes her aware of her wishes for love.

Rochester's bigamous proposal and the discovery of his marriage are similar to a countertransference-induced event in a treatment. There are moments in psychoanalysis when the analyst unconsciously acts in a way that is painful or deeply problematic for the patient. With careful work such events can be turned to therapeutic purpose (Levine, 1993). The Thornfield phase ends with an outburst of erotic feeling abetted by Rochester's misleading presentation of himself as available for marriage. It is followed by Jane's flight into asceticism. Like such events in treatment, this crisis has a potentially positive outcome. At Morton Jane uses her relationship with cousin St. John to work through the superego problem that has been stirred. Again, Jane *articulates to* St. John the inner consequences of accepting his proposal ("you would kill me. You are killing me now.") While Rochester and St. John, the foils who stimulate insight, do not have a conscious therapeutic intent, I have shown how their qualities have the effect of removing Jane's resistances to knowledge about herself and thus enable her to change.

It can be argued, of course, that these events occur for purposes of the novel's plot, that they have meanings and purposes independent of intrapsychic change. I would reply that it is in fact Brontë's depiction of Jane's growing insight that moves the plot along, and that plot movement in *Jane Eyre* is the fictional equivalent of therapeutic movement. Brontë could have resolved the problems of Jane's Thornfield phase much earlier and more easily, with the plot device of the fire and Rochester's release from Bertha Mason. The entire Morton phase can be seen as resolving the conflict between desire and conscience.

It is almost immediately after her final confrontation with St. John that Jane "hears" the call from Rochester. Externally she knows him as no different than before; internally, *her* alteration, resulting from an awareness of the devastating effects of guilt and self-punishment, allows her to seek him out again.

To summarize: transference, resistance, transference neurosis, countertransference, interpretation, and insight can all be found in *Jane Eyre*, allowing for the plot requirements of a novel. Missing is the conscious therapeutic intent of the foil, or foils, who serve as agents of change. Missing also is an initial wish for intrapsychic change on the part of the protagonist. These elements — aspects of *directionality* in my model — are provided by such "natural" motivations as desire, resentment, morality, or ambition. If analytic process is a special version of a natural process, we should expect such natural motives to function in place of the conscious wish to get better, or to help another get better. Indeed, careful consideration of motivations in analysis reveals that under the "therapeutic contract," on both sides, are different, more complex, transference-driven motives.

We can carry these observations further as an example of the sort of question that looking at change in a fictional text can raise: Is it possible that analytic process is, and should be, moved by more personal motivations? Does Anna Freud's (1936) prescription for the analyst's position — "equidistant from id, ego and superego" — mean a static, neutral position, or a more active, flexible one, in which the analyst or therapist, deliberately or intuitively, acts differently at different moments (Lohser and Newton, 1997). This idea is subject to the challenge of the shibboleth, "corrective emotional experience," that is, that to react differentially to the patient is manipulation, and no longer analysis. But it is also possible that, in a manner more like the novel's foils than the ideal of steady neutrality, analysts react and transmit these reactions to patients as a necessary part of therapeutic process. This idea is hardly new, as students of countertransference would be the first to point out, but its reappearance in this exploration of process affirms the value of further study of the analyst's emotional responsiveness, and particularly the ways in which the analyst's ego monitors affects stirred by the patient and modulates behavior toward the patient.

I do not mean to argue that the fictional relationship and the therapeutic relationship are identical, but that they are mutually informative because of their symmetry. One—therapy—actually happens, but is very difficult to describe and define because human interaction is so complex; therapy involves two personalities and their continuous impact on one another; it involves internal experience as well as observable behavior. The other—the novel—is created, but is a subject that "holds still," that is, it is static as a written text between the author's articulation of fantasy and the reader's evoked imaginative response.

This analysis of *Jane Eyre* has demonstrated that the novel describes a process of development, and of resolution of internal conflict through the impact of specific, dyadic interactions. In the most powerful relationships of *Jane Eyre* many of the elements of psychoanalytic process can be identified. Both Spence (1982) and Schafer (1983) have used narrative as a metaphor for analytic process, contrasting it particularly with Freud's earlier "surgical" metaphor (1912), in which the analyst acts as an uninvolved transference screen and interpretive voice to reflect the patient's transferences and resistances. The argument here builds on those of Spence and Schafer, and suggests that analytic process can be used to approach fiction, which in turn can tell us more about analysis. The usefulness of the schema I have employed for this study indicates the likelihood that there are universal elements that operate in intrapsychic change; the schema is a first step towards exploring these elements. Recent discussions of analytic process acknowledge the difficulty of defining it (Abend, 1990). It is my hope that the venture into nonanalytic data will help elucidate some of the elements of process by indicating where universal phenomena emerge.

SUMMARY

Examined from a psychoanalytic point of view, the novel *Jane Eyre* emerges as an interesting and rich depiction of (1) female development; (2) neurotic conflict in a young woman; and (3) the role of intense dyadic interaction in developmental progression and in resolution of intrapsychic conflict. The novel falls into five phases, roughly corresponding to the oedipal stage, latency, puberty, adolescence, and young adulthood. I propose a three-part model of intrapsychic change that occurs in dyads. This model forms a basis for examining way the heroine changes, and for comparing that change to change in psychoanalysis.

In treatment, change occurs within one relationship, with the analyst taking on meanings for the patient that are often a blend of multiple individuals, past and present. The relationship becomes a theater for enacting developmental issues, and projections of parts of the patient's past and inner experience. *Jane Eyre* makes use of similar condensations. In the novel, characters whom the protagonist encounters help her resolve multiple neurotic and developmental conflicts, often at the same time. Hopefully, this way of looking at a familiar novel suggests new perspectives both on a familiar text and on the unfinished exploration of how people change in psychoanalytic therapies.

Works Cited

Abend, S. M. (1990). The Psychoanalytic Process: Motives and Obstacles in the Search for Clarification. *Psychoanal. Quarterly* 59:532–549.

Almond, B. (1990). *The Secret Garden:* A Therapeutic Metaphor. *Psychoanal. Study Child* 45:477–494.

———. (1992) The Accidental Therapist: Intrapsychic Change in a Novel. *Literature and Psychology* 38:84–104.

———. (1991). A Healing Relationship in Margaret Drabble's Novel *The Needle's Eye. Annual of Psychoanalysis* 19:91–106.

Almond, R. (1989). Psychological Change in Jane Austen's *Pride and Prejudice. Psychoanal. Study Child* 44:307–324.

———. (1992). The Child as a Therapeutic Figure: *Silas Marner. Annual of Psychoanalysis* 20:171–190.

———. (1995). The Analytic Role: A Mediating Influence in the Interplay of Transference and Countertransference. *J. Amer. Psychoanal. Assn.* 43:469–494.

Bettelheim, B. (1976). *The Uses of Enchantment.* New York: Alfred A. Knopf.

Bird, B. (1972). Notes on Transference. *J. Amer. Psychoanal. Assn.* 20:267–301.

Bornstein, B. (1951). On Latency. *Psychoanal. Study Child* 5:279–285.

Brontë, C. ([1847] 1988). *Jane Eyre.* Toronto: Bantam.

Fraser, R. (1988). *The Brontës: Charlotte Brontë and Her Family.* New York: Fawcett Columbine.

Freud, A. (1936). Instinctual Anxiety During Puberty. *The Writings of Anna Freud,* 2:152–172. New York: International Universities Press, 1966.

———. (1936). *The Ego and the Mechanisms of Defense.* The Writings of Anna Freud, vol. 2. New York: International Universities Press, 1966.

Freud, S. (1900). The Interpretation of Dreams. *Standard Edition,* volumes 9–10.

———. (1908). Creative Writers and Day-Dreaming. *Standard Edition,* volume 9.

———. (1912). Recommendations to Physicians Practising Psycho-Analysis. *Standard Edition,* volume 12.

Levine, H. (1993). The Analyst's Participation in the Analytic Process. *Internat. J. Psychoanal.* 75:665–676.

Lohser, B., and P. Newton (1997). *Unorthodox Freud: The View from the Couch.* New York and London: Guilford.

Poovey, M. (1988). The Anathematized Race: The Governess and *Jane Eyre*. In *Uneven Developments: The Ideological Work of Gender in Mid-Victorian England.* Chicago: University of Chicago Press.

Renik, O. (1993). Countertransference Enactment and the Psychoanalytic Process. In *Psychic Structure and Psychic Change: Essays in Honor of Robert Wallerstein, M.D.,* ed. M. J. Horowitz, O. F. Kernberg, and E. M. Weinshel. Madison, Conn.: International Universities Press, pp. 135–158.

Rich, A. (1982). *Jane Eyre:* A Tale. In *On Lies, Secrets, and Silence.* New York: W. W. Norton.

Sarnoff, C. (1976). *Latency.* New York: Jason Aronson.

Schafer, R. (1983). *The Analytic Attitude.* New York: Basic.

Shapiro, T., and R. Perry (1976). Latency Revisited. *Psychoanal. Study Child.* 31:79–105.

Spence, D. P. (1982). *Narrative Truth and Historical Truth.* New York: Norton.

Williams, C. (1989). Closing the Book: The Intertextual End of *Jane Eyre*. In *Victorian Connections,* ed. Jerome McGann. Charlottesville: University of Virginia Press.

The Enigmatic Jewishness of Leopold Bloom

PAUL SCHWABER

At one moment early in the afternoon, Leopold Bloom, the amiable modern Odysseus of James Joyce's *Ulysses* (1922), panics. Walking on Kildare Street toward Dublin's National Library, he glimpses Blazes Boylan coming the other way: "Straw hat in sunlight. Tan shoes. Turnedup trousers. It is. It is" (8.1168). Boylan will cuckold him later that afternoon, he knows; so, heart sinking, he swerves right and rushes toward the entry gate of the museum for cover. Hurrying, he registers quick images and thoughts: cold statues of goddesses; quiet and safe there; handsome building Sir Thomas Deane designed; sunlight on Boylan—might he not have seen? Still not at the entrance, Bloom simulates looking for something in his pockets, recognizing by touch his handkerchief, purse, *Freeman's Journal*, amulet potato, and bar of soap. One item surprises him: "Agendath Netaim. Where did I?"*—the Zionist flier that Dlugacz, the pork butcher, wrapped meat with that morning. It advertised a planter's colony founded in Palestine by Moses Montefiore and invited subscriptions at a Berlin address. Leopold had taken one, read it and, apparently, pocketed it. "Nothing doing," he then reflected, "still an idea behind it," (4.200) and soon dismissed Dlugacz from his thoughts as an "enthusiast" (4.493). Yet unwittingly he kept the flier with him: a Jewish connection that, approaching the library and unnerved by seeing Boylan, he rediscovers—and, like his potato, newspaper, and lemon-smelling soap, uses in his improvised evasion.

*Joyce's error. It should be *Agudath* Netaim.

The exigency of Bloom's crisis is here dramatized. His wife and Boylan will become lovers and, far from preventing it, he is routed. What he has recurrently approached and deflected in his thoughts today will come to pass. It is extraordinary to see him unravel so, because as we have followed his cerebrations and interactions from early morning to now close to 2:00 P.M., he has maintained a remarkably calm and controlled public manner. Cautious of speech and action, he earns early the naughty epithet "prudent member" (12.211) Joe Hynes will assign him in Barney Kiernan's—alluding to more, of course, than his membership in the Masons. We, however, privy to his thoughts, have come to know the canny, ever-curious, irreverent, comical, vulnerable, and compassionate sensibility behind the prudent manner. In my experience most readers, having come to care companionably about Bloom, feel wrenched by this moment of his dismay.

His distress shatters his customary containment but, interestingly, it is restored quickly. For the arc of the disruptive experience, extreme as it is, exemplifies a defining rhythm of his psyche: that following a mood plunge or a perception or thought that could engender one, he will struggle back to equanimity, using characteristic mental maneuvers. At such moments, moreover, he will trust the very process of his thoughts and follow its lead. Leopold Bloom has an idiom of resilience. The startled, frightened shame he evinces on seeing Boylan suggests how poignant Molly's expected tryst is for him and how powerless he feels. Yet even as he flees, searching in his pockets to seem preoccupied, he is reclaiming his self-possession. Recognizing handkerchief, purse, newspaper, potato, and bar of soap, and puzzled by "Agendath," he reaches the entrance of the museum and simultaneously his closing thought of the chapter: "Safe!" (8.1193).

Thus, as if bearing touchstones of continuity in his pockets, he reconstitutes his composure. Furthermore, the objects he carries with him symbolize much that intrigues us about him. Guarded, neat, polite, and middle-class, he carries a handkerchief and purse, and notably among his peers in *Ulysses,* he actually works (see Sultan, 1964, p. 112). At noontime we have seen him scurry to place the Keyes ad while Simon Dedalus, MacHugh, O'Molloy, Lenehan, and others in the newspaper office loafed, joshed, talked nostalgia and politics, and prepared to drink or to continue to drink, and Myles Crawford, the editor, busy reminiscing and already drunk, had no time for him. "Flapdoodle to feed fools on" (8.382), Leopold later remarks tartly to himself about their talk. Just now he was hoping to find in the library the logo of crossed keys, with an "inuendo of home rule" (7.150)—that is, of Irish political independence from England—he wants for the ad. He often thinks pragmatically and commercially: what ad will work or won't; why a shop or pub at one location will attract customers but across the street will not; whether cattle for England's market could be sent to the docks by tram rather than allowed to obstruct traffic, as happened this morning to Dignam's funeral procession. He has much business experience and a practical and playful ingenuity.

With time for a public bath before Paddy Dignam's funeral, he purchased the soap at the chemist's and ordered a skin lotion Molly likes, for which he will have to return. He likes to do little services for her—like bringing her breakfast in bed, or selecting pornographic books for her to read. This morning he checked the *Freeman* for the time of the funeral (11:00 A.M.), and he will fume all day about the advertisement for Plumtree's Potted Meat placed grotesquely under the obituaries; but he has the newspaper still because when he offered it to Bantam Lyons, explaining that he was about to throw it away, Lyons bolted off to bet on the dark horse Throwaway in the Gold Cup

Race. Bloom keeps informed of public affairs and politics in a general way. He has attitudes and opinions about them—home rule sympathies, for example—that he usually keeps to himself, and he seems unfailingly interested in the workings of the human, natural, and physical world. Tossing a penny's worth of Banbury cakes to the gulls on the Liffey, he watches them swoop down, greedily feed, and flap away:

> No accounting for tastes. . . . I'm not going to throw any more. Penny quite enough. Lot of thanks I get. Not even a caw. They spread foot and mouth disease too. If you cram a turkey say on chestnut-meal it tastes like that. Eat pig like pig. But then why is it that saltwater fish are not salty? How is that?
> His eyes sought answer from the river. (8.81-7)

Similarly:

> Where was the chap I saw in that picture some-where? Ah yes, in the dead sea floating on his back, reading a book with a parasol open. Couldn't sink if you tried: so thick with salt. Because the weight of the water, no, the weight of the body in the water is equal to the weight of the what? Or is it the vol-ume is equal to the weight? (5.37-41)

Often he will seek an answer, though not necessarily a correct one, and move on.

Advertising canvasser, husband and father, responsive ob-server, inquiring and thoughtful—sometimes foolish—citizen, he also eccentrically and always, apparently, carries a potato with him, the meanings of which amplify later in the book. To now we assume it a good luck charm perhaps and, to be sure, very Irish in basic and catastrophic associations. The flier also

proves representative (although Bloom is no Zionist), as does—
we shall see—his tardy recognition of it. For unusually in the
Dublin of June 16, 1904 depicted in *Ulysses*, Leopold Bloom is
Jewish. That is, through much of the day he thinks of himself as and feels Jewish; and he is taken by the other persons in
Ulysses as Jewish. Later, nonetheless, it becomes clear that he is
not circumcised when his foreskin sticks to his pants after he
masturbates; and later still he admits to Stephen Dedalus that
he knows he isn't Jewish. Finally we learn that by Jewish tradition he isn't. Born of a Christian mother (it is not clear whether
Protestant or Catholic) and a Jewish father who converted, he
was baptized Protestant at birth and baptized again as a Roman Catholic in order to marry Molly (17.540–7, 1635–40). So
how this middle-aged Irish businessman and family man, who
today will be cuckolded, came to his felt Jewish soul, and what
bearing that representation of himself to himself might have
on the events and meanings of the day, merit attention.

II

Bloom's Jewishness, intricately woven into the pattern of his
thoughts, provides the first hint in the book that something
deeply troubles him. While he fixed breakfast, watching and
talking to the cat, reflecting that, "they understand what we say
better than we understand them," he thought to add the pun-
gent taste of kidney to his morning fare. We'd been told right
off that he "ate with relish the inner organs of beasts and fowls"
(4.1–27). Checking first whether Molly, who still was in bed,
wanted anything more than toast and tea, and recognizing her
"Mn" to be a sleepy "No," he walked to the pork butcher's—
obviously not an observant Jew—and contemplated the recent
spell of hot, dry weather. He thought of the suit he's worn for
the funeral: "Black conducts, reflects, (refracts is it?), the heat.

But I couldn't go in that light suit. Make a picnic of it." Beginning to bask in the sun's early warmth, he conjured a curiously strategizing youthful wanderer: "Makes you feel young. Somewhere in the east: early morning: set off at dawn. Travel round in front of the sun, steal a day's march on him. Keep it up for ever never grow a day older technically." He elaborated the fantasy: a strange land; a city he enters, moving "through awned streets. Turbaned faces going by. Dark caves of carpet shops, big man, Turko the terrible, seated crosslegged, smoking a coiled pipe. Cries of sellers in the streets." He imagined adventure, danger, then nightfall: "The shadows of the mosques among the pillars: priest with a scroll roled up. A shiver of the trees, signal, the evening wind. I pass on. Fading gold sky. A mother watches me from her doorway. She calls her children home in their dark language" (4.43–96). There is poetry to his thought.

He himself judged his revery the "kind of stuff you read." Yet the Orientalist imagery called up by an impulse to roam and never grow a day older fit the daydreaming of a middle-aged man about to attend a friend's funeral. It also connected to Molly: "High wall: beyond strings twanged. Night sky, moon, violet, colour of Molly's new garters. Strings. Listen. A girl playing one of those instruments what do you call them: dulcimers. I pass" (4.95–9). Even before his grim certainty that today his wife would commit adultery emerged to consciousness, he defended against it wishfully in fantasy. He could leave. The Ottoman setting of the daydream would refocus soon, when the advertisement for a Zionist settlement in Palestine would catch his eye at the pork butcher's.

In their brief interaction, Bloom and Dlugacz played cunningly round the recognition each had that the other too was a Jew. When he saw the "pile of cut sheets: the model farm at Kinnereth," Leopold instantly registered, "I thought he was" (4.186–7). Then paying, he almost spoke about it: "A speck of eager fire from foxeyes thanked him. He withdrew his gaze after an instant. No: better not: another time." Perhaps it is odd that Bloom has never done so, though he's suspected before that Dlugacz is Jewish. But in fact his own Jewishness does not seem to incline him to communality or easy friendliness with other Jews. He thinks of no currently close Jewish friends, for instance. To Moses Dlugacz, at any rate, he remained reticent — though his thoughts were anything but quiet as he waited for the young woman ahead of him to be served and hoped to leave swiftly in order to follow her:

> A kidney oozed bloodgouts on the willowpatterned dish: the last. He stood by the nextdoor girl at the counter. Would she buy it too, calling items from a slip in her hand? Chapped: washingsoda. And a pound and a half of Denny's sausages. His eyes rested on her vigorous hips. Woods his name is. Wonder what he does. Wife is oldish. New blood. No followers allowed. Strong pair of arms. Whacking a carpet on the clothesline. She does whack it, by George. The way her crooked skirt swings at each whack. (4.145–51)

While "the ferreteyed porkbutcher" prepared her order, snapping two sheets from the pile, Leopold Bloom, noting Dlugacz's Jewishness, merged the model farm depicted on the flier with his own memories of work in the Dublin Cattle market and of the nextdoor girl's captivating way of whacking a carpet:

> Farmhouse, wall round it, blurred cattle cropping. He held the page from him: interesting: read it nearer, the title, the blurred cropping cattle, the page rustling. A young white heifer. Those mornings in the cattlemarket, the beasts lowing in their

pens, branded sheep, flop and fall of dung, the breeders in hobnailed boots trudging through the litter, slapping a palm on a ripemeated hindquarter, there's a prime one, unpeeled switches in their hands. He held the page aslant patiently, bending his senses and his will, his soft subject gaze at rest. The crooked skirt swinging, whack by whack by whack. . . .

. . . To catch up and walk behind her if she went slowly, behind her moving hams. Pleasant to see first thing in the morning. Hurry up, damn it. Make hay while the sun shines. She stood outside the shop in sunlight and sauntered lazily to the right. He sighed down his nose: they never understand. Sodachapped hands. Crusted toenails too. Brown scapular in tatters, defending her both ways. The sting of disregard glowed to weak pleasure within his breast. (4.157–77)

Walking to the butcher shop, he had registered Jewishness as an honorific when delighting in a witty remark he recalled by the nationalist leader Arthur Griffith; he praised it to himself as "Ikey" (4.103)—that is, smart and Jewish (Gifford, 1988, p. 72). At the pork butcher's, Jewishness coexisted for him with a manifest appetite for pork and an inclination toward solitude, with his riveted voyeurism and distinct fascination with pleasurable pain "whack by whack by whack"—all of which condensed in his intense desire to walk behind the young woman's moving hams, and again in his glow of weak pleasure at the sting of her disregard.

Unable, however, to spot her when he left, he looked at the flier anew: "Orangegroves and immense melonfields north of Jaffa. You pay eighty marks and they plant a dunam of land for you with olives, oranges, almonds, or citrons. . . . Every year you get a sending of the crop" (4.194-7). He demurred ("Nothing doing"); but the girl, the white heifer, and the promised fruits of Palestine led to happy memories of Molly and him early in their marriage and the apparently Jewish friends they liked being with then: "Oranges in tissue paper packed in crates. Citrons too. Wonder is poor Citron still in Saint Kevin's parade. And Mastiansky with the old cither. Pleasant evenings we had then. Molly in Citron's basketchair." He recalled Moisel explaining the ritual function of citrons at the fall festival of *Sukkoth:* "Always the same, year after year. They fetched high prices too. . . . Arbutus place: Pleasants street: pleasant old times. Must be without flaw, he said. Coming all that way: Spain, Gibraltar, Mediterranean, the Levant" (4.204-12). Remembering good times and old friends when they had lived in the largely Jewish neighborhood of Dublin (Hyman, 1972, pp. 167-168, 182), he evoked pleasant recurrences and an image of sacramental perfection—the citron at *Sukkoth*—before suddenly plunging into a fantasy so frightening and forlorn that it taxed his considerable powers of recovery:

> A cloud began to cover the sun slowly, wholly. Grey. Far.
> No, not like that. A barren land, bare waste. Vulcanic lake, the dead sea: no fish, weedless, sunk deep in the earth. No wind could lift those waves, grey metal, poisonous foggy waters. Brimstone they called it raining down: the cities of the plain: Sodom, Gomorrah, Edom. All dead names. A dead sea in a dead land, grey and old. Old now. It bore the oldest, the first race. A bent hag crossed from Cassidy's, clutching a naggin bottle by the neck. The oldest people. Wandered far away over all the

earth, captivity to captivity, multiplying, dying, being born everywhere. It lay there now. Now it could bear no more. Dead: an old woman's: the grey sunken cunt of the world.

Desolation.

Grey horror seared his flesh. Folding the page into his pocket he turned into Eccles street, hurrying homeward. Cold oils slid along his veins, chilling his blood: age crusting him with a salt cloak. Well, I am here now. Yes, I am here now. Morning mouth bad images. Got up wrong side of the bed. Must begin again those Sandow's exercises. On the hands down. Blotchy brown brick houses. Number eighty still unlet. Why is that? Valuation is only twentyeight. Towers, Battersby, North, MacArthur: parlour windows plastered with bills. Plasters on a sore eye. To smell the gentle smoke of tea, fume of the pan, sizzling butter. Be near her ample bedwarmed flesh. Yes, yes. (4.218–39)

The vision appalls him: a devastated biblical landscape, grey and dessicated, bearing dead names: Sodom, Gomorrah, Edom; a ruinous history of exile, futility, and captivity; and the figure of an old woman's worn-out womb and *cunt*—the word bristling with rage and scorn. He hurries back home to Molly's live body, strenuously calming himself with physical explanations and nostrums ("Morning mouth bad images . . . Must begin . . . exercises") and his ongoing commercial puzzles until he is again able to affirm life kindly, "Yes." He seems to be venting usually-repressed feelings here that involve women and Jewishness, provoked apparently by thoughts of the girl and the Zionist flier, his memories of good times with Molly, and the sun disappearing behind a cloud—and roiled implicitly by his marital plight. Molly's incipient affair devastates him. He feels grey, dried up, like a despised old woman—perhaps unconsciously wishes she might be one. But in his consciousness the desolation is distinct from Molly. Her wished-for presence would comfort and renew him. The moment taps a well of depression, but his defenses hold.

Early on, then, Leopold Bloom's inner Jewishness proves crucial to who he perplexingly is. It provides a repository of signs for gratifying and radically distressing moments—filters to consciousness that enable even repressed terror and fury access to affect, however briefly. In his wasteland fantasy, his Jewishness links intriguingly to desolation in places and possibly persons of origin. It may connect by association, thereby, to the mother calling her children home in the more benign previous fantasy of ageless wandering. We have seen Bloom's Jewishness coexist with sexual fascinations, voyeurism, and masochistic pleasures. It serves too as a point of pride and standard of value ("Ikey touch that"). But as the ground of kinship to Dlugacz, it supports Bloom's holding back and remaining separate. More commonly, of course, being Jewish marks a boundary of distinctness between him and gentiles, across which they see him and he sees them as different. On this day of his cuckolding, we realize before very long that he enjoys responding mentally to women he stares at or feels drawn to. Passing the time before Dignam's funeral, he picked up a general delivery letter from Martha Clifford, with whom he has been corresponding under the pseudonym Henry Flower. Her letter revealed the lure of their epistolary flirtation: a chance for her to play cruel temptress and long for love, and for him to be a punished naughty boy. In her straining for refinement, she unintentionally showed her lower class status: "Henry dear, do not deny my request before my patience are exhausted" (5.253–4). A bit later, still waiting for the funeral, he sat in a church thinking of her desire that they meet:

> Meet one Sunday after the rosary. Do not deny my request. Turn up with a veil and black bag. Dusk and the light behind. She might be here with a ribbon round her neck and do the other thing all the same on the sly. Their character. That fellow that turned queen's evidence on the invincibles he used to receive the, Carey was his name, the communion every morning. (5.375–9)

"Their" in "their character" must mean Catholic: that's the sort of thing those Catholics do. Some moments further on, the same pronoun sweeps up all Irish Christians, when, asserting to himself that cricket is not played well in Ireland, he avers: "Donnybrook fair more in their line. And the skulls we were acracking when M'Carthy took the floor" (p. 71).

So Jewishness gauges Bloom's separateness and within himself secures a perch for judgment and for fantasies of romance, adventure, and horror. It is central to his identity, his gateway to feelings, his ground of prudence and safety, his locus of solitude. Whatever lonely isolation he feels, therefore, derives not alone from what others assume or do, or from fate, but from the inner demarcation he preserves, a sense of self that prominently includes himself as a Jew. As such, however, Jewishness contributes to his suffering, by meshing with the heavy losses he feels this day. His wife will commit adultery. Their daughter Milly, who delights him and who the day before turned fifteen, has left home to work in Mullingar. The death and funeral of Paddy Dignam, moreover, who seems more an acquaintance than a friend, has prodded his memories of "poor mamma" (p. 91) and of "poor papa with his hagadah book, reading backwards with his finger to me. Pesach. Next year in Jerusalem. Dear, O dear! All that long business about that brought us out of the land of Egypt and into the house of bondage *alleluia. Shema Israel*

Adonai Elohenu" (7.206–9). He recalls his father's suicide and his infant son's death. The good-hearted midwife Mrs. Thornton "knew from the first poor little Rudy wouldn't live. Well, God is good, sir. She knew at once. He would be eleven now if he had lived" (4.418–20). On June 16, 1904 Bloom's losses and deaths accompany him, no doubt fueling his wasteland terror and his passive helplessness about Molly's liaison with Boylan. The slip of memory is telling: "brought us out of the land of Egypt and into the house of bondage" suggests hopelessness.

He has received a letter from Milly, thanking him for the birthday gift he sent and mentioning a boy calling on her. Her fond father thinks protectively of her and of Molly:

> Milly too. Young kisses: the first. Far away now past. Mrs Marion. Reading, lying back now, counting the strands of her hair, smiling, braiding.
>
> A soft qualm, regret, flowed down his backbone, increasing. Will happen, yes. Prevent. Useless: can't move. Girl's sweet light lips. Will happen too. He felt the flowing qualm spread over him. Useless to move now. Lips kissed, kissing, kissed. Full gluey woman lips.
>
> Better where she is down there: away. (4.444–51)

He enacts his passivity and acceptance here, moving in thought between Milly and Molly, feeling regret flow down his backbone and issue in stasis, then flow again over all of him until he is enclosed in the sensation of "full gluey woman lips." Milly's coming of age and Molly's infidelity will actually happen. They cannot be prevented. So not preventing, he joins the experience, becomes vicariously both kisser and kissed, both male and female. Eschewing action, he identifies and thereby gains a muted joy akin to his pleasure at the porkbutcher's, when, looking at the flier and conjuring a palm smacking a hindquarter and the girl whacking a carpet, "he held the page aslant patiently, bending his senses and his will, his soft subject gaze at rest." He was enthralled.

This masochistic fulfillment doesn't last, and he pulls back to confirm that Milly is better off where she is, far from her parents' vagaries. Open to such joys of surrender, however, and feeling no anger at Molly, he may well be colluding unconsciously with her affair. For he confronts neither her nor himself about it; and we know that around 2:00 P.M. he will flee from meeting Boylan. Nor, though he thinks of it repeatedly, does he ever keep their appointed tryst in focus for long. That would be too painful. Thus he implicitly cooperates with his cuckolding, distancing himself and like Odysseus steering his course to adventures—albeit mainly mental ones—and finding what comfort he can by turning passivity into activity in fantasy.

Each time Molly's late afternoon rendezvous recurs in his thoughts—"afternoon she said," "at four she said"—he pushes it away:

> All kinds of places are good for ads. That quack doctor for the clap used to be stuck up in all the greenhouses [public toilets]. . . . Dr Hy Franks. Didn't cost him a red. . . . POST NO BILLS. POST 110 PILLS. Some chap with a dose burning him.
> If he . . . ?
> O!
> Eh?
> No . . . No.
> No, no. I don't believe it. He wouldn't surely?
> No, no.
> Mr Bloom moved forward, raising his troubled eyes. Think no more about that. (8.95–109)

But there are two other losses that pain him recurrently today, and with each he lingers longer: his father's suicide and his infant son's death. He first recalled "poor papa" when tarrying at a billboard announcing the performance of Mosenthal's *Leah*, with the American actress Mrs. Bandmann Palmer in the title role. His father, he remembers, impressed upon him the powerful truth of one scene in particular.

> Mr. Bloom stood at the corner, his eyes wandering over the multi-coloured hoardings. Cantrell and Chochran's Ginger Ale (Aromatic) Clery's Summer Sale . . . Hello. *Leah* tonight. Mrs Bandmann Palmer. Like to see her again in that. Hamlet she played last night. Male impersonator. Perhaps he was a woman. Why Ophelia committed suicide. Poor papa! How he used to talk of Kate Bateman in that. Outside the Adelphi in London waited all the afternoon to get in. Year before I was born that was: sixtyfive. And Ristori in Vienna. What is this the right name is? By Mosenthal it is. *Rachel,* is it? No. The scene he was always talking about where the old blind Abraham recognises the voice and puts his fingers on his face.
>
> Nathan's voice! His son's voice! I hear the voice of Nathan who left his father to die of grief and misery in my arms, who left the house of his father and left the God of his father.
>
> Every word is so deep, Leopold.
>
> Poor papa! Poor man! I'm glad I didn't go into the room to look at his face. That day! O, dear! O, dear! Ffoo! Well, perhaps it was best for him. (5.192–209)

The play involves a Jewish heroine persecuted by an apostate Jew named Nathan, who turned anti-Semitic (Gifford, p. 89). In a climactic scene Nathan is recognized by his dead father's close friend, Abraham. Rudolph Bloom's poignant retelling of the dramatic episode—"Every word is so deep, Leopold"—suggests torment of his own as a convert, a theme of betrayal and guilt that helps to account for Leopold's having absorbed Judaic lore and connection without formal schooling in it. His father, we eventually learn, married late and in old age returned, in attention at least, to Judaism. Apparently he talked about it often with his only child, when Leopold could have been no older than his early teens.

A guilty Jewish conscience, however, seems not to have been the precipitating cause of Rudolph's suicide. The note he left "To my dear son, Leopold," of which we learn snatches, asked that his dog Athos be cared for and mentioned a longing to be "with your dear mamma" again (17.1880-6). She had died evidently some time in the six years between Leopold's leaving high school and his father's death. There may also be an allusion to business reversals. As it turns out, the lonely old man poisoned himself some eighteen years ago, a year before Leopold met Molly. Today he is much on his son's mind:

> That afternoon of the inquest. The redlabelled bottle on the table. The room in the hotel with hunting pictures. Stuffy it was. Sunlight through the slats of the Venetian blind. The coroner's sunlit ears, big and hairy. Boots giving evidence. Thought he was asleep first. Then saw like yellow streaks on his face. Had slipped down to the foot of the bed. Verdict: overdose. Death by misadventure. The letter. For my son Leopold.

No more pain. Wake no more. Nobody owns.
(6.359-65)

The matter of suicide came up during the coachride through the city to Dignam's funeral. Jack Power offered that it was "the greatest disgrace to have in the family," and Simon Dedalus responded, "They say a man who does it is a coward." Martin Cunningham alone seemed to know about Bloom's father and tried to change the subject. Grateful to him, Leopold thought: "They have no mercy on that here or infanticide. Refuse Christian burial. They used to drive a stake of wood through his heart in the grave. As if it wasn't broken already" (6.334-48). His own sadness, his father's pain, and a troubled sense of self as Jewish draw the son to his father this day.

On the eighteenth anniversary of Rudolph's death, June 27, Leopold plans to be in Ennis, where his father died. Molly, who sings, will be touring the North with her impressario, Boylan, at the time—when Leopold will commemorate in his way the annual Jewish ritual of *Yahrzeit*.

The other loss he returns to repeatedly is that of his little son, who was named after Rudolph and who died eleven days after being born eleven years ago. Today Leopold recalled Rudy first when thinking pleasurably of Milly's sprightly charm and alertness, and again in the funeral coach to Glasnevin Cemetery, when he spotted Dedalus's son Stephen as they passed him in the street. Simon asked if "that Mulligan cad" was with him and then inveighed against his wife's family and Stephen's friends: "He's in with a lowdown crowd," he snarled—and ceased:

> Mr Bloom glanced from his angry moustache to
> Mr Power's mild face and Martin Cunningham's
> eyes and beard, gravely shaking. Noisy selfwilled

man. Full of his son. He is right. Something to hand on. If little Rudy had lived. See him grow up. Hear his voice in the house. Walking beside Molly in an Eton suit. My son. Me in his eyes. Strange feeling it would be. From me. Just chance. Must have been that morning Raymond Terrace she was at the window watching the two dogs at it by the wall of the cease to do evil. And the sergeant grinning up. She had that cream gown on with the rip she never stitched. Give us a touch Poldy. God, I'm dying for it. How life begins.

Got big then. Had to refuse the Greystones concert. My son inside her. I could have helped him on in life. I could. Make him independent. Learn German too. (6.72–84)

He could have taught Rudy the language of science and high culture, secured opportunities for him, handed something on. But Leopold also holds himself responsible for the boy's death: "Our. Little. Beggar. Baby. Meant nothing. Mistake of nature. If it's healthy it's from the mother. If not from the man. Better luck next time" (6.328–30).

However irrational, this puzzling notion occurs to him at Glasnevin Cemetery, as he ponders the little caskets of children. Something he wanted to hand on and couldn't—something in the male line of descent from his grandfather Virag to his father Rudolph (who left the home of his father and the faith of his father and changed the patronymic from Hungarian "Virag" to English "Bloom"), to Leopold and on to little Rudy—something has died, for which Leopold blames himself. Molly too seems to share that assumption: "a fine son . . . was he not able to make one it wasnt my fault" (18.1444–6). Moreover, when their infant son died a quality of Leopold's sexual arousal died with him, and that powerful source of guilt seems still to be Leopold's secret. In her silent soliloquy Molly doesn't appear to know it; she believes he must be sexually active elsewhere. Again, Bloom laments his lost heritage of male something after recalling better times, not long before he catches a glimpse of Boylan on Kildare Street and flees:

> I was happier then. Or was that I? Or am I now I? Twentyeight I was. She twentythree. When we left Lombard street west something changed. Could never like it again after Rudy. Can't bring back time. Like holding water in your hand. Would you go back to then? Just beginning then. (8.608–11)

"Could never like it again after Rudy." The conciseness of phrase obscures who couldn't—whether he, she, or they. But given the severed line of descent from grandfather to son, Leopold's de facto collusion with the impending adultery, his curious assumption of responsibility for little Rudy's death, and (what follows from never liking it again) eleven subsequent years of failed or disappointing sexual intimacy between husband and wife, a more composite if not yet clear picture of why this cautious and pleasant man will be cuckolded, why he feels guilty, and why he feels Jewish begins to emerge. For him both sexual disfunction and Jewishness touch on the severed male line of family.

III

Home-rulers commonly drew parallels between the Irish under Britain's governance and the ancient Israelites in Egyptian captivity; they compared their lost leader, Parnell, to Moses (Ellmann, 1959, pp. 32, 91n; Hyman, 1974, pp. 179–180; Nadel,

1989, pp. 85–92). When, in the newspaper office, MacHugh declaimed John F. Taylor's stirring speech on the revival of Gaelic that lauded the young Moses's prophetic vision, he roused Stephen Dedalus's envy and his love of language. Stephen's "Parable of the Plums" then alluded to Moses in its subtitle: "A Pisgah Sight of Palestine." Earlier, Haines at the tower and Deasy at the school had offered him anti-Semitic gambits, but Stephen joined in neither. Bloom himself reflected ambiguously on the moneylender Rueben J. Dodd, a Catholic (See Sultan, 1987, pp. 77–82): "Now he's really what they call a dirty jew" (8.1159). But the apposite actuality of Jews in Ireland becomes a matter for public disputation in Barney Kiernan's pub around 5:00 P.M., climaxing with Bloom being rushed to a cab by Martin Cunningham and shouting at the bigoted nationalist who is goading him: "Mendelssohn was a jew and Karl Marx and Mercadante and Spinoza. And the Saviour was a jew and his father was a jew. Your God." Then for good measure he adds: "Your God. Christ was a jew like me." The citizen, as the other is known, a former shot-put champion of Ireland, springs back to the pub to find something to throw, swearing: "By Jesus . . . I'll brain that bloody jewman for using the holy name. By Jesus, I'll crucify him so I will. Give us that biscuitbox here" (12.1804–11). The events at Barney Kiernan's are among the funniest and most distressing in *Ulysses*. They unforgettably depict an anti-Semitic scapegoating and Leopold Bloom's only act of sustained and open defiance.

He was to meet Cunningham and Power at Kiernan's pub and proceed with them to discuss with Paddy Dignam's widow her rights to the life insurance policy her husband had heavily mortgaged. At the cemetery, Bloom had contributed handsomely to the fund Martin took up for the family. Perhaps therefore he was asked to join the others advising Mrs. Dignam. Was the Jew invited, as Hugh Kenner suspects, because he would be thought to be good at finagling about money (1978, pp. 91, 117–118; 1980, pp. 102–103)? If so, that implicit slur would fit the tenor of the chapter, but the evidence is scanty. What is undoubted is that the citizen challenges Bloom's Irishness and maligns him as a Jew. "Those are nice things," he snarls, "coming over here to Ireland filling the country with bugs," and adds: "Swindling the peasants . . . and the poor of Ireland. We want no more strangers in our house" (12.1141–51). When asked his nation, Leopold replies: "Ireland . . . I was born here. Ireland" (12.1431). To which the citizen contemptuously says nothing and spits. Soon Lenehan avers—incorrectly—that Bloom has won the Gold Cup by betting on Throwaway at twenty to one, and the heat glows incandescent. That the Jew may have won and did not buy rounds for all the fellows is beyond bearing, and they turn on him.

The very form of the chapter, with its analogue between the citizen and Homer's one-eyed Cyclops, proffers expressive structure to extremity. The narrative alternates between two voices—the first belonging to a scurrilous and unnamed bill collector, a lowlife and a gossip. This first-person narrator seems to have damaging information about everyone and a nasty, vivid word for all. Of the citizen spitting, he says, for example, that he "cleared the spit out of his gullet and, gob, he spat a Red bank oyster out of him right in the corner" (12.1432–3); and of Bloom wondering at the others' anger, he says: "Mean bloody scut. Stand us a drink itself. Devil a sweet fear! There's a jew for you! All for number one. Cute as a shithouse rat. Hundred to five" (12.1760–1). This scoundrel, who meets Joe Hynes at the beginning of the chapter and accompanies him to Keirnan's to speak with the citizen, reports and comments on events there and thus provides the bitter common denominator for all reference and judgment. The chapter's second voice interpolates asides, often at considerable length, that slow the action but amplify distinct tones, attitudes, or styles of experience in turn—articulating each in an appropriate rhetoric—and pushing many of them, playfully and exuberantly, to absurdity. Thereby, the shaping rhythm of narration sustains a series of colorful modes as unvarying and fixed in their ways as the unnamed one is splenetic. In the riveting circumstances, any freshness, nuance, kindness, or grandeur has to struggle for breath, while the succession of perspectives accumulates to a laughing satire of all one-eyed certainties.

At Barney Kiernan's pub we see Leopold Bloom entirely and at length from the outside for the only time in *Ulysses*. And such externality befits him, because he operates there without his customary self-awareness or caution. The situation is hardly promising, to be sure: with a bibulous and rabid patriot holding court in a pub late in the day. As the first-person narrator winsomely puts it, "there, sure enough, was the citizen up in the corner having a great confab with himself and that bloody mangy mongrel, Garryowen, and he waiting for what the sky would drop in the way of a drink" (12.120–1). Everybody who enters Kiernan's, except Bloom—and, at the end, Cunningham—seems primed for raillery; and the citizen inveighs against Britain at every opportunity:

> To hell with them! The curse of a goodfornothing God light sideways on the bloody thicklugged sons of whores' gets! No music and no art and no literature worthy of the name. Any civilization they have they stole from us. Tonguetied sons of bastards' ghosts. (12.1197–1201).

After being urged by him to stop pacing back and forth outside, Bloom enters hesitantly. He refuses Hynes's offer of a drink but accepts a cigar—Hynes, we know, owes him money—and then joins the conversation with untoward insistence. One loaded topic leads to another—hangmen's letters, capital punishment, foot and mouth disease of Irish cattle, Gaelic sports, British naval discipline—and whatever, Leopold quietly argues the point. What has happened to his prudence?

> So they started talking about capital punishment and of course Bloom comes out with the why and the wherefor and all the codology of the business and the old dog smelling him all the time I'm told those jewies does have a sort of a queer odour coming off them for dogs about I don't know what all deterrent effect and so forth and so on.
> —There's one thing it hasn't a deterrent effect on, says Alf.
> —What's that? says Joe.
> —The poor bugger's tool that's being hanged, says Alf.
> —That so? says Joe.
> —God's truth, says Alf. I heard that from the head warder that was in Kilmainham when they hanged Joe Brady, the invincible. He told me when they cut him down after the drop it was standing up in their faces like a poker.
> —Ruling passion strong in death, says Joe, as someone said.
> —That can be explained by science, says Bloom. It's only a natural phenomenon, don't you see, because on account of the . . .
> And then he starts with his jawbreakers about phenomenon and science and this phenomenon and the other phenomenon. . . .
> . . . Phenomenon! The fat heap he married is a nice phenomenon with a back on her like a ballalley.
> (12.450–503)

Leopold's persistence irks this narrator, who has a hair-trigger temper. But what could he be about, discussing, debating, and trying to enlighten the incorrigible?

So then the citizen begins talking about the Irish language and the corporation meeting and all to that the shoneens that can't speak their own language and Joe chipping in because he stuck someone for a quid and Bloom putting in his old goo with his twopenny stump that he cadged off Joe and talking about the Gaelic league and the antitreating league and drink, the curse of Ireland. Antitreating is about the size of it. Gob, he'd let you pour all manner of drink down his throat till the Lord would call him before you'd ever see the froth of his pint. . . . (12.679–86)

So off they started about Irish sports and shoneen games the like of lawn tennis and about hurley and putting the stone and racy of the soil building up a nation once again and all to that. And of course Bloom had to have his say too about if a fellow had a rower's heart violent exercise was bad. I declare to my antimacassar if you took up a straw from the bloody floor and if you said to Bloom: *Look at, Bloom. Do you see that straw?* Declare to my aunt he'd talk about it for an hour so he would and talk steady. . . . (12.889–96)

—But, says Bloom, isn't discipline the same everywhere? I mean wouldn't it be the same here if you put force against force?

Didn't I tell you? As true as I'm drinking this porter if he was at his last gasp he'd try to downface you that dying was living. (12.1360–4)

Even if we allow for the intemperate reporter, Bloom here seems decidedly imprudent—pedantic and obdurate too, and inappropriate.

The mystery of his untoward behavior is easily solved, at least preliminarily, by way of a parapraxis he makes early on, when explaining his presence there:

> . . . As a matter of fact I just wanted to meet Martin Cunningham, don't you see, about this insurance of poor Dignam's. Martin asked me to go to the house. You see, he, Dignam, I mean, didn't serve any notice of the assignment on the company at the time and nominally under the act the mortgagee can't recover on the policy.
> —Holy Wars, says Joe, laughing, that's a good one if old Shylock is landed. So the wife comes out top dog, what?
> —Well that's a point for the wife's admirers.
> Whose admirers? says Joe.
> The wife's advisers, I mean, says Bloom.
>
> Then he starts all confused mucking it up about mortagor under the act like the lord chancellor giving it out on the bench and for the benefit of the wife and that a trust is created but on the other hand that Dignam owed Bridgeman the money and if now the wife or the widow contested the mortagee's right till he near had the head of me addled with his mortgagor under the act. (12.760–75)

The slip makes obvious a concurrent drama forcing its way to Bloom's consciousness. At this very moment at 7 Eccles Street Molly's admirer is with her, and they will have finished the preliminaries. Leopold is defending against anguish by diverting, through repression, his passion and anger and attending stoutly to matters at hand. Doing nothing to intervene at home, he aggresses in talk at Kiernan's, unconsciously looking for trouble with men who laugh at the "pishogue" husband Denis Breen and ask pointedly about Molly's coming tour. The manifestly political topics lead inevitably to national hatreds, which Leopold opposes ("Persecution, says he, all the history of the world is full of it. Perpetuating national hatred among nations"), and soon to his outrage as a Jew:

> —And I belong to a race too, says Bloom, that is hated and persecuted. Also now. This very moment. This very instant.
>
> Gob, he near burnt his fingers with the butt of his old cigar.
>
> —Robbed, says he. Plundered. Insulted. Persecuted. Taking what belongs to us by right. At this very moment, says he, putting up his fist, sold by auction in Morocco like slaves or cattle.
>
> —Are you talking about the new Jerusalem? says the citizen.
>
> —I'm talking about injustice, says Bloom.
>
> —Right, says John Wyse. Stand up to it then with force like men.
>
> That's an almanac picture for you. Mark for a softnosed bullet. Old lardyface standing up to the business end of a gun. Gob, he'd adorn a sweepingbrush, so he would, if he only had a nurse's apron on him. And then he collapses all of a sudden, twisting around all the opposite, as limp as a wet rag.
>
> —But it's no use, says he. Force, hatred, history, all that. That's not a life for men and women, insult

> and hatred. And everybody knows that it's the very
> opposite of that that is really life.
> —What? says Alf.
> —Love, says Bloom. I mean the opposite of hatred.
> I must go now, says he to John Wyse. Just round to
> the court a moment to see if Martin is there. If he
> comes just say I'll be back in a second. Just a mo-
> ment. (12.1467–87)

So he proposes a radical alternative that should be familiar to
these Christians but isn't, a message of love that suggests his
own struggle against fury at one remove—this very moment,
this very instant, plundered, insulted, persecuted, taking what
belongs to us by right—that is, not consciously about Molly but
about Jews and injustice, national and group hatreds. Touching
and overdetermined, his plea is dismissed in his brief absence
as unmanly palaver.

> —Do you call that a man? says the citizen.
> —I wonder did he ever put it out of sight, says Joe.
> —Well there were two children born anyhow, says
> Jack Power.
> —And who does he suspect? says the citizen.
>   Gob, there's many a true word spoken in jest.
> One of those mixed middlings he is. Lying up in
> the hotel Pisser was telling me once a month with
> a headache like a totty with her courses. Do you
> know what I'm telling you? It'd be an act of God
> to take a hold of a fellow the like of that and throw
> him in the bloody sea. Justifiable homicide, so it
> would. (12.1654–62).

The psychology of sexually fearful projection in scapegoating
could not be more clear, nor Bloom at the end more wondrous—almost:

When lo, there came about them all a great brightness and they beheld the chariot wherein He stood ascend to heaven. And they beheld Him in the chariot, clothed upon in the glory of brightness, having raiment as of the sun, fair as the moon and terrible that for awe they durst not look upon Him. And there came a voice out of heaven, calling: *Elijah! Elijah!* And he answered with a main cry: *Abba! Adonai!* And they beheld Him even Him, ben Bloom Elijah, amid clouds of angels ascend to the glory of the brightness at an angle of fortyfive degree over Donohoe's in Little Green street like a shot off a shovel (12.1910–18).

Nevertheless, defending the Jews, bringing light to the gentiles, and beloved of heaven, he has by this moment been cuckolded.

IV

"I sometimes think that it was a heroic sacrifice on their part when they refused to accept the Christian revelation," Joyce told his friend Frank Budgen about Jews. "Look at them. They are better husbands than we are, better fathers, and better sons" (1948, p. 23). He wanted those familial qualities for his modern Odysseus because he admired them; and for the most part the scholars and critics have approached the matter of his Jewish hero biographically, like Richard Ellmann (1959) pondering Joyce's affinity with Jews as fellow exiles, mental artists, and urbanized everymen never wholly of one time and place (S. Benstock, 1979; Fogel, 1979; Epstein, 1982; Levitt, 1982; Reizbaum, 1982; Hildesheimer, 1984; Nadel, 1986, 1989). As Frank O'Connor said: "Jewish literature is the literature of townsmen, and the greatest Jew of all was James Joyce" (1967, p. 198). These traits bear also on Bloom's appeal. Recently, Brian Cheyette (1993, pp. 206–34) and Niel R. Davison (1996) have pondered him a new and discerningly by way of English and European social constructions of "The Jew." But starting with Robert Martin Adams (1962, pp. 99–106), some commentators have doubted the adequacy of Bloom's Jewishness, pointing to the many ways he is not, by Jewish tradition, Jewish and stressing his apparent uninvolvement with the sturdy Jewish community of Dublin at the time. Erwin R. Steinberg made that case convincingly: Bloom was baptized not circumcised, never was a Bar Mitzvah, became a Catholic to marry Molly, and owns a burial plot in Glasnevin, a gentile cemetery, rather than in Dublin's Jewish cemetery. "In not a single rite of passage, past or future does Leopold Bloom qualify as a Jew" (1981, p. 29), he states, allowing, however, that Bloom may be metaphorically a Jew because he is rejected, persecuted, and alien even in his own land. Steinberg finds it hard to laud the exemplary family ties of a man who has denied his wife normal sexual relations for over a decade, sent his daughter away to ease his wife's affair, and in the early morning hours of June 17, 1904 tried to entice Stephen to their home by showing him an alluring photograph of Molly—and one cannot disagree. Finally, like many others, he notes the limited extent and quality of Bloom's knowledge about things Jewish. The honor roll Leopold flaunts to the citizen, as an instance, includes the composer Felix Mendelssohn, whose parents became Christians before he was born; Karl Marx, whose parents had him baptized and who himself wrote anti-Semitic tracts; Baruch Spinoza, who was excommunicated from the Amsterdam congregation for unorthodox views; Saverio Mercadante, a Catholic composer of operas and church music; and Jesus. Unintentionally, the list is ironic. Bloom, so attentive to facts, often gets them wrong. But his error also reveals a truth: that for him Jewishness is inclusive, because it includes Jews like him, who by tradition don't qualify.

Stereotypes about the familial ties of Jews and their dislike of drinking do not adequately define Bloom's consciousness, any more than biblical or rabbinical regulations do—though Molly remembers that he kissed her hall door (18.1406). His Jewishness registers continually with him nonetheless, and although still unaccounted for, it proves variously functional for him through the day and dependably part of his unfolding psychological being. It is, we have seen, a standard of value and a mode of continuity, self-recognition, and pride; a locus for displacement, defense, and widely ranging affect; an inner space in which to be lustful, voyeuristic, thoughtful, sensitive, and private, and in which to memorialize losses, especially those in the line of patriarchal descent severed since little Rudy's death except in Leopold's regretful memories and guilt. As was evident in Barney Kiernan's, Jewishness also symbolizes his social isolation and vulnerability. It should, then, be part of any understanding of his publicly cautious ways—as well as of their breakdown at Kiernan's.

To fathom what I have called Bloom's felt Jewish soul, we need to know not only how it is present and psychologically useful to him but how it came to be. For in light of the sizable number of Western European Jews who from the eighteenth century onward found it necessary or desirable to become part of the Christian majority, one must wonder about a non-Jew, who has not formally chosen to convert and has no apparent interest in theology, to merely *be* Jewish within himself—in one of the most Christian of cities to boot. To understand that we need the evidence of the "Nighttown" chapter, which provides entry to Bloom's encompassingly deep fantasies, and help from the penultimate chapter, for facts or near-facts about his life when he was younger.

Set in the red-light district of Dublin after midnight, the

"Nighttown" chapter presents experience in a style evocative of expressionist drama or film, of literary dreamscapes too by Goethe and Flaubert, the insidious clarity of Kafka, the infernal detail of the paintings of Hieronymus Bosch. It has the vividness and irrational feel of primary process (Freud, 1900, pp. 588–609). But it is not solely a realm of dream and fantasy because, as in every other chapter of the book, a continuing line of naturalistic events is discernible. Concerned about Stephen, who is desperate and drunk and has headed for Nighttown, Bloom follows. After surrendering his potato to Zoe Higgins, he enters Bella Cohen's whorehouse because Stephen is there. He conjures several extraordinary fantasies of his own, rallies then to reclaim his potato and take charge of Stephen's money before it is stolen, and then again to look after him when, knocked down by a British soldier and nearly arrested, Stephen lies out cold in the street.

There is a zany, illicitly sexual, and paranoid texture to Nighttown. Uneasy to be there and hardly sure why he is, Leopold proceeds with care. After the lad Tommy Caffrey (whom he observed earlier that evening) runs into him, he quickly searches his pockets to check that they haven't been picked. Such recurrences characterize the place, where comically, surprisingly, and metamorphically, persons, situations, and phrases from earlier in the book reappear like day residues. At one point having to jump out of the way of a sandstrewer, Bloom touches his potato, grateful for "poor mamma's panacea" (15.201–2). Shortly we will get our only direct view of his mother—and a very strange view it is. But first father Rudolph appears, stooped, bearded, and "garbed in the caftan of an elder of Zion." Yellow poison streaks his face. He is an exaggerated figure, a stage Jew whose son cringes and feels guilty with the father's own guilt. Crestfallen, Leopold hides the pig's crubeen and trotter he has bought:

Second halfcrown waste money today. I told you
not to go with drunken goy ever. So you catch
no money. . . .
What you making down this place? Have you no
soul? (*with feeble vulture talons he feels the silent face
of Bloom*) Are you not my son Leopold, the grand-
son of Leopold? Are you not my dear son Leopold
who left the house of his father and left the god of
his fathers Abraham and Jacob? (15.253–62)

Rudolph remembers a time in Leopold's teens when friends
brought him home drunk and muddied: "What you call them
running chaps?" he asks. Leopold replies quietly: "Harriers,
father. Only that once"—while his own garb instantly transforms:

> (*In youth's smart blue Oxford suit with white vest-
>   slips, narrowshouldered in brown Alpine hat, wear-
>   ing gent's sterling silver Waterbury keyless watch
>   and double curb Albert with seal attached, one side
>   of him coated with stiffening mud.*)
>   RUDOLPH
> Once! Mud head to foot. Cut your hand open.
>   Lockjaw. They make you kaputt, Leopoldleben.
>   You watch them chaps.
>   BLOOM
> (*weakly*) They challenged me to a sprint. It was
>   muddy. I slipped.
>   RUDOLPH
> (*with contempt*) *Goim nachez!* Nice spectacles for
>   your poor mother! (15.269–79)

Crucial themes are vented here in extreme form, themes
sounded throughout "Nighttown" and centrally in Bloom's ex-

perience: a stark, guilt-provoking contrast between Jews and goyim; the boy's disheartened effort to find a more inclusive, independent, stylish, and contemporary way; the father's almost frenzied sense of danger, which serves to introduce even more shrill hysterics of the "poor mamma":

> (*in pantomime dame's stringed mobcap, widow Twankey's crinoline and bustle, blouse with muttonleg sleeves buttoned behind, grey mittens and cameo brooch, her plaited hair in a crispine net, appears over the staircase banisters, a slanted candlestick in her hand, and cries out in shrill alarm*) O blessed Redeemer, what have they done to him! My smelling salts! (*She hauls up a reef of skirt and ransacks the pouch of her striped blay petticoat. A phial, an Agnus Dei, a shrivelled potato and a celluloid doll fall out.*) Sacred Heart of Mary, where were you at all at all? (15.283–90)

This is startling and hard to integrate. Ellen Bloom too is pictured as a stage figure, from the traditional English family entertainment, the Christmas pantomime. The Widow Twankey is Aladdin's mother (Gifford, p. 457)—and Bloom, of course, like Aladdin and Odysseus before him, has adventures. But this mother seems to be a Roman Catholic, with her phrases of prayer and Agnus Dei medal, although Leopold himself was baptized Protestant (see Benstock, 1979); or to her Jewish son she seems wildly frightened, superstitious, infantile, and crazily, exceedingly Christian—in the only extended thought he has about her during all of Bloomsday. What else might she have under her skirt? Pantomime Dames are notoriously rambunctious, bawdy, and forceful; they are always played by middle-aged men, with a broad, bisexual humor. They are never easily contained. So this is most curious testimony, that bears on Bloom's characterological caution, his vulnerability to depression, his puzzling identity, and his watching, sympathizing with, loving, yearning for, and fantasizing about women.

Immediately, another stunning event occurs. Molly appears in a Turkish outfit of jacket and trousers and treats him with teasing condescension. Last night he dreamt of her wearing trousers, and waking he has wondered whether she wears the pants in their home. His mother, meanwhile, has vanished — as, during the day, she has been almost totally missing from his thought. In a day so full of memories and losses, that is noteworthy. Does Molly, who figures as male and female to him, often camouflage and cover his mother in his thoughts?

If we take this bizarre vision of mother, father, son, and wife as a disguised but important clue, in the manner of a dream, and the rest of "Nighttown" and indeed of *Ulysses* as associations thereto, a new, developmental entry into Bloom's dilemmas will, I think, be opened. He has very few memories of mamma but repeated thoughts of Molly and a ready fascination with women generally. His relation to them can suggest its beginnings with mother: at some level terrified and terrifying, superstitious, explosive, very fragile, and yet very powerful — at least in the hold such a mother can have on a child, requiring of him precocious care, attention, cooperation, patience, and no answering explosiveness: the very qualities Leopold displays in the present crisis with Molly. To this day he carries a potato with him, as his mother did, a fetish to augment the phallic forcefulness he could not claim with her and to symbolize basic supplies he did not get from her. This suggests that young man Leopold — who cut an attractive figure with the ladies and courted Molly with Byron's poems and his own passion, married her, and fathered two children with her, one of them possibly conceived before the marriage — had not yet, despite appearances, sufficiently secured his adult masculinity before it was doubly traumatized. The two devastating losses he suffered in adulthood that prey on his mind—his father's suicide when Leopold was twenty, and his little son's death seven years later—upset, with Rudy's death, his psychosexual equilibrium, most tellingly in his inability thereafter to have complete intercourse with his wife. As the mathematical narrator of the "Ithaca" chapter puts it: "there remained a period of 10 years, 5 months and 18 days during which carnal intercourse had been incomplete, without ejaculation of semen within the natural female organ" (17.2282–4).

Molly's tryst with Boylan staggers him anew and he can do nothing to prevent it. In "Nighttown" he descends first into several elaborate fantasies—he is accused of sexual crimes, for example, and punished for them by hanging. Martha Clifford charges breach of promise. The Blooms' former serving girl Mary Driscoll claims assault: "I had more respect for the scouringbrush, so I had. I remonstrated with him, Your lord, and he remarked: keep it quiet" (15.892–3). Mrs. Yelverton Barry, Mrs. Bellingham, and finally, The Honourable Mrs. Mervin Talboys accuse him of more perverse twists:

> This plebeian Don Juan observed me from behind a hackney car and sent me in double envelopes an obscene photograph, such as are sold after dark on Paris boulevards, insulting to any lady. I have it still. It represents a partially nude senorita, frail and lovely (his wife, as he solemnly assured me, taken by him from nature), practising illicit intercourse with a muscular torero, evidently a blackguard. He urged me to do likewise, to misbehave, to sin with officers of the garrison. He implored me to soil his letter in an unspeakable manner, to chastise him as he richly deserves, to bestride and ride him, to give him a most vicious horsewhipping.

She intends to start immediately:

> (*stamps her jingling spurs in a sudden paroxysm of fury*) I will, by the God above me. I'll scourge the pigeonlivered cur as long as I can stand over him. I'll flay him alive.

And he likes the idea: "(*his eyes closing, quails expectantly*) Here? (*he squirms*) Again! (*he pants cringing*) I love the danger" (15.1064–86). J.J. O'Molloy tries to defend him: "I shall call rebutting evidence to prove up to the hilt that the hidden hand is again at its old game. When in doubt persecute Bloom" (15.974–6). But the tide of disapproval is too strong. He is that guilty and self-punishing.

When Zoe Higgins, a young whore—who turns out uncannily to have his mother's maiden name (17.537)—suggests sarcastically that Bloom give a stump speech, he launches another extended fantasy of himself as a reformer and great leader. Made Lord Mayor, proclaimed Leopold the First, and adored as Parnell's successor, he prophesies the New Bloomusalem and gives speeches in Hebrew and English:

> Aleph Beth Ghimel Daleth Hagadah Tephilim Kosher Yom Kippur Roshaschana Beni Brith Bar Mitzvah Mazzoth Askenazim Meshuggah Talith ... (15.1623–5)
> I stand for the reform of municipal morals and the plain ten commandments. New worlds for old. Union of all, jew, moslem and gentile. Three acres and a cow for all children of nature. Saloon motor hearses. Compulsory manual labor for all. All parks open to the public day and night. Electric dishscrubbers. Tuberculosis, lunacy, war and mendicancy must now cease. General amnesty, weekly

carnival with masked licence, bonuses for all, esperanto the universal language with universal brotherhood. No more patriotism of barspongers and dropsical impostors. Free money, free rent, free love and a free lay church in a free lay state. . . . Mixed races and mixed marriage. (15.1685–93)

But again he is toppled, like Parnell for sexual misconduct, but also for being an Episcopalian, Caliban, Jack the Ripper, a condom user, and the false Messiah. Pronounced "bisexually abnormal" (15.1775–6) by Mulligan and "a finished example of the new womanly man" (15.1798–9) by Dixon, he gives birth to "eight male yellow and white children" (15.1821–2) before being put to flame by the Dublin Fire Brigade. Leopold Bloom may well represent a pacific and androgynous transformation of the hero in Western literature, but at this moment in "Nighttown," however comically, he is scorned.

When the whoremistress Bella Cohen appears, striking and hard, Bloom follows out the path of his masochism. "Powerful being," he says. "In my eyes read that slumber which women love." The fan she is tapping replies, "We have met. You are mine," and Bloom, cowed, answers, "Exuberant female. Enormously I desiderate your domination." Before his eyes Bella transforms to Bello, a man, while Bloom manages merely to mumble, "Awaiting your further orders we remain, gentlemen":

BELLO
(*with a hard basilisk stare, in a baritone voice*) Hound of dishonour!

BLOOM
(*infatuated*) Empress!

BELLO
(*His heavy cheekchops sagging*) Adorer of the adulterous rump!

BLOOM

(*plaintively*) Hugeness!

BELLO

Dungdevourer!

BLOOM

(*with sinews semiflexed*) Magmagnificence!
(15.2834–45)

Soon Bello squats on Bloom's face, reading the newspaper, quenching his cigar in Bloom's ear, and farting. "Not man," Bloom recognizes, "Woman," and Bello pronounces:

No more blow hot and cold. What you longed for has come to pass. Henceforth you are unmanned and mine in earnest, a thing under the yoke. Now for your punishment frock. You will shed your male garments, you understand. Ruby Cohen? and don the shot silk luxuriously rustling over head and shoulders. And quickly too! (15.2964–8)

He will be a young girl, to pander to men's Gommorahan vices. Bello taunts him:

What else are you good for, an impotent thing like you? (*he stoops and, peering, pokes with his fan rudely under the fat suet folds of Bloom's haunches*) Up! Up! Manx cat! What have we here? Where's your curly teapot gone to or who docked it on you, cockyolly? Sing, birdy, sing. It's as limp as a boy of six's doing his pooly behind a cart. Buy a bucket or sell your pump. (*loudly*) Can you do a man's job? (15.3127–32)

The only counterthrust during these articulations of Bloom's inner state comes with the sudden arrival of grandfather Lipoti Virag, whose verbal abandon matches his sexual exhilaration.

"Stop twirling your thumbs and have a good old thunk," Virag lectures his quiescent gandson. "See, you have forgotten. Exercise your mnemotechnic" (15.2383–5). He urges vigor and primeval impulse:

> Woman, undoing with sweet pudor her belt of rushrope, offers her allmoist yoni to man's lingam. Short time after man presents woman with pieces of jungle meat. Woman shows joy and covers herself with featherskins. Man loves her yoni fiercely with big lingam, the stiff one. (*he cries*) *Coactus volui.* Then giddy woman will run about. Strong man grapses woman's wrist. Woman squeals, bites, spucks. Man now fierce angry, strikes woman's fat yadgana. (*he chases his tail*) Piffpaff! Popo! (*he stops, sneezes*) Pchp! (*he worries his butt*) Prrrrht! (15.2549–56)

But it is to no avail at that moment.

Bloom, who was drawn to Zoe, gave her his potato when she asked for it—he called it a talisman and heirloom—and exposed himself thereby to the depths of his fearful wishes: for exhibitionistic fame and martyrdom, for anal erotism, perversion, and soiling, for voyeurism, masochistic bondage, homosexual submission, bisexual realization, and continued castration. And having displayed himself to himself, having dramatized his regressive degradation, impotence, and guilt, he had enough, and more than enough. The Nighttown chapter seems to embody Freud's original assumption about psychotherapeutic relief, that bringing conflicted material to consciousness would itself bring about change. Leopold springs into action, first of all getting his potato—"a relic of poor mamma"—back: "There is a memory attached to it. I should like to have it" (15.3520). Consolidated again that much, he acts more effectively than he has all day. He protects Stephen's money, refuses Bella's charge for damages from it, tries to keep Stephen out of a fight, and finally takes charge of the fallen lad. Bending over him and soon to sober him up and offer him a place to sleep, Leopold has a final vision, inspired by Si Dedalus's son. He sees his own:

> (. . . *Against the dark wall a figure appears slowly, a fairy boy of eleven, a changeling, kidnapped, dressed in an Eton suit with glass shoes and a little bronze helmet, holding a book in his hand. He reads from right to left inaudibly, smiling, kissing the page.*)
>
> BLOOM
>
> (*wonderstruck, calls inaudibly*) Rudy!
>
> RUDY
>
> (*gazes, unseeing, into Bloom's eyes and goes on reading, kissing, smiling. He has a delicate mauve face. On his suit he has diamond and ruby buttons. In his free left hand he holds a slim ivory cane with a violet bowknot. A white lambkin peeps out of his waistcoat pocket.*) (15.4956–67)

It is so poignant, so fondly idealized and too sweet. But as it reminds us of Bloom's unassuaged grief, it also reveals much about what he, the son of an immigrant father and an Irish mother, had hoped for, for his lost son and for himself: an integration of cultures and opportunities, a sensitive and even feminine sweetness. Rudy wears Cinderella's shoes, a stylishly appointed Eton jacket, Mercury's bronze hat, and holds his phallic but nice ivory cane. Is that a Christian lambkin peeking from his pocket? And of course Rudy is literate. He reads from right to left, inaudibly, in a Hebrew prayer book, and kisses the page. At eleven he might have begun to prepare for his Bar Mitzvah (see Levitt, 1972).

This is a diaspora idea of assimilation, with Jewish identity and connection a handsome part of it—what the views we get of Bloom in his late teens and twenties would suggest. Before and for a while after marrying Molly, he lived in the southern, heavily Jewish section of the city (Hyman, pp. 167, 182). His peers were Jews and non-Jews. He had friends—some of them older, more his dead father's age: Matt Dillon, Luke Doyle, and Alderman John Hooper, all of whom gave them wedding presents. He was thought perhaps to have a chance in politics (see 18.1186-7, 16.1579-85). For a couple of hours before Leopold and Stephen part, they walk and talk about a range of subjects trivial and searching, rarely agreeing but comfortable enough to linger with one another. Neither has had any such companionship all day, and Bloom, we learn, hasn't had any such for a decade.

> Had Bloom discussed similar subjects during nocturnal perambulations in the past?
> In 1884 with Owen Goldberg and Cecil Turnbull at night on public thorough-fares between Longwood avenue and Leonard's corner and Leonard's corner and Synge street and Synge street and Bloomfield avenue. In 1885 with Percy Apjohn in the evenings, reclined against the wall between Gibraltar villa and Bloomfield house in Crumlin, barony of Uppercross. In 1886 occasionally with casual acquaintances and prospective purchasers on doorsteps, in front parlours, in third class railway carriages of suburban lines. In 1888 frequently with major Brian Tweedy and his daughter Miss Marion Tweedy, together and separately on the lounge in Matthew Dillon's house in Roundtown. Once in 1892 and once in 1893 with Julius (Juda) Mastiansky, on both occasions in the parlour of his

(Bloom's) house in Lombard street, west, (17.46–59)

From 1884 to 1893 many, but after 1893, when they moved to another section of Dublin and Rudy died, none. Nor has he talked again this way with Molly. His infant son's death precipitated a regression that held until today. He was more withdrawn, more cautious, more Jewish, yet removed from that community too. His vulnerable masculinity had given way, and he became sexually inhibited. His felt Jewishness, then, is restitutive, a sign, even as it expresses his weakness and isolation, of his continued attempt to find and be accompanied by his anguished father, to regain his manhood. Jewishness has held him together for the last decade. And like the Agendath flier, he recognized it late but had had it with him.

Leopold Bloom's Jewish identity opens up every developmental level of his masculinity, from its shaky roots to its postadolescent synthesis, leading to its breakdown for a decade in adulthood, and its possible retransformation today into a more assertive and connected idiom. The nadir of his regression is reached in "Nighttown"; and there, having been assertive as a Jew at Kiernan's, and having wishfully extended the paternal line back to an actively sexual grandfather, he begins to reclaim more proximally his phallic power and aggression. In adulthood, Bloom's inner sense of Jewishness has served to define and to bolster his dynamically regressed masculinity, and now by way of a transient son-substitute, it may serve the bare possibility of sexual and familial renewal with Molly.

Bibliography

Adams, R. M. (1962). *Surface and Symbol: The Consistency of James Joyce's Ulysses.* New York: Oxford Univ. Press.

Benstock, S. (1979). Is He a Jew or a Gentile or a Holy Roman? *James Joyce Quarterly*, 16: 493–497.

Budgen, F. (1941). James Joyce. In *James Joyce: Two Decades of Criticism*, ed. S. Givens. New York: Vanguard, 1948, pp. 19–26.

Cheyette, B. (1993). *Constructions of "The Jew" in English Literature and Society: Racial Representations, 1875–1945*. Cambridge: Cambridge Univ. Press.

Davison, N. R. (1996). *James Joyce, Ulysses, and the Construction of Jewish Identity: Culture, Biography, & "The Jew" in Modernist Europe*. Cambridge: Cambridge Univ. Press.

Ellmann, R. (1959). *James Joyce: New and Revised Edition*. New York: Oxford Univ. Press, 1982.

Epstein, E. L. (1982). Joyce and Judaism. In *The Seventh of Joyce*, ed. B. Benstock. Bloomington: Indiana Univ. Press, pp. 221–224.

Fogel, D. M. (1979). James Joyce, The Jews and *Ulysses*. *James Joyce Quarterly*, 16: 498–501.

Freud, S. (1900). The Interpretation of Dreams. *Standard Edition*, vols. 4 and 5.

Gifford, D. with R. J. Seidman (1988). *Ulysses Annotated: Notes for James Joyce's Ulysses*. Second edition, revised and enlarged, of *Notes for Joyce*, 1974. Berkeley: Univ. of California Press.

Hildesheimer, W. (1984). *The Jewishness of Mr. Bloom / Das Jüdische an Mr. Bloom: English / Deutsch*. Frankfurt: Suhrkamp.

Hyman, L. (1972). *The Jews of Ireland: From Earliest Times to the Year 1910*. Shannon: Irish Univ. Press.

Joyce, J. (1922). *Ulysses: The Corrected Text*, ed. H. W. Gabler with W. Steppe and C. Melchior. New York: Random House, 1986.

Kenner, H. (1978). *Joyce's Voices*. Berkeley: Univ. of California Press.

———. (1980). *Ulysses: Revised Edition*. Baltimore: Johns Hopkins Univ. Press, 1987.

Levitt, M. P. (1972). The Family of Bloom. *New Light on Joyce from the Dublin Symposium*, ed. F. Senn. Bloomington: Indiana Univ. Press, pp. 141–148.

———. (1982). The Humanity of Bloom, the Jewishness of Joyce. In *The Seventh of Joyce*, ed.B. Benstock. Bloomington: Indiana Univ. Press, pp. 225–228.

Nadel, I. B. (1986). Joyce and the Jews. *Modern Judaism*, 6: 301–310.

———. (1989). *Joyce and the Jews: Culture and Texts*. London: Macmillan.

O'Connor, F. (1967). *The Backward Look: A Survey of Irish Literature*. London: Macmillan.

Raleigh, J. H. (1977). *The Chronicle of Leopold and Molly Bloom:* Ulysses *as Narrative.* Berkeley: Univ. of California Press.

Reizbaum, M. (1982). The Jewish Connection, Cont'd. In *The Seventh of Joyce,* ed. B. Benstock. Bloomington: Indiana Univ. Press, pp. 229–237.

Steinberg, E. R. (1981). James Joyce and the Critics Notwithstanding, Leopold Bloom Is Not Jewish. *Journal of Modern Literature,* 19: 27–49.

Sultan, S. (1964). *The Argument of Ulysses.* Columbus: Ohio State Univ. Press.

———. (1987). *Eliot, Joyce and Company.* New York: Oxford Univ. Press.

Unconscious Fantasy in
Jane Eyre and *Ulysses*

COMMENT ON ALMOND AND SCHWABER

JEROME A. WINER

It is hard to think of two more different characters in all of literature than Jane Eyre and Leopold Bloom, nor two more different novels than *Jane Eyre* and *Ulysses*. As I began to prepare the discussion of the contributions by Richard Almond and Paul Schwaber, I also felt that two papers demonstrating how Freud has affected our reading of literature could not be farther afield. But, in fact, upon careful study, commonality emerges. Both papers deal with the enormous effect the fear of genital sexuality and procreation has on determining character and motivating action. In addition, Almond is explicit about a process whereby characters can effect change upon each other even in this core conflictual area. Schwaber, too, implicitly suggests this is possible but does not elaborate a specific mechanism. I wish to discuss each paper's arguments first and then return to these unintended commonalties.

Richard Almond notes that the relationship between psychoanalysis and literature has a long history. The relationship between psychoanalysis and *Jane Eyre,* however, has practically no history in the mainstream psychoanalytic literature. My search of the writings of clinical psychoanalysts yielded but one article on Charlotte Brontë and that a half-century old (Friedlander, 1943). Psychoanalytic literary critics, on the other hand, have found Charlotte Brontë and *Jane Eyre* of great interest and I will draw upon their contributions. Almond serves us well then to study a major novel neglected from a clinical perspective. Almond has proposed a fascinating framework for viewing intrapsychic change in novels [based on three stages: a sense of *engagement* that makes two characters highly significant to each other; a powerful pattern of *mutual influence* with consequent reciprocal alterations in the characters' behavior; a resultant change that has a positive *directionality* toward resolution of conflict, growth, and adaptation. He believes these stages parallel the analytic process. *Engagement* is like the development of transference, by which I think he means the transference neurosis. *Mutual influence* parallels the interplay of transference and countertransference, resistance and interpretation. *Directionality* corresponds to the clinical principle of the special attitude of the analyst to ensure that the atmosphere is constructive. Almond seems to say that in literature this third factor can come from either partner of a dyad where in the clinical situation it resides largely in the analytic attitude of the analyst. At any rate, Almond clearly views analysis as a two-person circumstance, not one where the analysand projects transference onto a blank screen.

Almond mainly focuses on the elements and patterns of interpersonal interaction in Jane's development that are crucial to conflict resolution. The positive outcome allows Jane to form a successful sexual-affectional bond. Almond divides Jane's life into five phases: childhood, latency, puberty, adolescence, and young adulthood. He believes he can locate in the novel how Jane's defenses shift at each developmental level. He names each section with the name of the place where Jane resides. Interestingly, an earlier writer (Cowart, 1981) also coordinates Jane's psychological development with these geographic locales but uses the traditional psychosexual developmental phases: anal (Gateshead and Lowood School), phallic/oedipal (Thornfield), latency (Morton), and genital mature sexuality (Ferndean).

When we meet ten-year old Jane at Gateshead, she is sadistically treated by her widowed aunt, Mrs. Reed. Both Jane's parents and her mother's brother, Mr. Reed, are dead. Almond claims that Mrs. Reed, in her negative way, catalyzes Jane's psychic development. Mrs. Reed, like the wicked stepmother in Cinderella, proves to Jane that there is no hope of ever having a parent's love or satisfaction of wishes within the family. Almond believes that Mrs. Reed's bad parenting solidifies within Jane's superego her dedication to psychological and moral truthfulness and her idealization of her own self-concept. I have some trouble drawing a parallel with the analytic process at this point, as does Almond himself, because of Mrs. Reed's cruelty and narcissism. The blindness of her seeing eye (Freud, 1895) and the hypocrisy with which she moralizes certainly may contribute to Jane's having a superego strongly opposed to instinctual gratification. But this would happen because of the years of limited chance for expression of and heightened stimulation of Jane's aggressive drive. Jane's honesty is in good measure propelled by Mrs. Reed's falseness because Jane's aggression toward Mrs. Reed is largely turned toward herself (Freud, 1930; Hartmann and Loewenstein, 1962). Almond omits the poignant incarceration of Jane by Mrs. Reed after Jane's rebellion. She orders Jane to be locked alone in the "red room," the room where Jane's uncle died. Her panic in the red room when she feels that Uncle Reed's ghost will come to claim her has been viewed as projection of her oral greed as a motherless child (Cowart, 1981) or as a primal guilty desire for the father (Smith, 1965; Sadoff, 1982). The latter view buttresses Almond's position that banishment to Lowood School is a representation of forced relinquishment of hopes for incestuous gratification.

But in Jane's interior monologue, she states "I dared commit no fault: I strove to fulfill every duty." She then considers suicide by depriving herself of all food and drink, a typical example of hatred turned against the self.

Almond has a different emphasis, one that does not privilege aggression and largely tracks the path of Jane's libidinal development. He stresses Jane's banishment to boarding school as symbolizing her entry into latency even though Jane is ten years old. The text has no evidence supporting a prolonged oedipal period in Jane but Almond feels that this episode represents the early post-oedipal relinquishment of parental love and the transfer of interest to homoerotic peer love. I do not think that Almond takes enough account of Jane as an early parent loss case. Bernstein (1985) sees the tremendous losses Jane suffers early in life as responsible for the coldness that reigns inside and outside her. Analytic research (Fleming, 1972; Altschul, 1988) has demonstrated that analysands who have lost a parent early in life cannot proceed with the establishment and resolution of a transference neurosis until the analyst provides certain replacement parenting activities. Certainly Mrs. Reed fails to do this. Miss Temple will do some. Much will fall to Rochester and the Rivers sisters.

Returning to the oedipal framework, I tend to agree with Cowart, who finds more oedipal material at Thornfield, where Jane competes for Rochester with Blanche Ingram and with his wife, than at Gateshead, where Almond locates the oedipal. Her renunciation of the married Rochester and her ascetic flight to and with St. John Rivers at Morton more convincingly suggest latency phase than does the Lowood School period. Almond's notion of an adolescent reworking of the oedipal at Morton is plausible however, particularly in light of the asceticism described by Anna Freud and cited by Almond. At any rate, Jane is sent to Lowood, a Spartan environment under the directorship of Mr. Brocklehurst, whom Almond rightly calls greedy, punitive, and depriving. But there too is Miss Temple, the head teacher, who is warm, giving, gentle, and kind—the first such person with whom Jane has had an ongoing relationship. Here she also lives with Helen Burns, an empathic fellow student a bit older with whom Jane finds support and companionship. Miss Temple supplies cake and Helen models reading as a mode of incorporation easily available to a parentless child.

After eight years at Lowood, Jane, in Almond's view, is still functioning like a latency child, with resentment aimed at the "bad father" Brocklehurst. Love is turned toward Miss Temple and other females. Angry competition with Mrs. Reed is replaced by idealization and identification with Miss Temple, other teachers, and students, especially Helen Burns. The oedipal love object is replaced by homoerotic peers. I do not believe it is worth belaboring an examination of Jane's actual oedipal years because we have no evidence in the text about her at that age. We know only that she is an orphan who came while still nursing to her uncle, Mr. Reed, and his wife. Mr. Reed was kind, feeding her himself at times. Jane was the child of his beloved sister. Almond neglects to tell us that the dying Mrs. Reed informs Jane that her husband cherished Jane more than his own children. In his last illness, he had insisted that Jane be brought to him repeatedly. Such a child, if she knew about the tender uncle, could make him the desired oedipal male. Mrs. Reed then easily falls into place as the interfering hated rival. Of course Jane's own father, whom Mrs. Reed despised, could also serve similarly as the real world figure for the desired father of the unconscious oedipal fantasy. If Almond feels that her protracted entry into latency is because of her having no male object other than Brocklehurst, he is not explicit in saying so.

The place where Almond's key argument—that interpersonal interaction between characters in a novel can resemble the analytic process—must be put to the test is Thornfield. When Miss Temple marries and leaves Lowood, Jane leaves also, putting herself into a position to likewise establish a heterosexual relationship. It is true, as Almond avers, that Rochester, like a therapist, encourages Jane to voice her thoughts and feelings without revealing his own. Rather than neutrality, however, Rochester's stance is one of sarcastic imperatives, bitterness, and constant interrogation. I can accept that Jane arrives at Thornfield a postpubescent early adolescent, although eighteen. The frequent statements that Jane is physically short can be viewed as allusive evidence of developmental arrest in the psychological sphere as well. We are again forced by the textual hiatus of six years of Jane's life to speculate about causes of arrested development. Jane spent the years between ten and sixteen becoming first in her class and the next two as a teacher at fifteen pounds per annum. All vacations were spent at Lowood so that outside interpersonal heterosexual relationships could not develop.

Let us look closely at Almond's schema, particularly as depicted in diagram 1. Rochester *is* the external stimulus for weakening of Jane's latency defenses and the emergence of desire. His prior marriage and the fact that he is twenty years older (which Almond does not mention) plausibly give him an incestuous (father) meaning to her. Her desire *is* aroused but conflicted. He is incessant in pursuing her. Jane must flee. The engagement is intense, the mutual influence undeniable.

In diagram 2 Almond presents the process of mutual influence during the Thornfield phase in detail. He categorizes Jane's "problem" (i.e., conflicts). He describes the manner in which a "response" from Rochester reflects the mutual influence and how he modifies her behavior and its underlying psychological structure. It is often said that no analyst conducts an analysis to termination without undergoing personal change.

But the responses Rochester gives to Jane's "problems" present some problems themselves. Rochester's "basic goodheartedness" may be seen as an attribute of most analysts but "his real need for love" that alters her basic mistrust is not expectable behavior for an analyst. Certainly his goodheartedness might resemble the growth-enhancing attitude (Loewald, 1960; Stone, 1961) of the analyst. With respect to his need for love, however, an analyst's need at the intensity Rochester exhibits must remain out of the clinical situation. When it cannot, a transfer of the case is indicated. I am not unmindful of the flashes of erotic or loving countertransferences that occur in most analyses. Rochester's response is far more intense and sustained than those, however. Malcolm (1987) wisely states that when Freud gave his female patients permission to fall in love with him psychoanalysis proper was underway. "But it was Freud's genius to presently see (as none of his predecessors had seen) that for sex to be kept at bay in therapy only *one* member of the therapeutic pair — namely, the doctor — has to behave himself" (p. 96). But that one member of the dyad must and Rochester does not. Like an analyst with his or her patient, Rochester treats Jane with the respect due an emotional equal. This does have an ameliorative effect on Jane's masochistic submissive style, but is it more of a "corrective emotional experience" (Alexander and French, 1946) than the achievement of analytic insight? Rochester, as Almond sensitively describes, also sees Jane's pride as defensive and confronts her accordingly with good result. Confrontation is a respected analytic intervention.

With the value he places on expressiveness Rochester does facilitate Jane's overcoming inhibition, through a kind of "manipulation" not regarded as inappropriate by psychoanalysts (Bibring, 1954). His own comfort with sexuality helps Jane overcome her denial of her own body and the repression of her libidinal desires. His sensuality, on the other hand, is not a modality for analytic progress but more in the area of a nonanalytic influence productive of change through transference love.

When he turns to directionality Almond could say more. Do Rochester's motives include helping Jane mature so that she is free to love (and work) or is he exclusively seeking to provide himself with a partner free of the madness of his wife and the narcissism of Blanche Ingram and her circle? The analyst works to bring an analysand to the fullest affirmation of his/her own inchoate self, fulfilling only one of the analyst's needs—to earn a living.

Almond feels the Thornfield phase brings Jane to puberty, where oedipal issues resurface. Her libidinal attachment to Rochester is fraught with incestuous meaning—he feels like "a relation" to her. It will take the Morton phase to give Jane an adolescence. Jane's flight into asceticism gives way to intimacy with the Rivers family. Jane can engage with them because of the psychological growth that has occurred. Now Jane can both achieve intimacy and be giving. Circumstances, youth, and her own undeveloped capacity for object relations had made that impossible earlier. Almond concludes that St. John's proposal makes Jane aware of the fact that further suppression of libidinal attachment would be unthinkable.

I was disappointed that Almond did not choose to discuss the Ferndean section to any appreciable degree, given the heuristic quality of his basic thesis. I concur that Jane's hearing Rochester's voice calling to her at Morton is an externalization of her new inner freedom. It would have been rewarding to watch Almond apply his ideas to the resolution of a transference neurosis and the establishment of mature love. Brontë did not help him by again inserting a hiatus of ten years between rapprochement and final state, where Jane is "bone of his bone and flesh of his flesh" (p. 431). Whether this is mature object love or some kind of primitive pre-oedipal merger transference (Kohut, 1971) remains unsettled. I would have liked to see Almond take up the working-through aspect of the parallel analysis as well. If Jane is "bone of his bone and flesh of his flesh" and she and Rochester spend almost every waking moment together, they cannot be two independent centers of initiative (Kohut, 1977), but instead we have some sort of primitive narcissistic fusion. St. John Rivers ends the book heading for heaven, Jane knows heaven on earth. I wonder how long it lasts.

Despite certain gaps in the suitability of *Jane Eyre* for Almond's formulation, he has a valuable framework to explain characterological change in literature. To further demonstrate its utility, I will apply Almond's paradigm to the relationship between Leopold Bloom and Stephen Dedalus after discussing Paul Schwaber's work. At the very beginning of this discussion, I claimed that the fear of genital sexuality and procreation affects not only Bloom but Jane Eyre as well. When Jane learns Rochester has a wife, she flees from the arrangement to live as man and wife that he proposes. She also rejects St. John's importunity to marry. Only when Rochester has lost his sight and his hand can she consent to be his wife. I believe this is possible because Jane changes the role Rochester plays in her unconscious fantasy life. He stops being the oedipal paternal figure ("my relation") because he is symbolically castrated and in actuality regressed. He is in need of her maternal care on a moment to moment basis, much like an infant. In fact, one can view him in an even more regressed mode, of being narcissistically experienced as part of herself. An infant does not threaten oedipal incest, nor does someone fused into one's representation as a part of a merger transference (Kohut, 1971). Jane's most likely predominant unconscious fantasy is mother taking care of her child (Rochester). She can then go on to have real children because the oedipal unconscious fantasy has been superseded by regression. Jane's own fantasy of being nurtured by the mother she never knew is operative with the roles reversed. Her fear of genital sexuality and procreation has been overcome by a change in her central organizing unconscious fantasy.

Let us turn to the other paper. As one plunges into *Ulysses* with psychoanalytic curiosity, one soon feels like poor Clarence drowned in a butt of malmsey, but of very good vintage. Schwaber has bravely taken on the enigmatic Jewishness of Leopold Bloom. He believes that Bloom, by reaffirming his inner sense of Jewishness, defines and bolsters his dynamically regressed masculinity. Unfortunately, Schwaber never defines or makes clear precisely what he means by Jewishness. His argument would be strengthened also if he took stock of the fact that Bloom's reclamation of Jewishness allows him to change predominant unconscious fantasies. I believe that there is evidence to substantiate the view that Bloom moves from a regressive state with both oral and anal features to the primal scene as his central organizing fantasy and then to the unconscious fantasy of a strong father caring for his vulnerable son. I agree with Schwaber that stimuli having to do with Jewishness catalyze the ultimate change in Bloom. It is, in contrast to Jane, a move toward a higher developmental level rather than to one governed by more regressed unconscious fantasies.

Schwaber begins in medias res with the description of Bloom's glimpse of Blazes Boylan on Kildare Street and consequent rush for the museum's entry gate to avoid an encounter. Boylan is Bloom's wife's concert manager and Bloom knows that Molly and Boylan's first assignation is planned for that very afternoon. In a frantic search through his pockets, Bloom finds the Zionist filer he took away from the Jewish pork butcher earlier that morning when he purchased the famed kidney that he then fried for his breakfast. The Zionist flier adumbrates the role Jewishness will have in Bloom's transformation. Although

Bloom favored mutton kidney, that morning he chose to go to Dlugacz, the pork butcher. Thursdays were not good mornings for buying mutton kidneys. Eating pork at the beginning of his day serves to demonstrate how far from Jewishness Bloom is at the beginning of *Ulysses*. It also serves to demonstrate his oral preoccupation.

It is Bloom's habit at all times to carry a potato in his trousers pocket, an overdetermined symbol, one meaning of which is oral and one which is phallic. Schwaber glosses over the fact that when Bloom fingers the objects in his pockets, pretending to be preoccupied with finding something, but really to avoid confronting Boylan, Bloom is reassuring himself that he still possesses his potato. Bloom wants to know that he, the Jew challenged by the robust Catholic male, is not castrated. Later we will learn that Bloom's weak Jewish father passionately warned him to avoid competition with gentiles. His feigned search for a lost object to cover his hasty retreat from Boylan gives him a chance to reassure himself that his prevailing rival has not already damaged his genitals. The castration concern at that moment, I contend, is intimately involved with an underlying fantasy of the primal scene viewed as violent. Bloom suddenly seeing Boylan and his subsequent fantasy of Boylan and Molly having sex is analogous to a child abruptly discovering the parents involved in intercourse. When Bloom left to buy the kidney, he felt in his hip pocket for his latchkey (which he did not have) and his potato (which he did). To be Bloom at the beginning of *Ulysses* is to fear competition, to be castrated, to have only a substitute for what is missing and to be an outsider.

In the pork butcher's shop, Bloom's thoughts had been stimulated by the hips of the female customer in front of him and he had hoped to follow her on the street to be stimulated by the movement of her "hams." Earlier he had remembered the

Dublin cattle market where men with switches in their hands whacked the hindquarters of animals. His next association is to his neighbor woman whacking carpets, her crooked skirt swinging with each effort. It is not much of a leap to Bloom's being whipped upon the buttocks but he is well defended against this and instead experiences gratification at her disinterest. The sting of her disregard paradoxically "glowed to weak pleasure within his breast" (Joyce, 1922 p. 49). Bloom, much like the Wolf Man (Freud, 1918), has a major erotic interest in women's buttocks. And, like the Wolf Man, under the influence of castration fear Bloom has retreated to anality and masochism. In being rejected there can be pleasure. One cannot help but think of "A Child is Being Beaten," in which Freud (1919) describes the impotent male who finds gratification in masturbation with the fantasy of being beaten by a woman who represents the mother. The fantasy derives from an underlying passive fantasy of being loved by the father. The fact that the beater is a woman disguises the underlying homosexual wish. The woman, however, is usually endowed with masculine attributes (see Bloom's mother; Molly in Turkish Trousers; Bella/Bello Cohen below). Regression from the oedipal phase to the anal sadistic one with role reversal explains why the passive sexual wish is it to be beaten. The Wolf Man's analysis also included a beating fantasy as well as a central primal scene fantasy.

The Wolf Man was not Jewish, however, and Schwaber's interest is in Bloom's Jewishness and how it figures in the workings of Bloom's mind. Joyce, despite his explicit dislike of Freud's ideas (Ellmann, 1982, p. 436), was very much interested in the flow of mental associations and their interconnectedness. The word Jewish itself is a kind of "switch word" (Freud, 1900), analogous to a siding on a railroad track that leads to many other meanings. Schwaber points out that despite the fact that Bloom is taken by persons in *Ulysses* as Jewish and thinks of himself as Jewish, he admits to Stephen Dedalus that he knows he is not Jewish. Only his father was, not his mother, as is necessary in matrilineal descent. Bloom was baptized as both a Protestant and a Catholic, and he was not circumcised. Yet his coming "to his Jewish soul" on June 16, 1904 is worthy of Schwaber's central attention and I believe ours as well, because aspects of Jewishness are important clues to understanding Bloom's unconscious fantasies.

Schwaber does not always explicate what he means by Jewishness but there are many rich and readily available connotations to the word. It is the Jew who is the consummate outsider who must watch life from the periphery, the wanderer trying like Ulysses to come home. Such meanings of the word Jew suggest the primal scene fantasy. It is also the Jew, however, who has a special role chosen to be an ethical light unto the nations, a moral exemplar, a teacher, a paterfamilias. These connotations suggest an underlying fantasy of the strong father helping and protecting his son. In Judaism, Moses, a representation of the father (Freud, 1938), is the central figure. Abraham, the first Jew, was instructed by God not to sacrifice his son but to nurture him in order to become the father of a nation with a population as numerous as the sands on the sea or the stars in the heavens. Whether it be Abraham, Moses, or God as the father, a central unconscious fantasy in Jewishness is the strong father nurturing his son, rescuing him, leading him out of bondage, supplying him with the fullness of life. Thus, getting in touch with his Jewishness can help Bloom move from more regressed to more developmentally advanced unconscious fantasy.

The use of unconscious fantasy by analysts studying Jewishness is not unprecedented. Arlow (1951) has studied the Bar Mitzvah and the prophets in the scriptures using unconscious fantasy as a generator of meanings. Abend (1979) discusses the unconscious fantasy of a patient to whom Jewishness represented care and nurturance because his beloved nanny had a Jewish first name (Esther). Bergmann (1988) has written about the psychoanalytic understanding of unconscious representations of a father's aggression toward his son in the Jewish religion and the Christian religions.

When Schwaber talks of Bloom's association to the Zionist pamphlet, he cites Bloom's pleasant memories of the early days of his marriage with Jewish friends in a Jewish neighborhood, memories of the father-like Moisel explaining the ritual function of citrons at the fall festival of Sukkoth. This paternal function is the role Bloom desires but fears. He cannot hold onto this organizer of experience, however, and his stream of associations plunges into a frightening forlorn fantasy of "barren land, bare waste, . . . dead sea . . . Sodom, Gomorrah, Edom, bent hag . . . the oldest people . . . Dead: an old woman's: the grey sunken cunt of the world. Desolation." These terrible images of a desiccated land, not one of milk and honey, are banished as Bloom recalls Molly; "Be near her ample bedwarmed flesh. Yes, Yes" (p. 50). Bloom's image of a parched Promised Land, dead, alone, withered, is what life is when unmitigated regression in response to castration threat leads to the possibility of an objectless internal world. It is far better to come to rest with the mother of the oral period who strokes and feeds, and whose warmth passes from skin to skin. This is the Molly whom Bloom loves, the one to whom he relates and is attached, not as an outsider, not as a witness to the primal scene, not as a Jew. Reaction formation leads to Bloom feeding *her* breakfast in bed. The faint smell of urine in his own breakfast is also infantile, for the mother's feeding and changing the baby often leads to mingled odors.

I strongly agree with Schwaber that Bloom's renewed Jewish identity reopens Bloom's development toward masculinity. I would elaborate that it is preceded by a traumatic primal scene enactment with Molly and Boylan taking the parental roles that disturb his regressed pre-oedipal positions. Bloom's perverse defenses against primal scene stimulation are enacted in Nighttown. The Jew as progenitor, modeled by his grandfather, changes Bloom's central organizing unconscious fantasy to one of a far higher level of development and he becomes ersatz father to a living son, Stephen.

Prior to that, however, Bloom reacts to the death of Paddy Dignan by longing for his Jewish father ("poor Papa with his hagadah book"), a suicide, and his infant son, who died eleven years ago. Schwaber believes that Molly's imminent infidelity and their fifteen-year-old daughter's approaching sexual activity lead Bloom in his passivity to identification with the female as well—to become "both kisser and kissed, both male and female." I would like to emphasize that it is an integral part of the primal scene fantasy for the child/observer to identify with both partners. Bloom not only must contend with looking in on Molly and Boylan, but on his daughter and her potential partner as well. Since the Blooms' baby son, Rudy (named after Leopold's dead father Rudolph), died, the Blooms have not had a satisfying sexual relationship. "Could never like it again, after Rudy." Schwaber believes that for Bloom, "broken Jewishness and sexual dysfunction touch on the severed male line of family." Bloom feels he somehow killed Rudy by fathering him imperfectly (p. 79) and Molly agrees (p. 640). He will not take that risk again.

The whole conflict comes close to consciousness because of Boylan's imminent intercourse with Molly and daughter Milly's letter reporting a boyfriend. Ellmann believes that despite Molly's premarital promiscuity this is only her second adulterous encounter and the first to be fully consummated (Ellman, 1982, p. 377). And that only after not having adequate sexual relations with her husband since she was twenty-two. It is thus Molly's refusal to remain Gaea Tellus, the earth mother, the pre-oedipal mother of warm breast and buttock that forces Bloom to again face the reality of genital intercourse, of adult heterosexuality. Death is made all the more real, however, by the recent death of Paddy Dignan. It is far safer for Bloom to be "kisser and kissed, both male and female," and thus identified with both parents as only an observer, rather than to father dead sons.

Schwaber points out that Bloom's uncharacteristic aggressiveness in Barney Kiernan's pub occurs at the very hour that Boylan and Molly are having sex. Bloom's verbal slip of "wife's admirers" for "advisers" shows his preoccupation with the tryst. Bloom says "I belong to a race [Jews] . . . that is hated and persecuted. Also now. This very moment. This very instant" (p. 273). The phrase "This very moment" certainly ties his affect to the interaction between Boylan and Molly but also is included in the thought that begins with his belonging to a persecuted and hated race. "Plundered. Insulted. Persecuted. Taking what belongs to us by right. At this very moment, says he putting up his fist, sold by auction in Morocco like slaves or cattle" (p. 273). To be cuckolded is to be furious, to be overstimulated, to be frightened—the feelings of the child witness to the primal scene. The child usually regards the parental intercourse as a violent encounter and may identify with either partner or both (Freud, 1908; 1918). Bloom's predominant identification at this particular moment is with the helpless onlooker. In his harangue it is the Jew who is attacked, abused, and humiliated, and Bloom, the Jew, who must helplessly and furiously watch his own kind be abused.

The parallel chapter in *The Odyssey* is that where Ulysses blinds the Cyclops Polyphemus, another primal scene derivative, the scoptophilic aspect being highlighted by the eye. The blinding condenses castration and penetration. Bloom nearly burns himself waving "the butt of his old cigar." This time a cigar is not just a cigar. It is a butt. A routed and castrated Bloom must plunge deep into wish-fulfilling fantasy to ascend like Elijah to heaven in a chariot of fire answering heaven's voice with Abba, the Hebrew for father. Schwaber says only that Bloom is defending Jews and could not be more wondrous, although by this moment he has been cuckolded. He does not comment on the castration symbolism, the regression to magical thinking, the transcendence of death anxiety (Elijah never died but ascended to heaven in a chariot of fire!), and the wish to submit to the father. Even the ascent to heaven "like a shot off a shovel" suggests Boylan's ejaculation. Bloom as a belligerent Jew has had to flee—to his heavenly father. The Old Testament God is a pretty strong father, however. Turning to the Jewish deity adumbrates Bloom's transformation as well. He will later abandon the primal scene as his primary organizer in favor of an unconscious fantasy of himself as strong father to a son. The ascent to heaven at this point leaves Bloom a son (Elijah) ascending to the father, God.

Schwaber asks the fascinating question of why Bloom, actually a non-Jew, a twice-coverted Christian, living in one of the most Christian of cities, is Jewish to himself. He uses evidence from the "Nighttown" chapter because it provides "entry to Bloom's encompassing deep fantasies," and from the penultimate chapter, which informs us about Bloom when he was younger. (Obviously I feel much is available about such "deep fantasies" considerably earlier in the text, but too much malmsey makes the head swirl.) He aptly compares "Nighttown" to the irrational feel of primary process and dream. Bloom's father appears garbed in the caftan of an elder of Zion. Schwaber discusses the father's almost frenzied sense of danger that comes from competition with Christian males. He then turns to the even more shrill hysterics of Bloom's mother. She appears dressed as a stage figure, the Pantomime Dame, from the traditional English family Christmas pantomime. This role was traditionally played bawdily by middle-aged men. From under her shirt comes a phial, an Agnus Dei medal, a shriveled potato, and a celluloid doll. Schwaber asks what else might be covered by her shirt but there is already enough: a phial (vagina), Agnus Dei medal (the embodiment of the primal scene), a shriveled potato (penis), and a celluloid doll (child onlooker). Edelheit (1974) has elaborated what he calls the primal scene schema, where the child has a double identification either alternating or simultaneous with the copulating parents. The crucified Jesus (as represented by the medal) represents the combined image of both parents and at the same time the helpless observing child (Edelheit, 1974). The bisexuality of the Pantomime Dame also suggests the primal scene couple embodied in one individual. Schwaber states that Nighttown is where Bloom goes through the nadir of his regression. I believe that this happens because of a change in central organizing fantasy from primal scene with its dual roles — active and passive, sadistic and masochistic, male and female — to an unconscious fantasy of strong father protecting his son.

Molly appears next, dressed in Turkish trousers. Schwaber asks if Molly, who figures as male and female to Bloom, often camouflages and covers the mother in his thoughts. The answer has to be yes, particularly in view of Freud's concept of psychic determinism, where two consecutive episodes in a dream must certainly be associated. Molly appears directly after Bloom's mother and after his father. The woman in trousers is still bisexual, although she is more female than the pantomime lady. The primal scene still governs with both partners condensed into one. Schwaber then turns to Bloom's potato, claiming it symbolizes the phallic forcefulness he could not claim with Molly and basic supplies he did not get from her. I am reminded of the joke where a fool complains women will not pay much attention to him. A friend advises him to put a potato into his pants. When they next meet, the fool laments that the women are avoiding him totally. The friend shouts "I meant in front, you idiot!" As with the fool in the joke there is an anal twist to Bloom's avoidance of phallic assertiveness, nicely alluded to by Schwaber in his discussion of the sadomasochistic fantasies that excite Bloom in the sequence that follows.

Zoe Higgins, a young prostitute who bears Bloom's mother's maiden name, is a critical figure. Zoe suggests sarcastically that Bloom give a "Stump speech" *after she puts his potato into her pocket*. Without his potato, he has only a stump—like his cigar. Bloom's speech not only finds him Lord Major Leopold the First and Parnell's successor, but speaking Hebrew as well as English. But like Parnell he is toppled for sexual misconduct— the oedipal temptation first inflates Bloom and then brings him down. As Mulligan says, Bloom is "bisexually abnormal." He cannot transcend the oedipal conflict and be generative—yet. Dr. Dixon says that Bloom is a finished example of the new womanly man. This is Bloom at the nadir organized by the primal scene fantasy—identified with both partners, incapable of procreation and fatherhood. And then Bloom gives birth to "eight male yellow and white children!" I believe the yellow alludes to the poison stain on his father's face after his suicide. Bloom is giving birth himself, overcoming the terror of procreation, transcending the need for a father, on the road to becoming one again.

Although he has followed Zoe, Bloom never consummates the act with her. His grandfather appears and eventually Bella Cohen, the whoremistress, who turns into Bello, a man. Bloom is to be used like a woman despite being urged to be phallic by his grandfather, the manifest Jew. Schwaber claims that by giving Zoe his potato, Bloom makes manifest all his fearful wishes for exhibitionism, anal eroticism, perversion and soiling, voyeurism, masochistic bondage, homosexual submission, bisexual realization, and continued castration. Zoe Higgins/Ellen Higgins Bloom as sexual object brings Bloom to the depths of regression from the primal scene, with perversions as the result. Perversion in response to primal scene stimulation when the parents have marital problems is well documented (Freud, 1918; Esman, 1973; McDougall, 1972; Peto, 1975; Chasseguet-Smirgel, 1984). Schwaber continues that the Nighttown chapter embodies Freud's early view that bringing conflicts to consciousness produces change. Regardless of cause, from that point on Bloom is a changed man. Schwaber could say more, however, about how Bloom's restored Jewish identification accomplishes the change. Bloom is decisive, he can be a father to Stephen and free of jealousy with respect to Molly. By the end of the night Bloom has refound his latchkey.

Let me return to Almond's paradigm at this point, because I believe it is apposite. There is something in the relationship between Bloom and Stephen that taps into the universal capacity for therapeutic involvement and change. First, there is a sense of *engagement* that makes the figures highly significant to each other. Bloom's concern about the desperate and drunk Stephen made Bloom follow him to Nighttown in the first place. Bloom rallies and reclaims his potato and begins to protect and care for Stephen. Second, Almond cities *mutual influence;* each character must facilitate alteration in the behavior of the other. Clearly Bloom has become a successful father and Stephen, the son. Bloom reclaims his potato, protects Stephen's money, refuses Bella's charge for damages, tries to help Stephen out of a fight, and finally takes charge of him when he has fallen. Bloom's actual son Rudy appears, reading from a Hebrew prayer book in the Hebrew manner from right to left. Stephen has had enough impact on Bloom to produce the vision of his own son alive at age eleven. Third, Almond believes the interaction must have a *positive directionality,* a pull toward conflict resolution and growth. Stephen's becoming son to Bloom's father has restored Bloom and saved Stephen. Bloom has not had such conversation and companionship in a decade, in essence, since Rudy died. Schwaber hopes that Bloom's restored masculinity may serve sexual and familial renewal with Molly. We will never know.

If Schwaber believes that Bloom's new strength comes from his restored Jewishness, and certainly Rudy is portrayed as an eleven-year-old *Jewish* boy, how then does Bloom get from pervert to strong unambivalent male to whom the primal scene (Molly's adultery) is no longer of great consequence? Surely it is Stephen's need that catalyzes Bloom's development. As Schwaber claims, Jewish Grandfather Virag also has his role. The God of Noah and later of Abraham commands, "Be fruitful and multiply." The Jewish scriptures narrate tale after tale of strong father and beloved son. It is the enactment of this underlying fantasy that proves crucial to Bloom's change, in my view.

References

Abend, S. (1979). Unconscious fantasies and theories of cure. *Journal of the American Psychoanalytic Association* 27:579–596.

Alexander, F., and French, T. (1946). *Psychoanalytic Therapy.* New York: Ronald Press.

Altschul, S. (1988). *Childhood Bereavement and Its Aftermath.* Madison, Conn.: International Universities Press.

Arlow, J. (1951). A psychoanalytic study of a religious initiation rite: Bar mitzvah. In *Psychoanalysis: Clinical Theory and Practice.* Madison, Conn.: International Universities Press.

Bergmann, M. (1988). The transformation of ritual infanticide in the Jewish and Christian religions with reference to anti-semitism. In *Fantasy, Myth, and Reality,* ed. H. Blum, Y. Kramer, A. K. Richards, and A. D. Richards. Madison, Conn.: International Universities Press.

Bernstein, S. (1985). Madam Mope: The bereaved child in Brontë's *Jane Eyre. Child and Youth Services* 7:117-129.

Bibring, E. (1954). Psychoanalysis and the dynamic psychotherapies. *Journal of the American Psychoanalytic Association* 2:745-770.

Chasseguet-Smirgel, J. (1985). *Creativity and Perversion.* London: Free Association.

Cowart, D. (1981). Oedipal dynamics in *Jane Eyre. Literature and Psychology* 31:33-38.

Edelheit, H. (1974). Crucifixion fantasies and their relation to the primal scene. *International Journal of Psychoanalysis* 55:193-199.

Ellmann, R. (1982). *James Joyce.* Revised edition. New York: Oxford University Press.

Esman, A. (1973). The primal scene: A review and reconsideration. *Psychoanalytic Study of the Child* 28:49-81.

Fleming, J. (1972). Early object deprivation and transference phenomena: The working alliance. *Psychoanalytic Quarterly* 41:23-49.

Friedlander, K. (1943). Charlotte Brontë: A study of a masochistic character. *International Journal of Psychoanalysis* 24:45-53.

Freud, S. (1895). Studies in hysteria. *Standard Edition,* 2.

———. (1908). On the sexual theories of children. *S.E.,* 9.

———. (1918). From the history of an infantile neurosis. *S.E.,* 17.

———. (1919). A child is being beaten: A contribution to the study of the origins of sexual perversions. *S.E.,* 17.

———. (1930). Civilization and its discontents. *S.E.,* 21.

———. (1938). Moses and monotheism. *S.E.,* 23.

Hartmann, H., and Lowenstein, R. Notes on the superego. *Psychoanalytic Study of the Child,* 17:42-81.

Joyce, J. (1922). *Ulysses: The Corrected Text,* ed. H. W. Gabler with W. Steppe and C. Melchior. New York: Random House, 1986. All quotations from *Ulysses* are from this edition.

Kohut, H. (1971). *The Analysis of the Self.* New York: International Universities Press.

———. (1977). *The Restoration of the Self.* New York: International Universities Press.

Loewald, H. (1960). On the therapeutic action of psycho-analysis. *International Journal of Psycho-analysis* 41:16-33.

Malcolm, J. (1987). J'appelle un chat un chat. *The New Yorker,* April 20, pp. 84-102.

McDougall, J. (1972). Primal scene and sexual perversion. *International Journal of Psychoanalysis,* 53:371-384.

Peto, A. (1975). The etiological significance of the primal scene in perversions. *Psychoanalytic Quarterly* 44:177–190.

Sadoff, D. (1982). *Monsters of Affection: Dickens, Eliot and Brontë on Fatherhood.* Baltimore: Johns Hopkins University Press.

Smith, D. (1965). Incest patterns in two Victorian novels. *Literature and Psychology* 15:135–162.

Stone, L. (1961). *The Psychoanalytic Situation.* New York: International Universities Press.

4
ART

A Century of Silence

ABSTRACTION AND WITHDRAWAL

IN MODERN ART

LYNN GAMWELL

*An age of silence has settled on art. It renders works of art obsolete.
But while they do not speak any longer, their silence speaks all the
more loudly.*
—Theodor Adorno, *Aesthetic Theory*

*In the other room, Rateau was looking at the canvas, completely
blank, in the center of which Jonas had merely written in very small
letters a word which could be made out, but without any certainty
as to whether it should be read* "solitaire" *or* "solidaire."
—Albert Camus, *The Artist at Work*

What are you building?
*I want to dig a subterranean passage. Some progress must be made.
My station up there is much too high.
We are digging the pit of Babel.*
—Franz Kafka, *The Pit of Babel*

Whether or not one can directly experience reality—either external, natural reality or ultimate, divine reality—and whether
reality can be represented in visual imagery or the spoken word
has been debated for centuries. The ineffability of absolute
reality and the superiority of abstraction over sensory experience have long been manifested in religious iconoclasm and the
mystical tradition. But by the end of the nineteenth century,
the hierarchy of terms in this old, largely theological debate
had collapsed, and amid its ruins began new deliberations in a

century characterized by a more radically abstracted art and a population more severely alienated and withdrawn than previously known.

A core of genuine art in this century is drained dry: the canvas is blank, the actor stutters, the musician falls silent. Advanced psychotherapy is also an impoverished landscape where doubts about the ability of language to communicate threaten the "talking cure." Modern man, following the ancient admonition to "know thyself," turns away from traditional religion toward the new cultural sanctuaries and professional priesthoods, where he encounters the silent artist and the silent analyst.

This essay asks why this has been a century of silence and is illustrated with examples from twentieth-century visual and performing arts that manifest abstraction and a sense of withdrawal. The question obviously has multiple and complex answers, and I will comment on two topics that would be part of any response: the concepts of reality peculiar to this century, and modern attitudes toward the power of symbols to communicate that reality. I will join Theodor Adorno and others[1] in arguing that art in this century is silent (blank, empty, enigmatic, unintelligible) because certain artists have experienced modern scientific, social, and political conditions as threats and have turned inward, away from the world of shared experience toward a psychologically isolated inner core. In previous cultures centers of meaning shifted, for example, from the supernatural to the natural, resulting in art forms that alternately were more idealistic or realistic; modern culture is characterized by a loss of meaning in all realms and an overwhelming distrust of communicative codes of any kind. Specifically, certain modern artists have both withdrawn from society's public realities and remained mute on the subject of their private psyches, resulting in the creation of a defensive art which is, if not completely silent, intentionally obscure on all fronts.

The most revolutionary advances of modern physics, such as the splitting of the atom and the development of the theory of relativity, present highly abstracted views of the universe and are based on the indirect detection of phenomena not perceivable by humans. While these intellectual concepts of abstract, imperceivable realities have certainly led some artists in a non-representational direction, it is the social impacts of modern scientific and technological advances that have constituted assaults on the psyche and precipitated the psychological withdrawal cited above. Notable examples include the rise of the secular, scientific intellectual environment with the concomitant decline in religion, the mass communication surfeit, and, most ominously, the threat of nuclear annihilation.

The psychological impact of the replacement of religious doctrine of scientific theory can be appreciated by remembering Freud's discussion of these topics in "The Future of an Illusion." There he wrote that the goal of science is "to gain some knowledge about the reality of the world" no matter how unpleasant or painful that might be.[2] Religion lulls believers away from knowledge by comforting them with infantilizing illusions, such as that they will enjoy eternal lives of bliss beyond the grave, or that they are the special children of an omnipotent deity who will protect them.

While new scientific explanations of the universe might be intellectually satisfying, even fascinating, the decline of religion has meant that secular adults now face hostile elements without these illusions. According to Freud's family model of religion, the psychological converse of an adult who feels protected by parental deities is the atheist who faces the terrors of nature, the cruelty of fate, and the power of the state with the dread of an abandoned child.[3]

The rapid pace of change and the emphasis on clarity and verifiability in the scientific world, which have so diminished the power of religion over people's lives, have also been a threat to the aesthetic realm, which has traditionally been understood as transcendent of the material universe. The primitive psychological realm to which the artist withdraws is a haven from secular stoicism, a place where the rules of rationalism are not enforced and where illusions of artistic autonomy can be maintained.

The inescapability of endless information from the media and the culture industries endows modern artists with a historical consciousness which obviates the unself-conscious creation of anything. Withdrawal to a silent realm provides the artist with what Susan Sontag has called the desired "cultural clean slate."[4] But, alas, the slate itself has inevitably been assigned an accession number in the contemporary museum of blank canvases. In this mediated culture, renunciation itself can become trendy and produce art that has been minimalized without a sense of loss.

Nuclear annihilation and other forms of mass destruction have shattered the syntax of art that even indirectly addresses these topics; there is something loathsome about presenting Hiroshima or Auschwitz as subjects in a traditional artistic format. Giving the unthinkable a rational forum, expressing agony in an aesthetic context, elevates atrocities as themes in a culture's artistic heritage. As Adorno has written, "By turning suffering into images, harsh and uncompromising though they are, it wounds the shame we feel in the presence of the victims. For these victims are used to create something, works of art, that are thrown to the consumption of a world which destroyed them."[5]

Confronted with annihilation and genocide, many artists

have taken up posts in the bunker of irrationality. A good example is the treatment of mass destruction by Samuel Beckett in *Endgame*. Or is that the topic? The audience is never told exactly why there is no life outside the window. Beckett uses trivial and disjointed chatter in place of articulate dialogue to promote the audience's ominous feeling that something is dreadfully wrong—could it be that the game is ending? The play does not state a political theme; rather it resonates a primordial babble, or as Adorno has put it, "the violence of the unutterable is mimed by the dread of mentioning it."[6]

The psychological withdrawal from society by modern artists has superficial similarities to Eastern mysticism, but unlike that ancient tradition, the silent art of this century is essentially secular, even when artists themselves encourage a mystical interpretation. Their art moves progressively inward, to the solemn chant of aestheticism, and does not lead anywhere truly transcendent.[7]

Artists who withdraw exist in a kind of limbo. To become truly silent they would have to stop making art, as Marcel Duchamp did when he turned to chess. That master of irony taught us that when objects or events occur in an artistic context, an audience is inescapable. Much has been written about the ongoing battle between modern art and its public; Adorno, for example, has described the battle regarding music:

> The opinion that Beethoven is comprehensible and Schoenberg incomprehensible is an objective deception. The general public, totally cut off from the production of new music, is alienated by the outward characteristics of such music. The deepest currents present in this music proceed, however, from exactly those sociological and anthropological foundations peculiar to that public. The dis-

sonances which horrify them testify to their own conditions; for that reason alone do they find them unbearable.[8]

What about the audience which is not horrified but returns for the next concert because only dissonance rings true? Silent artists and their audiences share a bizarre bond; both find meaning in the absence/presence of the other. Defensive, dissonant art offers its audience the meager comfort of knowing that it is not being lied to, that it is being addressed in an authentic, though muted, voice.

The artist who has withdrawn from modern society is like the psychologist's "silent patient;" one who has retreated to the noncommunicative core of his or her psyche for protection in times of stress.[9] D. W. Winnicott has written that "at the center of each person is an incommunicado element; this is sacred and most worthy of preservation."[10] The silent center of the psyche is pre-verbal and infantile in its lack of connection to the rational world. Withdrawal from everyday experience need not be pathological; indeed, Winnicott sees the capacity to be alone as "a highly sophisticated phenomenon" which is "closely related to emotional maturity."[11]

Psychologists differ as to whether and by what means hidden aspects of the personality are knowable. Freud, describing his discovery of the unconscious realm of the psyche, which by definition is not perceivable, wrote that "reality will always remain unknowable."[12] It can, however, be known indirectly: "How are we to arrive at a knowledge of the unconscious? It is only, of course, as something conscious that we know it, after it has undergone transformation or translation into something conscoius. Psychoanalytic work shows us every day that translation of this kind is possible."[13]

Freud's faith in the communicative power of words, so fundamental to the psychoanalytic method, is manifest in his characterization of Moses, in *Moses and Monotheism*, as a prophet who verbally communicated his ideas to the chosen people of God. Yosef Hayim Yerushalmi has contrasted Freud's anachronistic "verbal optimism" with the "verbal pessimism" of Freud's Viennese contemporary Arnold Schoenberg, who expressed his modern distrust of the capacity of words to communicate absolute reality in his opera *Moses und Aron,* in which "Moses, the servant of the Absolute, is inarticulate; Aron, who cannot really share his brother's vision, is the man of words, overflowing with eloquence."[14]

This modern distrust of words, along with images and other symbolic codes, surfaced in the arts in the late nineteenth century and continues today. The following quotations from cultural critics give a sense of the communication crisis: "Modern music sees absolute oblivion as its goal. It is the surviving message of despair from the shipwrecked."[15] And: "The poetry of modernism is a matter of structured debris: from it we are made to envision, to hear the poem that might have been, the poem that will be if, when, the word is made new."[16] But perhaps the dilemma has been best described by poets:

> What an age is this anyway where
> A conversation about trees is almost a crime
> Because it entails being silent about so many misdeeds?
> —Bertolt Brecht (1933–38)[17]

> A leaf, treeless
> for Bertolt Brecht:
>
> What times are these
> when a conversation

is almost a crime
because it includes
so much made explicit?
—Paul Celan (1971)[18]

This communication crisis has raised doubts about psychotherapy and the analytic situation, which is essentially a speech
relationship that places an overwhelming valuation on verbal
articulation. As George Steiner has noted, "There is in Freud's
refusal to deal with psychosis a terror before the inchoate, before
the semantically closed."[19] The crisis has led to reformulations
of classical Freudian theory on broader linguistic and symbolic
foundations, including structural linguistics and transforma-
tional and generative grammars along with nonverbal semiotic
systems.[20] It also has caused a reevaluation of the meaning of
silence in the psychoanalytic hour; whereas Freud and his early
followers interpreted silence as resistance, later analysts have
come to view silence as a goal because it is a sign that the
patient is taking responsibility for his or her inner world and
does not need to spill everything out.[21] On the other hand, the
ideal of the silent analyst has changed very little in this century,
from Freud's 1912 "Recommendations to Physicians Practicing
Psychoanalysis"[22] to late twentieth-century studies of analytic
technique such as Reed Brockbank's "On the Analyst's Silence
in Psychoanalysis," which states: "The analyst's silence can be
a more potent stimulus to the patient's unconscious fantasies
than any verbal interpretation he could make."[23]

Donald Kuspit has related the obscurity of much modern art
to the kind of psychological retreat described above by Winnicott: "At the core of unintelligible abstract art is a sense of true
self, that is, a self that is really human—only it is in an incommunicado condition."[24] Silent artists who have withdrawn in a
gesture of self-protection to the core of their psyches (their true

selves, their human essence) share this incommunicado stance. Winnicott has described the necessity of that protective position if the self is to remain whole: "Rape, and being eaten by cannibals, these are mere bagatelles as compared with the violation of the self's core, the alteration of the self's central elements by communication seeping through the defenses."[25] One can easily imagine that many artists would be wary of psychoanalysis and its ability to erode the defenses, as Freud proudly claimed: "He that has eyes to see and ears to hear may convince himself that no mortal can keep a secret. If his lips are silent, he chatters with his fingertips; betrayal oozes out of him at every pore. And thus the task of making conscious the most hidden recesses of the mind is one which it is quite possible to accomplish."[26] It is well to remember that therapeutic gains in an analytic situation come at a price of self-disclosure, which is often unassessed. As Steiner has warned: "Though it claims as its therapeutic aim the reconstruction of a proper economy of internal resources, psychoanalysis, by virtue of its process, erodes the autonomous energies of inward dictum and plenitude. . . . where a secret has been dislodged and published, a kind of malign emptiness remains."[27]

The arts were given to mankind, along with fire, by the Greek god Prometheus. Zeus, enraged that man had been empowered with these gifts, chained Prometheus to a rock and sent a savage eagle to tear out his liver; Zeus would free Prometheus only if he would reveal a secret. In the face of this suffering, Prometheus remained silent, keeping the secret within himself.[28]

Silent, defensive art is enigmatic, uninterpretable. Withdrawn from shared social realities and incommunicado about his or her personal core, the silent artist remains most profoundly human in a state of solitude.

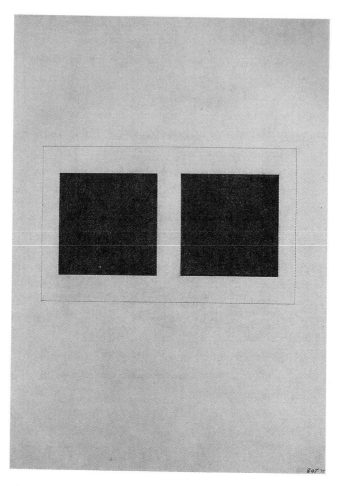

Kasimir Malevich, *Suprematist Elements: Two Squares*, 1915, pencil on paper, 19³/₄ × 14¹/₄ in. Museum of Modern Art, New York. © 1998 Museum of Modern Art.

In 1913, Malevich painted the first completely blank, black square. Looking back on the evolution of modern art, Adorno wrote: "If works of art are to survive in the context of extremity and darkness, which is social reality, and if they are to avoid being sold as mere comfort, they have to assimilate themselves to that reality. Radical art today is the same as dark art. . . . The ideal of blackness is, in substantive terms, one of the most profound impulses of abstract art" (*Aesthetic Theory*, p. 58).

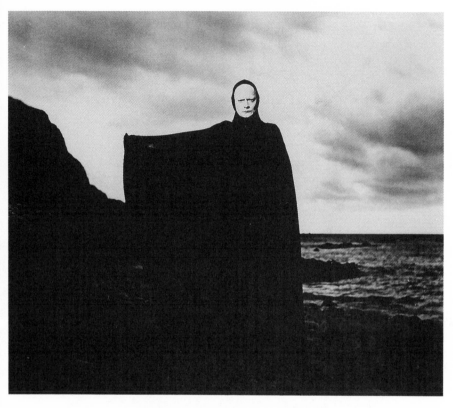

Ingmar Bergman, *The Seventh Seal,* 1956, black and white film, sound, 96 minutes. Museum of Modern Art, New York.

Death (Bengt Ekerot), shown here in his black cape, comes for a knight, who challenges him to a game of chess. Throughout the game, the knight tries to demonstrate to Death the basic goodness of mankind.
But in the end, Death takes them all.

Knight: I want knowledge, not faith, not suppositions, but knowledge. I want God to stretch out his hand toward me, reveal himself and speak to me.
Death: But he remains silent.
Knight: I call out to him in the dark but no one seems to be there.
Death: Perhaps no one is there.

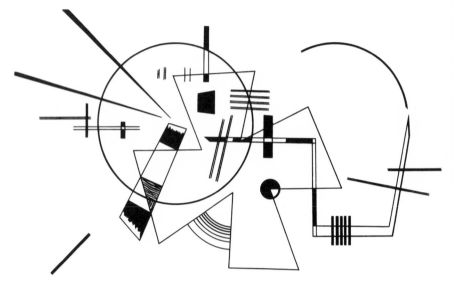

Wassily Kandinsky, *Composition,* 1925, lithograph, 15³/4 × 10⁵/8 in.
Collection of the State University of New York at Binghamton, gift of
Dr. and Mrs. Samuel Finkelstein.

On the eve of World War I in Munich, Kandinsky created a style of
abstract art based on the analogy between painting and music, both
communicating their spiritual content through abstract elements such as
color, form, chord, and tempo. Kandinsky had heard the music of
Schoenberg for the first time in 1911 and had written to the composer:
"In your works you have realized what I, albeit in uncertain form, have so
greatly longed for in music. The independent progress through their own
destinies, the independent life of individual voices in your compositions,
is exactly what I am trying to find in my paintings."

Arnold Schoenberg, *Moses and Aaron,* begun 1932, first performed in 1957,
unfinished at the composer's death in 1951; photograph from the
New York City Opera performance of 1991. Martha Swope
Associates, New York.

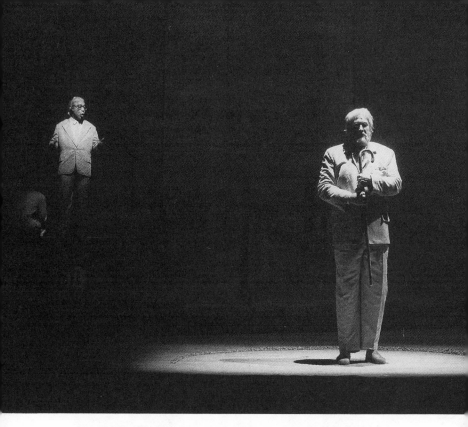

Arnold Schoenberg began composing *Moses und Aron* in 1932. It was unfinished at his death in 1951 and was first performed in Zurich in 1957. This photograph is from the 1991 New York City Opera production with Thomas Young and Richard Cross. In addition to composing, Schoenberg also painted nonobjective art; thus it is not surprising that he was drawn to biblical prohibitions against imagery and the theme of how to communicate an abstract idea of divinity. It is perhaps fitting that the composer left his work on the theme of expressing the inexpressible unfinished.

Moses: Inconceivable God!
Inexpressible, many-sided idea, will you let it be so explained?
Shall Aaron, my mouth, fashion this image?
Then I have fashioned an image too, false, as an image must be.
Thus I am defeated!
Thus, all was but madness that I believed before, and can and must not be given voice.
Oh word, thou word, that I lack!

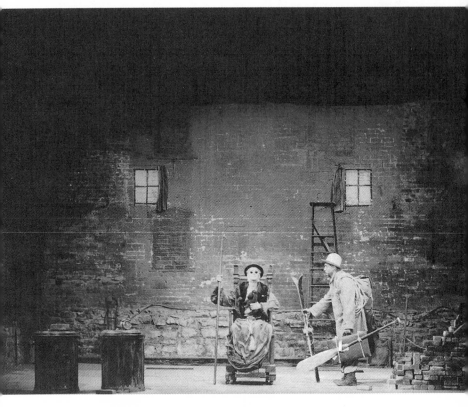

Samuel Beckett, *Endgame,* first performed in 1957; photograph from the 1958 performance at the Cherry Lane Theater in New York. Billy Rose Theater Collection, New York Public Library for the Performing Arts, Astor, Lenox, and Tilden Foundations.

Samuel Beckett's *Fin de Partie* was first performed in London in 1957. A 1958 performance of the dramatist's English translation, *Endgame,* at the Cherry Lane Theater in New York is shown here. Lester Rawlins played Hamm, the blind cripple in the wheelchair, and Alvin Epstein his companion, Clov.

Hamm: Did your seeds come up?

Clov: No.

Hamm: Did you scratch round them to see if they had sprouted?

Clov: They haven't sprouted.

Hamm: Perhaps it's too early.

Clov: If they were going to sprout they would have sprouted. (*Violently*) They'll never sprout.

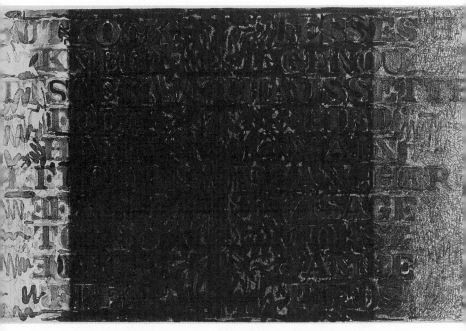

Jasper Johns (with Samuel Beckett), *Words*, 1975–76, etching, lift-ground
aquatint and burnishing, 10⁹/₁₆ × 17¹/₂ in., plate vii/x from
Foirades/Fizzles (New York: Petersburg Press, 1976). Courtesy of the
artist and Petersburg Press S.A.

Foirades/Fizzles combined a text by Beckett and a suite of prints by Johns.
Beckett wrote *Foirades* in French, the language of his adopted homeland,
and translated it into his native tongue, English, as *Fizzles*. In the print,
Johns used a list of seven words (names of body parts in his painting
Untitled, 1972) printed in such a way that they suggest the density of the
Beckett text. On the left, the darker English words are printed over the
burnished, reversed French; on the right the darker French words are over
the burnished, reversed English.

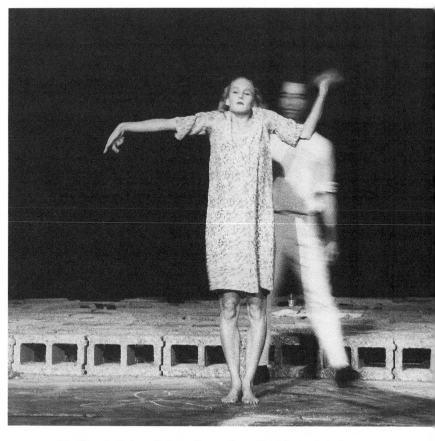

Pina Bausch, *Palermo/Palermo*, first performed in Palermo, Italy, in 1991;
photograph from the 1991 performance at the Brooklyn Academy of
Music. Martha Swope Associates, New York.

The 1991 performance at the Brooklyn Academy of Music began with the
collapse of a cinder-block wall, shown lying in the background, on the
ruins of which the dancers then performed. In this episode from Act I
the woman repeatedly demands that the man hold her, then she shakes
herself free of him, demands again, and so on.

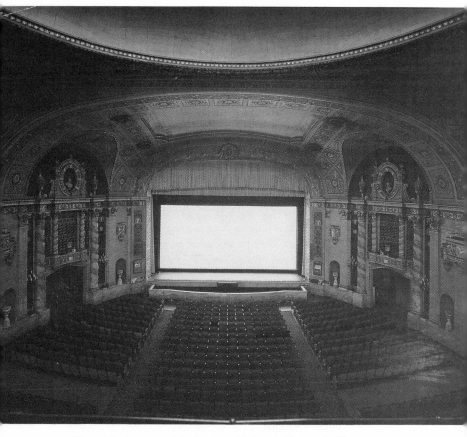

Hiroshi Sugimoto, *U.A. Walker, New York,* 1978, black and white
photograph, ed. of 25, 20 × 24 in. Sonnabend Gallery, New York.

This is from Sugimoto's haunting series of black and white photographs
of old movie houses, which he creates by making a time-lapse exposure
of the darkened theater during the projection of a film. The
glowing screen and highlights of the darkened interior
are the visual "memory" of the film.

Notes

1. Especially Donald Kuspit, Susan Sontag, and George Steiner, whose works are cited below.

2. Sigmund Freud, "The Future of an Illusion" (1927), in *The Standard Edition of the Complete Psychological Works of Sigmund Freud* (hereafter referred to as *S.E.*), ed. and trans. by James Strachey in collaboration with Anna Freud, 24 vols. (London: Hogarth, 1953–74), vol. 21, pp. 55–56.

3. On the psychology of secularism and its philosophical roots, see Patrick Masterson, *Atheism and Alienation* (Dublin: Gill and Macmillan, 1971).

4. Susan Sontag, "The Aesthetics of Silence," in *A Susan Sontag Reader* (New York: Farrar, Straus, and Giroux, 1982), pp. 189–90, 192; on a related topic, see also Sontag's "Against Interpretation," in the same volume, pp. 95–104.

5. Theodor W. Adorno, "Commitment" (1962), trans. Francis McDonagh, in *Aesthetics and Politics* (London: Verso, 1986), p. 189.

6. Theodor W. Adorno, "Towards an Understanding of *Endgame*" (1958), in *Twentieth Century Interpretations of "Endgame"*, ed. B. G. Chevigny (Englewood Cliffs, N.J.: Prentice-Hall, 1969), p. 86. On the effects of genocide on language, see Andre Neher, *Exile of the Word: From the Silence of the Bible to the Silence of Auschwitz,* trans. David Maisel (Philadelphia: Jewish Publication Society of America, 1981); it is hard to concentrate on even such an excellent study as this without hearing the echo of Adorno's remark, "All post-Auschwitz culture, including its urgent critique, is garbage," (*Negative Dialectics,* trans. E. B. Ashton, [New York: Continuum, 1973], p. 367).

7. For a thoughtful attempt at incorporating the tradition of Eastern meditation into contemporary psychotherapy, see Mohammad Shafii, "Silence in the Service of the Ego: Psychoanalytic Study of Meditation," *International Journal of Psychoanalysis* 54 (1973), pp. 431–42. Adorno has questioned whether this link can be made in the atomic age, when annihilation "has become the total Apriori, leaving a bombed-out consciousness no place from which it could meditate" ("Towards an Understanding of *Endgame,*" p. 86).

8. Theodor W. Adorno, *Philosophy of Modern Music* (1948), trans. A. G. Mitchell and W. V. Blomster (New York: Seabury, 1973), p. 9.

9. The extensive literature on the silent patient, which begins with Theodore Reik's seminal paper "The Psychological Meaning of Silence" (1926), *Psychoanalytic Review* 55 (1968), pp. 172–86, is summarized in Stephen A. Kurtz's "On Silence," *Psychoanalytic Review* 71, 2 (1984), pp. 227–45.

10. D. W. Winnicott, "Communicating and Not Communicating Leading to a Study of Certain Opposites" (1963), in *The Maturational Processes and the Facilitating Environment* (Madison, Conn.: International Universities Press, 1965), p. 187. Others with a similar view include R. Laing, *The Self and Others* (London: Tavistock, 1961).

11. D. W. Winnicott, "The Capacity to be Alone" (1958), in *The Maturational Processes and the Facilitating Environment*, p. 36.

12. "Outline of Psychoanalysis" (1938), *S.E.*, vol. 23, pp. 196–97.

13. "The Unconscious" (1915), *S.E.*, vol. 14, p. 166.

14. Yosef Hayim Yerushalmi, "The Moses of Freud and the Moses of Schoenberg: On Words, Idolatry and Psychoanalysis," *The Psychoanalytic Study of the Child* 46 (New Haven: Yale University Press, 1992), p. 6.

15. Adorno, *Philosophy of Modern Music*, p. 133.

16. George Steiner, *After Babel* (New York: Oxford University Press, 1975), pp. 181–82; for a discussion of the possible social and linguistic causes of the crisis, see George Steiner's *Language and Silence: Essays on Language, Literature and the Inhuman* (New York: Atheneum, 1967).

17. "An die Nachgeborenen," in *Gesammelte Werke* (Frankfurt, 1967), vol. 9, p. 723, quoted in Theodor W. Adorno, *Aesthetic Theory*, trans. C. Lenhardt (London: Routledge, 1984), pp. 58–59.

18. *Poems of Paul Celan*, trans. M. Hamburger (New York: Persea, 1988), p. 331.

19. George Steiner, "A Note on Language and Psychoanalysis," *International Review of Psychoanalysis* 3 (1976), p. 254.

20. For an overview see Paul Ricoeur, "Image and Language in Psychoanalysis," in *Psychoanalysis and Language*, ed. Joseph H. Smith (New Haven: Yale University Press, 1978), pp. 293–324. Ricoeur especially stresses nonverbal models: "The universe of discourse appropriate to psychoanalytic discovery is not so much a linguistic one as that of fantasy in general" (p. 311).

21. Silence is seen as a defensive strategy in Freud, "The Dynamics of Transference" (1912), *S.E.*, vol. 12, p. 101, and in Sandor Ferenczi, "Silence is Golden" (1916), in *Further Contributions to the Theory and Technique of Psychoanalysis* (London: Hogarth, 1927), pp. 250–51. Silence is seen as an accomplishment of the patient in Winnicott, "The Capacity to be Alone," and in Didier Anzieu, "Éléments d'une Théorie de l'Interprétation," *Revue française de psychanalyse* 34 (1970), pp. 755–844.

22. *S.E.*, vol. 12, pp. 111–20.

23. *International Journal of Psychoanalysis* 51 (1970), pp. 457–64.

24. Donald Kuspit, "The Will to Unintelligibility in Modern Art," *New Art*

Examiner (May 1989), p. 29; on a related topic see Kuspit's "A Freudian Note on Abstract Art," *Journal of Aesthetics and Art Criticism* 47, 2 (Spring 1989), pp. 117–27.

25. Winnicott, "Communicating and Not Communicating," p. 187.

26. "Fragments of an Analysis of a Case of Hysteria" (1905), *S.E.*, vol. 5, pp. 77–78.

27. Steiner, "A Note on Language and Psychoanalysis," p. 257.

28. On the topic of the heroic nature of silence, see Ellen Handler Spitz, "Promethean Positions," in *Freud and Forbidden Knowledge*, ed. Peter L. Rudnytsky and Ellen Handler Spitz (New York: New York University Press, 1994).

Primary Art Objects

PSYCHOANALYTIC REFLECTIONS
ON PICTURE BOOKS FOR CHILDREN
ELLEN HANDLER SPITZ

It has long since become common knowledge that the experiences of a person's first five years exercise a determining effect on his life, which nothing later can withstand. Much that deserves knowing might be said about the way in which these early impressions maintain themselves against any influences in more mature periods of life.
—Sigmund Freud, "Moses and Monotheism"

Recent scholarship in the humanities has questioned the narrow range of cultural objects that fall under serious interpretive scrutiny. This paper responds to that critique by examining a relatively neglected category of such objects, namely, the picture book. In addition, psychoanalysis, in postulating such universal constructs as drive, ego, and early object relations as primary influences on the child's psyche, wrestles only intermittently and marginally with the impact of cultural context. This interdisciplinary study aims to address that gap by demonstrating the impact of such artifacts as the picture book on the developing child's mind and to urge the need for interpreting them. Highly charged and subtly coded, reprinted and experienced by generations of children, the classic texts discussed here are worthy of consideration by researchers and educators in the field of early childhood, clinicians, and scholars interested in image-text relations.

A tradition for such exploration was established by the pioneering work of Anna Freud, who advocated the application of psychoanalytic insights into early childhood to realms that extend beyond the clinic but, in turn, impinge on it. More proximally, however, the questions that have motivated my work stem from suggestive papers by Winnicott (1966) and Greenacre (1957). Both of these papers address the child's initial experiences with the arts and culture but in highly speculative modes. Like theirs, my own work is principally interpretive rather than empirical, yet it differs in attempting to ground theory by the use of concrete examples. Drawn from the repertoire of picture books available in the United States, these examples have been chosen for their longevity (lasting in one case over a half-century). Such longevity speaks to the ongoing capacity of these and similar artifacts to enthrall not only children but adults and to stimulate the latter to recapture and share their own earliest moments of fantasy and illusion.

My topic, precisely, is the initiation of young children into the arts and culture by means of artifacts designed expressly for their use. Among the spectrum of such artifacts, I have chosen the picture book because of its hybrid form: it combines the two great sign systems of image and text in a physical object (i.e., a book) that carries enormous cultural signification; its temporal and spatial coordinates allow it to be perceived and handled intimately and repetitively and thus to be preserved and cherished or mutilated and destroyed. It serves as a prototype for various highly differentiated aesthetic objects that the child will encounter as he or she matures.

Parallel to the psychoanalytic construct of advancing from primary to secondary process is the notion, deeply implanted in our cultural heritage, of a necessary turning from (pictured) images to (written) words. While programmatically (in our educational system, for example) we have valued words over images and elevated reason above imagination, we know that to deny our daydreams and fantasies altogether would be to lose touch with complementary aspects of our human nature. Parenthetically, it is interesting to note that the prevalence of television and other visual media seems in our time to be effecting an alteration in, or perhaps even a reversal of, this accepted direction.

Nevertheless, the movement away from images and toward the preeminence of words (reflected in some religious as well as developmental and historical contexts) can be interpreted, psychoanalytically speaking, partly in terms of a fear of regression—a viewpoint paralleled by the twin notion that when we do value the *imagery* of art, the *spectacle* of theater, and the *illusions* conjured up by poetic texts, we do so in no small part because they foster and permit a pleasurable, safe, and limited regression. To employ this model is to comprehend in part the fascination of the picture book. Enjoyed by children from less than a year to about five years of age, it is an object designed to traverse the border between image and word at precisely that juncture in the life span when intrapsychic bridges between these realms are being constructed. In negotiating the gap between experience, perception, and the written word, children use picture books as a transitional form—but a form that is, in its own right, quintessentially an art.

In addition, it is essential to stress the role of the reading adult, whose own engagement over time with both artifact and child is fundamental. As in the Suzuki approach to learning violin (McDonald, 1970), it is human relationship that must initially contextualize cultural object, infusing it with richness and layered meanings that resonate with a lasting vibrato, empowering young minds to take the next step, which is toward rewarding solitary experiences with cultural objects.

II

Piping into inner fantasy life often at very deep levels, the picture book simultaneously transmits ethical values, aesthetic values (tastes), and basic cultural knowledge. Many of its most enduring messages are, as I shall endeavor to show, subliminally conveyed (for a fascinating recent discussion of subliminal visual stimulation, see Fisher, 1988). It assists children in forming concrete and symbolic connections between space and time, nature and culture, inside and outside, self and other. Partaking in a mini-tradition—namely, an iconographic and literary tradition with interconnecting references—the genre establishes modes of pictorial and verbal citation; in so doing, it initiates young minds into the realm of cultural cross-reference and builds a foundation for future interpretive activity.

One of the finest picture books, *Goodnight Moon* (by Margaret Wise Brown and Clement Hurd, originally published in 1947), for example, begins with visual references to both a favorite nursery rhyme, "The Cow Jumped over the Moon," and a beloved nursery tale, "The Three Bears." These pictorial quotes (given as framed decorations on the wall of a bunny-child's bedroom, the frames serving as emblematic equivalents of quotation marks) are later anchored in the text with verbal labels. When, however, a direct address is made to the cow ("Goodnight cow jumping over the moon"), the image is released from its frame and liberated to become a signifier for more than the words of the rhyme. Flying through the air with a page all to herself, the leaping cow is free to evoke associations for the child as an image. Yet, important among these

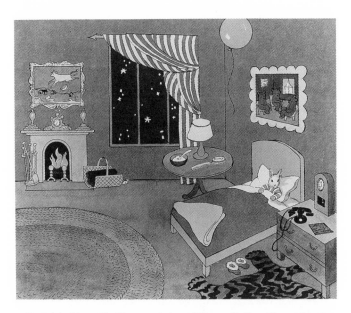

Goodnight Moon. Used by permission of HarperCollins. Illustration ©
renewed 1975 by Edith T. Hurd, Clement Hurd, John Thacher Hurd,
and George Hellyer, as Trustees of the Clement Hurd 1982 Trust.

associations, whether available to consciousness or not, are the
child's previous experiences of having heard, shared, and repeated the rhyme. Thus, encounters with one picture book may
call up, through such citation, encounters with other cultural
objects so that connections among books, imagery, poetry, and
shared good feelings can be established and reinforced. (The
three bears, incidentally, who are at least potentially frightening at bedtime, remain, unlike the friendly cow, confined *within*
their frame: they are bid "good night" while securely contained
within clearly bounded limits.)

In an essay devoted principally to a detailed interpretation
of one picture book (Spitz, 1988), I have discussed the ways in
which this genre simultaneously urges children toward words,
language, and secondary process while at the same time vali-

dating and privileging their inner worlds of fantasy. I have also used a theatrical metaphor to emphasize its performance aspect. The child, unable as yet to read, listens to the voice of an adult, who serves rather like a violinist translating the notes of a score into audible sound and whose accuracy, interpretive skill, enthusiasm, timing, and contact with the listener all affect the reception of the music. Like a musical or theatrical performer, the mother (or other adult) must mediate between child and cultural object. She is, of course, also a listener herself and not unaffected by the "music." (Note, for a description of this, Plato's Ion, whose eyes fill with tears, hair stands on end, and heart throbs when he is called upon to speak certain lines.) Further, just as the musician "holds" his or her audience, so also the picture book reader sits comfortably close to and often holds the child in his or her lap.

We may theorize about the role of the adult reader by evoking Winnicott's concept of the "holding environment." Our knowledge of the course of cognitive and psychosexual development teaches us that young children can only gradually separate fantasy from reality and that, in the years when picture books are used, representations are not yet easily distinguished from objects of representation. (The belief common to small children, for instance, that persons visible to them on the television screen actually exist inside the set and can be directly addressed has been exploited to great effect by such programs as *Mister Rogers' Neighborhood*, where the host, Fred Rogers, engages in "dialogue" with his youthful audience.)

Thus, we must expect that picture books will occasionally elicit anxiety, regressive fantasy, or hostile impulses. Both because of the immaturity of their audience and because, like other works of art, they necessarily call forth vivid moments of identification and projection, picture books require a containment that their given formal elements may not always prove adequate to provide. This additional contextualization must come from the reading adult, who creates precisely what can be called an extended "holding environment." Reading adults serve as editors and improvisers—explaining vocabulary, pointing out pictorial details, elaborating a theme, and occasionally censoring the text by substitution or omission; they expand the boundaries of the object to include a legacy of shared experience. The significance of this role is manifest when we consider the fate of children who suffer its absence. Left to experience cultural artifacts on their own, such children miss an essential step in the initiation process. They may experience motivational difficulties in learning to read or, in some cases, fail to develop a deep love for books. Each time, however, a small child is helped by an adult (or older child) to undergo the rising and falling of narrative tension and the stunning, immediate effects of color and graphics, his or her heightened achievement of mastery and pleasure marks a way station on the path of intiation into the realm of arts and culture.

In a recent lecture to a group of first-time mothers, I asked them to try to recall frightening images from books that were read to them in their own early childhoods. With gentle prodding, many divulged such memories—often of oral aggression (e.g., the toothy, disembodied grin of the Cheshire cat in *Alice's Adventures in Wonderland;* the huge, gaping mouth of Monstro the whale from *Pinocchio*) or the death of a parent (e.g., the page in *Babar* where a "wicked hunter" has shot the young elephant's mother). A propos this last example, however, I have discovered that many adults, while fondly recalling the Babar of their childhood, fail utterly to remember his mother's violent death at the start of the story. However, in recalling their own anxiety, often readily accessible despite the passage of years, many of these mothers were sensitized, at least momentarily, to the powerful impact of pictorial imagery on the psyches of their own children.

Asked to recall what techniques they had invented to cope with their fear, several remembered anticipating the offending page and turning it over quickly. Others reported having closed their eyes while peeking furtively. In general, avoidance was the most frequently reported defense. None could remember (or admit) tearing or mutilating a disturbing page or scribbling over an especially troubling picture. These more extreme, iconoclastic measures, when resorted to, signal a conversion of terror into rage and, by provoking parental response, may serve to bring a child's secret fear into the open. In so serving, such destructive nonverbal responses to imagery may be counted as communication in the sense that Winnicott (1956) described it.

Just as parents (or other caretaking adults) in their mediating and interpreting roles respond according to vicissitudes of their own, as well as their assessment of the child's needs, so it is with the child. Different developmental stages, for example, dictate new agendas or altered patterns of response to well-loved picture books. In one case, a two-year-old boy searched obsessively for the moons in *Where the Wild Things Are* (by Maurice Sendak, originally published in 1963) and asked for the moon on each page where it is not represented. Later, at four years of age, loving the book still, the same boy had no interest in moons but expressed anxiety during the wild orgy depicted in the center pages, where pictures completely supersede written text (Spitz, 1988). In the absence of further data, one might speculate on the basis of developmental stage theory that whereas separation had preoccupied him at the time of his initial encounter with the book, the control of sexual and aggressive impulses had, by age 4, come into prominence as a theme of greater moment. Of special interest here is that the desire to see the image of the moon may also be linked to the child's relationship to a specific pictorial convention (as I shall show). Also notable is the salient fact that, in spite of all the changes that had occurred in his life between the ages of two and four, one picture book remained capable of sustaining his interest, keeping up with him, so to speak, and symbolizing the major motifs of his ongoing developments—a testament to the power of the genre.

III

Oldest historically, and among the earliest developmentally, among the different types of picture books is the alphabet primer. Juxtaposing a picture with its name and initial letter in expectable sequence, the primer affords a model of language acquisition based on the priority of noun or name. As an imitative, static model of learning, the primer locks into nonreversible hierarchical order not only its terms—i.e., image and text—but the relative positions of reader and listener. Even here, however, the message may be amplified and/or subverted. Bright pictures (of wild animals, for instance) can leap out of the pages to haunt young minds and spark extended fantasy. This tendency on the part of images to escape being controlled by words, like the unruly tendency of primary process to erupt into reasoned discourse, crops up, therefore, even in this most predictable of formats. Its best examples are those, like *Brian Wildsmith's ABC* (winner of the Kate Greenaway Award, 1963), that openly strive to extract aesthetic response and carry children—by innovative color, scale, gesture, and design—far beyond the fixedness of prescribed arrangement. In such cases, each noun seems to engender a verb, every picture gives birth to story, and staid primers blossom into works of art.

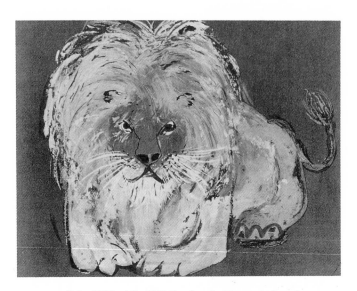

Brian Wildsmith's ABC. Reprinted with permission of
Oxford University Press.

IV

Even prior to the primer, children still in the crawling stage
may encounter picture books like *Pat the Bunny,* which conjoin
the perceptual and verbal with kinesthetic, olfactory, and tactile
experience, strongly prioritizing the latter. Such objects emphasize the physicality, the materiality of art—qualities which,
as adults acculturated into a universe of abstract codes, we learn
early on to decathect. Yet, touching, holding, loving, all intimately related for the small child, are transferable, displaceable,
by means of these transitional forms, to physically more remote
encounters later on with sophisticated cultural objects.

Pat the Bunny (by Dorothy Kunhardt, originally published
in 1942) conveys cultural myths and values of enduring significance to children often too young either to walk or to speak in
complete sentences. The first page addresses its naïve spectator

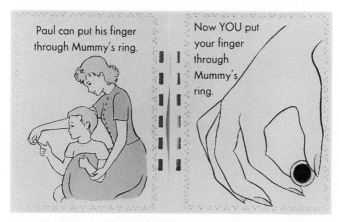

Pat the Bunny. Reprinted with permission of Golden Books
Publishing Company.

in the second person and explicitly invites him or her to identify with its characters. Two blond children, the boy taller than
the girl, are pictured on the facing page. Without placing undue emphasis on this particular image, it is worthwhile to consider how many girls feel ashamed and embarrassed years later
if they grow taller than boys and to consider the beauty ethic
innocently implicit in this picture. The final page is a repetition
of this one with variations. Paul and Judy wave good-bye, and
the boy protects or restrains the girl in a gesture that indicates
a certain element of control.

Explicitly, the imagery of this simple book sets up for the
pre-oedipal child the positive oedipal situation as a paradigm:
the mother encourages her son to insert his finger into the hole
of her ring while the father, holding his daughter against his
body, invites her to touch his unshaven face. Like the children,
the mother is blond. Thus, pictorially, the book conveys that
little girls can stay the way they are and grow up to resemble
mother whereas boys, resembling the mother at this stage, must
radically differentiate themselves from her if they are (later

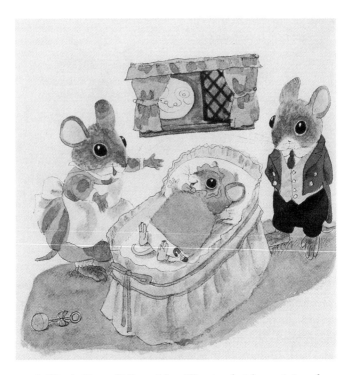

Is This the House of Mistress Mouse? Reprinted with permission of
Golden Books Publishing Company.

on) to resemble the dark father. In terms of the reading-as-
performance metaphor I have evoked above, the child in relation to this tactile-type book becomes an actor in the drama
and participates directly with the reading adult.

A slightly more advanced and complex version of this tactile-
type picturebook is Richard Scarry's *Is This the House of Mistress Mouse?* (originally published in 1964) in which the child
repeatedly inserts his or her forefinger into a hole to feel a
furry substance that turns out to be the hide of several different
(frightening) animals before it can be interpreted as belonging
to the house of the (friendly and maternal) title character and

being, in fact, the fur of her new baby. Here, libidinal, ego, and object-related issues call forth a gamut of emotions ranging from anticipation to pleasurable satisfaction by way of anxiety, dread, surprise, bewilderment, and delight.

Repetitive encounters with the book confer a sense of mastery: the child's wish for a happy ending is threatened but always finally achieved. The happy ending, however, involves not merely fulfillment of the original wish (Mister Mouse finds Mistress Mouse) but the surprise appearance of their new baby. Entirely unheralded in the text, a complete mystery to its parents, this baby is greeted with unmitigated joy and then the book abruptly ends. Thus, image and text collaborate here to foreclose the intense curiosity and ambivalence stirred up by this event. This is an excellent example of a case in which additional parental contextualization seems warranted. Parenthetically, the book closes with the baby's crib placed under a window through which a moon shines—an image that is gradually building in its associative value for the child-reader. This picture also encodes gender difference by depicting the mother dressed in the same color as the baby and as rushing toward the crib with arms extended toward the child; Father Mouse admires baby from a distance, his hands behind his back.

V

Some picturebooks seem targeted at specific developmental themes. I shall mention four currently available examples. *Goodnight Moon* (see above) ranks supreme and was eulogized in a *New York Times* editorial (Feb. 14, 1988) when its gifted illustrator died. Speaking directly to every small child's fear of the dark and the recurrent anxieties surrounding bedtime separation from primary objects, this book, with elegance and simplicity, offers itself to sleepy toddlers as a primary art object.

In visual terms, it soothes and comforts by creating a solid and cozy space that, as its pages are rhythmically turned, grows progressively darker, while, instead of disappearing, all the child's familiar things—comb, brush, mittens, dollhouse—remain securely in place, and, with unwavering constancy, a moon shines in through the window.

Noodle (published originally in 1937, reissued in 1965) is a book for upper age-range toddlers who can later on read it to themselves. Its long record is a tribute to the inspired collaboration of author Munro Leaf (famous for his *Story of Ferdinand* of 1936) and artist Ludwig Bemelmans (originator of *Madeline,* 1939). Noodle is a dachshund whose short front legs make it hard for him to dig holes because the dirt flies up and hits him in the tummy. One day, after much labor, he digs up a wishbone and expresses the desire to be some other size and shape than he presently is. Visited by an unforgettable dog fairy (who arrives onomatopoetically in "a whirr and a buzz and a flip-flap of wings"), Noodle learns that he will be granted his wish but must choose the new size and shape in just a few hours. After visiting the nearby zoo and interviewing other animals concerning their size and shape, Noodle returns home to eat and nap. When the dog fairy returns to grant his wish, he tells her he has decided to remain "just exactly the size and shape [he is] *right now.*"

In her classic paper "Early Physical Determinants in the Development of a Sense of Identity," Phyllis Greenacre (1958) persuasively argues that children's awareness and acceptance of their own bodies must serve as a basis for all future identity formation and reality testing. *Noodle* symbolically digs up this *bedrock* issue and the inevitable disappointments, longings, and conflicts surrounding it. Adumbrated here are wishes to be the sex one is not (to have both male and female genitalia) as well as to alter the details of one's body image. Digging down into the

earth (at the cost of considerable discomfort), the little dachshund comes up with, of all things, a *wishbone* (with protuber-
ances and hollows that are repeated in various guises throughout the book and convey a vague bisexuality). Even without
a detailed analysis of format and style, we can note the occa-
sional strategic matching of the shape of the printed text on the
left-hand page with that of the image on the right—a schema
that underscores the theme of bodily size and shape. Stylistically, the drawings convey a spontaneous whimsy associated
often with children's own linear art. Psychosexual innuendoes
abound (such as the picture of Noodle poking his nose into the
hollow earth to smell the bone), and older children can readily
associate to other tales involving wishes and fairies. Poetic devices such as onomatopoeia and alliteration reinforce the impact of theme and variations as Noodle visits in turn a male
zebra, a married female hippopotamus, an unmarried female
ostrich, and finally a male giraffe.

Where's Wallace? (by Hilary Knight, author of *Eloise,* published originally in 1965 and recently reissued) concerns a mischievous orangutan who repeatedly escapes from his cage in a
zoo and thus forces his keeper (and the child-reader) to find
him. Because the fumbling keeper (aptly named Mr. Frumbee)
absentmindedly leaves Wallace's cage door ajar, the child can
perceive the adult as a collaborator in Wallace's thrillingly dangerous game of running away, hiding, and being found. The
terror of actually being lost is mitigated even further because,
in addition to rigging the cage, the keeper (and child-reader)
always have advance knowledge of the limited milieu (page-
space) in which the creature is bound to be hiding and thus
found. In this way, the format of the book provides multiple
roles for the child, who can identify simultaneously and serially
with hider, seeker, finder, and the one found.

Each locale into which Wallace disappears (e.g., department

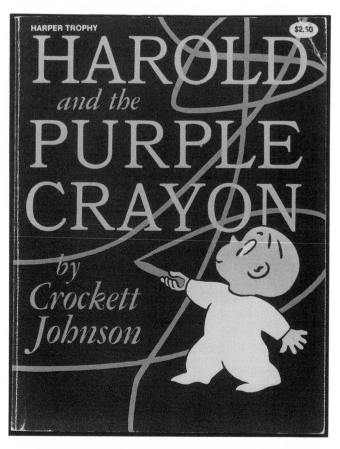

Harold and the Purple Crayon. Used with permission of HarperCollins.
© 1955 by Crockett Johnson, © renewed 1983 by Ruth Krauss.

store, museum of natural history, circus, ocean beach, amusement park) is delineated in minute graphic detail and includes
repeated unnamed figures—a runner, a baby, a knitting lady,
a man with a bass viol, and a naughty little girl with pigtails
whose mother is always depicted as gesturing frantically. These
provide a thread of visual continuity in locales that are, in any
case, never entirely foreign to the child-reader. Thus, while di-

rectly addressing the themes of separation anxiety and object constancy, *Where's Wallace?* concurrently explores a number of environments of cultural significance for the child. Parenthetically, this is also the case with another brilliant picture book, *Madeline,* where the narrative is set against backgrounds that depict Nôtre Dame, Sacre Coeur, the Place Vendôme, the Eiffel Tower, and the like, so that the child who loves this story becomes visually acquainted with the city of Paris.

My last example in this series is *Harold and the Purple Crayon* (by Crockett Johnson, originally published in 1955). This physically minute book of purple line drawings calls upon children to identify directly with its creator, to become, as it were, artists and authors of their own invented worlds. It valorizes the realm of make-believe and models the creation of bedtime fantasies: little Harold draws one himself before our eyes with his purple crayon. After giving it form and projecting into it his private wishes and danger situations, after pleasing, exciting, scaring, and rescuing himself, he ingeniously finds his way back to the safety of his bedroom. In the last picture, he lies snugly in bed with the moon shining through his window. After drawing [*sic*] the covers up, his purple crayon drops to the floor, and Harold drops [*sic*] off to sleep—these verbal puns serving as analogues for the visual puns that have carried the story along from page to page in a witty and wonderful secondary elaboration of the unpredictable associative links of the primary process.

Again in this book, the moon plays a central role. In fact, it is Harold's memory of the moon shining through his bedroom window that enables him, when lost, to find his way back to familiar surroundings. I wish to underline the potent effect of *quotation* here—the point that young children preconsciously associate to Harold's empowering memory their own prior experiences with picture books such as *Goodnight Moon.* In this way, a repertoire of cultural reference is gradually accumulated.

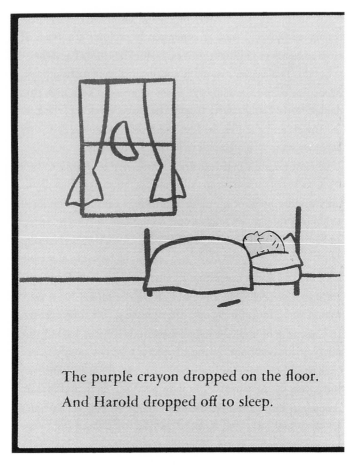

The purple crayon dropped on the floor.
And Harold dropped off to sleep.

Harold and the Purple Crayon. Reprinted with permission of HarperCollins.

To sharpen my point, the referent for "moon" is never simply the one out there in the sky but all the *pictured moons* the child has known and loved. Parenthetically, the most brilliant children's book to deploy this symbol is probably James Thurber's *Many Moons* (1943), a masterpiece that deserves a separate essay of its own.

Before going on, I would like to address the possible meanings to the young child of the repetitive symbolism of moon shining through window, a visual trope consistent in the picture books discussed thus far. Clearly, the moon figures in part as a maternal symbol, not only because of its roundness, suggestive of the breast, but perhaps also because of its repetitive cycles: like the mother, the moon disappears gradually and predictably reappears—changing shape but always recognizable. Illuminating the darkness, it, again like the mother, serves as a beacon in the frightening realm of the unknown. Associated by the child with bedtime and thus separation, its predictable presence stands as a constant, a bulwark against the fear of strangeness and boundlessness that loss of parental objects betokens. In this sense, the moon shining through the window may be seen as a pictorial representation of the very "holding environment" instantiated by the reading of the picture book itself in the company of a caretaking adult.

Furthermore, as depicted in these texts, the moon shining in through a window can be seen as mirroring the child's own face as he or she looks at the pictured scene from the other side. A fine example may be found in Tomi Ungerer's *Moon Man* (1967), where the beholder is meant to identify with the soft, round-faced title character, whose envious narrative ends in a peaceful return to familiar surroundings. Thus, in keeping with Paulina Kernberg's (1987) studies of the young child's conflation of self and maternal object in the mirror, we might interpret the presence of the moon as representing not only the maternal object per se but perhaps a form of transitional or self object. According to this interpretation, the window through which the moon is visible figures both the door through which the mother appears and disappears and, likewise, the frame of a mirror.

VI

Now I shall turn to a unique artifact: a small collection of picture books by Maurice Sendak originally published in 1962 and entitled *The Nutshell Library*.[1] After a glance at its general format, I shall focus on one of its four volumes. Compact enough in size to turn even the smallest child into a giant, this novel work can be taken as paradigmatic of the primary art object in all the senses I have attempted to convey. Moving zestfully in two directions, it fosters fantasy while turning inexorably toward secondary process, ego autonomy, mastery, and object permanence. Metaphorically it focuses on oral themes: growing up (it teaches) means filling up, nourishing the self with good things for both mouth and stomach, eye and mind. It conveys the message that growing up entails growing into a culture; that in order to achieve this one must both eat and read, activities that confer comfort and pleasure as well as genuine power and mastery.

The four tiny volumes in *The Nutshell Library* each measures a scant three-by-four inches. These volumes are not packed in any foreordained sequence, as the end leaf of each lists the order differently. They are as follows: a counting book, *One Was Johnny;* a book of months, *Chicken Soup with Rice;* an alphabet primer, *Alligators All Around;* and an ethical tract, *Pierre.* Thus, each conveys a different kind of knowledge to the young mind, and, because their order is unfixed, they subtly teach that no one kind of knowledge may be prized or prioritized over any other. All are important, all equally valid.

The slipcase instantiates the very nutshell that is imprinted upon its every side, its contents, the volumes themselves, thus being its nourishing and delicious nutmeats. (One thinks, parenthetically, of the collegiate expression "to crack a book.")

Each of the three sides of the slipcover is designed like a miniature stage set with a small white curtain overhead inscribed with Sendak's name. Thus, they participate in the metaphor of theater, spectacle, and performance established earlier in this essay. However, whereas I spoke earlier of the reading adult as a performer-artist with respect to a child-audience, *The Nutshell Library* dramatizes its themes somewhat differently: here, the metaphor shifts to a direct, unmediated relationship between child and book: *the book will stage itself for the child*. Masquerading characters in each of the volumes serve to underscore this trope and assert that imagination (make-believe) is central to all learning.

Each miniature stage depicted on the slipcover is flanked by columns decorated with oak leaves and topped by fluted acorn capitals. Supporting these columns are blocks with smiling faces suggesting traditional masks of comedy (no tragedy). An acorn and a silver crown adorn the top of the slipcase. Joining the anonymous Latin quotation that translates as "Tall oaks from little acorns grow" with Francis Bacon's "Knowledge is power" ("Nam et ipsa scientia potestas est"), we may interpret the iconography as saying that small children, like acorns, can become powerful, like oak trees, through the acquisition of knowledge, the imbibing of culture.

This theme is graphically portrayed on the back of the slipcase, where, onstage, face to face, sit two characters from the books inside: the little boy from *Chicken Soup* licks his lips and spoons up steaming liquid from his bowl, while a happy alligator from *Alligators All Around* reads from an open book. The parallelism here equates these two kinds of consumption and depicts them both as deeply satisfying. Interestingly, these figures are upstaged by a cat and rat (characters from *One Was Johnny*), whose story of hunt and chase seems ready to begin —

the cat looking smug with back arched, the mouse poised, sniff-
ing, about to run. Thus, suspense links the theatrical metaphor
with the acts of reading and taking in.

Other characters from the books inhabit stages on the slipcover front and the binding. Pierre reads face to face with
his lion (who is also reading), and, on the binding, the monkey from *One Was Johnny* reads peacefully under the chandelier
from which he swings wildly in his book. All these characters,
if interpreted as reading about themselves in their own books,
express by analogy the pleasure of children who can relive (and
eventually sublimate) their own silliness, naughtiness, disorder,
and disobedience through their symbolic representation in cultural objects.

In addition to their visual elements, all four books build ingenious bridges between a toddler's joy in experimenting with
sound, early language play, and sophisticated devices of poetic
diction. Simple repetition is used not only in pictures but in
refrains. In *Chicken Soup with Rice* the refrain is reiterated on
every page of the text, as is very nearly the case in *Pierre*, where
the title character continually chants, "I don't care!" *Alligators
All Around* features alliteration, a form of repetition used not
only by masters of poetic language but by infants practicing
with word-sounds. Thus, this alphabet primer strengthens a
child's grasp of the sound of letters by offering phrases such as
"B bursting balloons," "G getting giggles," "M making maca-
roni," and "Y yacketyyacking." In *Chicken Soup with Rice,* alliteration is unforgettably the major trope for the month of January: "In January / it's so nice / while slipping / on the sliding
ice / to sip hot chicken soup / with rice./ Sipping once / sipping
twice / sipping chicken soup / with rice."

Celebrated throughout the year, chicken soup is symbolic of
basic oral comfort, a restorative to which the child can repair

in every kind of weather—weather standing here as a metaphor for the child's varied and mercurial inner states. A figure for love, it is analogized by image and text with cultural experience. As pointed out above, the book of months and the counting book, whose protagonists are visually interchangeable, suggest that being alone with a book, like having a bowl of hot chicken soup, can enable one to feel loved, nourished, sustained.

With regard to the theme of quotation, the counting book offers a nose-pecking blackbird, undoubtedly one of the four-and-twenty baked in a pie from the nursery rhyme "Sing a Song of Sixpence." This pecking blackbird also figures in Sendak's own self-reflexive iconography; it appears, for example, in *Hector Protector* and *As I Went Over the Water* (1965). The tiger selling old clothes, also a character in the counting book, inescapably refers by reversal to the tale of "Little Black Sambo," where the tigers *take* the little boy's *new* clothes; furthermore, whereas those tigers threaten to eat the child up, here it's the little boy who tells the animals that if they don't leave him alone he will devour them! A small white dog, another Sendak creation, appears in *The Nutshell Library;* it also stars in *Higglety Pigglety Pop!* (1967) and plays a walk-on (or, perhaps, a run-on) role in *Where the Wild Things Are.*

VII

Psychoanalytically speaking, the meatiest nut in the shell is *Pierre,* subtitled *A Cautionary Tale in Five Chapters and a Prologue.* Self-confessedly literary in its format, this book is the ethics primer of the set. Its deliberate stylization (the prologue is a limerick) serves not only to introduce formal elements but also, because the content is frightening (a little boy is eaten by a lion), to alienate and defend the child-reader from its impact. Likewise, the foreign name of its protagonist (Pierre as opposed to Peter) functions to distance the title character and forestall too immediate an identification (Torsney, 1988).

Pierre's drama is that of a little boy who responds to his mother's affection, offer of breakfast, etc., by repeating the words: "I don't care!" The mother soon leaves, and the father appears. To each of the latter's commands, threats, bribes, and entreaties, the child reiterates his response: "I don't care!" Mother and father now both depart, and a hungry lion arrives. To all the lion's questions, such as whether Pierre would like to die, whether he realizes that the lion can eat him up, and whether, finally, he has anything else to say, Pierre produces his classic retort. On the page following this interchange, we find a conspicuous gap: Pierre is missing! The lion, filling the entire space occupied previously by both figures, looks smug: the accompanying text is terse: "So the lion ate Pierre."

Arriving home, the mother and father find a lion sick in Pierre's bed. Suspecting the worst, they assault him and inquire about their son. Classically, the lion replies, "I don't care!" On the next page, a doctor shakes the lion upside down, whereupon Pierre falls out onto the floor.[2] After being hugged by his mother and queried by his father, the little boy reassures them both, and together they all ride home astride the lion. Pierre, perched on the lion's head, finally shouts, "Yes, indeed I care!" The lion remains with them as a "weekend guest," and, as in all true fables, the last line informs us of the moral, which is: "CARE!"

A truly memorable creation, Pierre's lion condenses many aspects of a child's inner life. He represents previously disowned aggression turned now against the self, aggression for which the parents first serve as both willing and unwilling objects; in addition, he represents the parental introjects themselves combined into a punitive, primitive superego forerunner—an active version of the passive aggression expressed by the child's behavior. For Pierre does not attack the parents directly; in adopting a typically oppositional stance, he aggresses against them by contrarily *not* doing, *not* responding. He *won't* eat, *won't* go to town, and in fact turns the milk pitcher, bowl, broom, and himself quite literally upside down.

This upside-down motif figures prominently in the drama. A small panel of drawings frames the book, ornamenting both the table of contents and the final page. In sequence, these drawings depict Pierre performing a headstand; the last of them, however, in which he actually stands on his head, shows his right arm rising from the ground and his right leg bending as if to indicate that he is about to flip over again and come right side up. Thus, a process is indicated: the drawings suggest that although a child may indeed turn himself upside down, he can right himself as well. This motif also signifies in the dramatic action: not only does Pierre infuriate his father by talking to him from a feet-up posture early on, but later the lion, having swallowed Pierre, must in turn be turned upside down in order to release him.

The lion, we note, comes onstage only after Pierre's parents leave. In abandoning their (dependent) young child, parents may become, in that child's fantasy, bad and threatening, for they display, as it were, their trump card: their ultimate power to desert. In this (Kleinian) sense, the lion represents also the projected badness of the abandoning parents. In addition, their absence leaves Pierre without external objects on whom to vent his aggression; thus, it now turns against him and must be confronted. In keeping with the oral theme of *The Nutshell Library* and the developmental imperatives of its young readers, the lion not only threatens (with words) but actually eats Pierre (Pierre disappears from the page). Before this, however, Pierre is informed that, after being eaten, he will be *inside* the lion;

in other words, things will be *inside out:* the child's projected aggression will consume him. Thus, the upside-down motif extends to encompass that of inside-out.

Significantly, when the parents return, they do not hesitate to aggress directly against the lion (the mother pulls his hair and the father lifts a chair to strike him). At no point in the story previously, however, did either parent attack Pierre. It is the child's triumphant aggression, his bad introject they attack, not the child himself. This important distinction is made by both sign systems, image and text. It powerfully implies the ongoing love of these parents for their child and the survival of that love in the face of developmentally induced negativity.

Verbally and pictorially, both parents conform to conventional gender stereotypes: mother calls Pierre "darling," offers him food, cries and hugs him when he emerges from the lion; father disciplines him, criticizes, commands, reasons, bargains, and asks him if he is all right when he reappears. Thus, typical roles inscribed by our culture are reinforced by the picture book. Mother wears high heels, a fur-trimmed coat, and a whimsical hat; father sports a mustache, an overcoat, and a fedora.

In the end, not just Pierre but also the parents are shown riding home on the lion, thus indicating that mastery of aggression is an issue not only for children but for entire families. Riding—as a symbol for control and mastery—occurs again, parenthetically, in *Where the Wild Things Are,* where Max (a visual double for Pierre) rides one of his introjects in the wild orgy scene. (One also recalls Freud's 1923 metaphor of the ego riding the forces of the id.) Finally, it matters that Pierre's lion does not depart ignominiously but, rather, stays on with the family. Thus, aggression is portrayed as an ongoing theme that will not vanish but must be continually addressed.

VIII

My effort in this paper has been to indicate, with the aid of psychoanalytic developmental theory, the impact of the picture book on young minds, its role in the process of acculturation, and its value for interdisciplinary studies.[3] Deceptively simple, this genre establishes—by means of image, text, performing adult, and attentive child—a space in which fantasy blossoms, psychological issues are symbolically enacted, and the roots of cultural knowledge pleasurably implanted.

"Culture" derives from the Latin *colere* which means "to till, to husband, to raise, to nurture." If we view culture in the light of this etymology, as a nurturing matrix for the growth of symbolic and semantic structures, it comes into sharp focus as a setting for early drive and object relations. Thus, while Greenacre (1957) has proposed the notion of "collective alternates" in the life of the gifted child, we may wish to extend her usage and accord a higher priority to significant artifacts in the lives of all children—especially to those artifacts uniquely designed to appeal to them, indoctrinate them, and expand their mental function. In closing, it is well to add that an essay such as this inevitably raises larger questions as to the deep impact of culture on psyche—its inextricability, perhaps, from biologically derived determinants.

Notes

Versions of this paper were given as Child Psychiatry Grand Rounds at New York Hospital-Cornell Medical Center, Westchester Division, and at the Gardiner program in Psychoanalysis and the Humanities, Yale University. I wish to thank Drs. Albert Solnit and Paulina Kernberg and the members of their respective groups for stimulating discussions that led to revisions of this paper. Also, I wish to acknowledge the support of the National Endowment for the Humanities Summer Institute on

"Image and Text" (1988) under the direction of Michael Fried and Ronald Paulson of Johns Hopkins University.

1. I am indebted to the perceptive literary insights of Cheryl Torsney (1986) and gratefully acknowledge her permission to draw on them.

2. The text says, curiously, that when Pierre fell out, he "laughed because he wasn't dead." In keeping with the Judaic motifs that interweave Sendak's works (e.g., the Yiddish expression *wilde chaye*—wild animal—which underlies his marvelous conception of the "wild things," and the stars of David in both *In the Night Kitchen* and *Dear Mili*, where Hebrew letters are engraved on the tombstones), Pierre's particular laughter at this moment of survival can be interpreted as evoking the biblical Isaac (Yitzchak, "One who laughs"). Pierre, like Yitzchak in the Akedah (the binding, Genesis 22: 1–19) survives what could only be experienced by a child as the extremity of parental aggression and abandonment.

3. A propos this impact, picturebooks designed with avowedly ideological aims deserve at least a mention here. In a recent lecture, Professor Yosef Yerushalmi (1988) presented repugnant examples of widely circulated Nazi picturebooks for children from the 1930s. These depict the Jew as a fox or, in one book, as a poisonous mushroom. In the latter book, blond German youngsters are shown distinguishing Jews from Aryans as noxious fungi that must be differentiated from safe, edible species. Sparks of bigotry and hatred, thus kindled, are not in later years easily extinguished.

References

Bemelmans, L. (1939). *Madeline*. New York: Simon & Schuster. (More recent edition, Penguin, 1987.)

Brown, M. W., and Hurd, C. (1947). *Goodnight Moon*. New York: Harper & Row.

Fisher, C. (1988). Further observations on the Poetzl phenomenon. *Psychoanal. Contemp. Thought*, 11: 3–56.

Freud, S. (1923). The ego and the id. *Standard Edition*, 19: 3–66.

———. (1939). Moses and monotheism. *S.E.*, 23: 3–137.

Greenacre, P. (1957). The childhood of the artist. In *Emotional Growth*. New York: Int. Univ. Press, 1971, vol. 2, pp. 479–504.

———. (1958). Early physical determinants in the development of a sense of identity. In *Emotional Growth*, vol. 1, pp. 113–127.

Johnson, C. (1955). *Harold and the Purple Crayon*. New York: Harper & Row.

Kernberg, P. (1987). Mother-child interaction and mirror behavior. *Infant Mental Health Journal*, (Winter) 8: 4.

Knight, H. (1964). *Where's Wallace?* New York: Harper & Row.

Kunhardt, D. (1942). *Pat the Bunny*. Racine, Wis.: Golden.

Leaf, M. (1937). *Noodle*. New York: Four Winds.

McDonald, M. (1970). Transitional tunes and musical development. *Psychoanal. Study Child*, 25: 503–520.

Plato. *The Dialogues of Plato*, trans. B. Jowett. New York: Random House, 1937.

Scarry, R. (1964). *Is This the House of Mistress Mouse?* Racine, Wis.: Golden.

Sendak, M. (1962). *The Nutshell Library*. New York: Harper & Row.

———. (1963). *Where the Wild Things Are*. New York: Harper & Row.

Spitz, E. H. (1988). Picturing the child's inner world of fantasy. *Psychoanal. Study Child*, 43: 433–447.

Thurber, J. (1943). *Many Moons*. New York: Harcourt Brace Jovanovich.

Torsney, C. B. (1986). *The Nutshell Library* as literary primer. Unpublished essay, read to the Modern Language Association.

Ungerer, T. (1967). *Moon Man*. New York: Harper & Row.

Wildsmith, B. (1962). *Brian Wildsmith's ABC*. Oxford: Oxford Univ. Press.

Winnicott, D. W. (1956). The antisocial tendency. In *Collected Papers*. New York: Basic, 1958, pp. 306–315.

———. (1966). The location of cultural experience. *Int. J. Psychoanal.*, 48: 368–372.

Yerushalmi, Y. (1988). Alisa in Wonderland: The book and the Jewish child. Lecture at the Jewish Theological Seminary, December 7.

Pimping and Midwifery

REFLECTIONS ON ART AND
PSYCHOANALYSIS
RICHARD KUHNS

A natural connection between history and psychoanalysis would seem to stem from several sources: the emphasis in psychoanalysis on the early childhood of the individual, the assumption that every symptom has a history, and the high value placed by psychoanalysts on art and culture. Moreover, psychoanalytic thought has, from its beginning, looked to ancient Greek, Elizabethan, and Romantic works of art for examples and inspiration. And yet with all its dedication to the past, psychoanalytic theory has seemed surprisingly and paradoxically ahistorical. By that I mean that the inquiries of art historical scholarship and literary history are more often than not ignored or neglected in psychoanalytic interpretations of art and of artists. Rather, the early psychoanalytic interpretations concentrated on the psychobiography of the artist, neglecting the larger historical context within which the artist lived and worked; an approach we might characterize as names without history, as contrasted with the opposite pole—history without names. And yet, the founders of psychoanalysis and the psychoanalytic theory of art—Freud himself, Ernest Jones, Otto Rank—were hardly ignorant of history, and were steeped in the cultural tradition in which they were writing. So one might suppose that they could readily have added the dimension of historical context to their interpretations.

This neglect of historical context has inspired acrimonious attacks on psychoanalytic interpretations and is one of the reasons why on a more benign level academic and psychoanalytic clinical researchers simply fail to meet on common ground. Academically trained art historians and literary critics—even today when theory that denigrates "history" is all the rage—display a historical interest that the psychoanalytically trained theorists ignore or override, as if they were deconstructionists *avant la lettre*, or on the other hand analytical philosophers working in the positivistic tradition of the twenties and thirties. And yet we know that the psychoanalysts and the deconstructionists ignore history for opposite reasons. The deconstructionist cannot "know" the reality of the past; meaning can only be determined in the present moment. For the psychoanalyst meaning is essentially timeless. In *The Interpretation of Dreams* Freud (1953a) writes: "Shakespeare's *Hamlet* has its roots in the same soil as *Oedipus Rex*. But the changed treatment of the same material reveals the whole difference in the mental life of these two widely separated epochs of civilization: the secular advance of repression in the emotional life of mankind. In the *Oedipus* the child's wishful phantasy that underlies it is brought into the open and realized as it would be in a dream. In *Hamlet* it remains repressed." Though the conscious manifest expression reflects the conditions of the contemporary cultural setting, the underlying meaning is unchanging and timeless. This position is also highlighted in the controversy around the criticism directed to Freud's study of Leonardo da Vinci. Meyer Schapiro (1941), who faulted Freud's study for not taking account of some of the iconographic conventions of the period, was answered by Kurt Eissler (1961). In replying to the accusation of psychoanalytic blindness to the historical, Eissler argued that not only is the psychological dimension of art always relevant whatever the historical realities may be, but further that the validity of the psychological interpretation is established independently of the historical context.

This psychoanalytic indifference to the historical contexts within which works of art and culture exist has resulted in reductionist analysis and limited conceptions of these objects. However, those of us who continue to take a psychoanalytic interest in art and culture wonder whether an interpretation which is historically richer yet remains insightfully psychoanalytic cannot be established. An incidental but significant benefit would be that psychoanalytic approaches to art would become a more integral part of academic endeavors, and would come forward to meet objections to psychoanalytic interpretations often directed against them by philosophers, and by art and literary historians. While today the history of art and literature occupies a central position in the university, it is a disappointing but not surprising fact that the psychoanalytic is merely stitched into the fringes of the departmental tapestry, remaining virtually isolated from the resources and training of traditional academic scholarship. I propose that if we begin by looking at psychoanalytic theory and these early psychoanalytic studies of art and culture from the vantage point of philosophy, we can see that in the original formulations there was a profound but often unnoticed philosophical influence on early psychoanalytic theorizing. I refer to the philosophic thought of Hegel, about which I shall say a few words.

Freud grew up in a Hegel-dominated cultural universe. Though we have no record that Freud read Hegel, that was unnecessary, for Hegel's thought defined an important part of the philosophical world in which Freud's thinking developed. The lectures Hegel presented at Berlin in the 1820s were during Freud's lifetime being transformed into the discipline we call art history. If we add to that the importance and excitement of the archeological uncoverings of Schliemann at Troy and the discovery of the Cro-Magnon caves at Altimara and elsewhere, we establish further the events that riveted the attention of Freud's intellectual world. Psychoanalysis incorporated these cultural speculations and actual digs into the past into its *Weltanschauung*. And these events provided the well-known metaphor employed by Freud in his description of the psychoanalytic method of investigation and treatment. However, Freud (1964) said that the Weltanschauung of psychoanalysis was that of modern science, and he failed, it would seem, to formulate the broad philosophic elements of the cultural setting that more silently shaped his own thinking.

Turning to the interpretation of history and art generated by Hegel, in those lectures I have already referred to, Hegel's thought was this: that the story of art could be told with a new structure that the idealistic philosophy of Hegel established, a structure that organized the total past into one evolutionary-developmental narrative. In that narrative art itself forms one chapter, to be followed by chapters on religion and philosophy, reflecting a sequence of development, for art evolves into those later, more encompassing, theory-generating cultural products whose ultimate expression is philosophy. It is philosophy that now interprets art for *art is at an end*. That is one of Hegel's disturbing conclusions, one that is today much argued over. What does it mean, and how has it come to influence psychoanalytic thinking? We might ask, how Hegelian was Freud?

To ask that question is to open up a complex inquiry that in itself requires historical reconstruction; my answer is but a bit of that totality. In its most basic hermeneutical structure Freud's method of interpretation, as laid out in *The Interpretation of Dreams,* can be said to be Hegelian in this sense: the distinction between manifest and latent content mirrors, whether or not it was conscious on Freud's part, the distinction Hegel maintains between historical description and inner spiritual meaning. Like Hegel, Freud regarded his theory as defining a method whereby the moves from manifest to latent and back again can be made. Further, Freud's view of history and the ways in which the past is to be interpreted shares with the Hegelian philosophical theory certain basic points of view. One is that modernity can now reinterpret the past and understand it under a new theory, the psychoanalytic theory. The second is that the past falls into eras or periods which are clearly distinguished one from another on both conscious and unconscious levels of thought. Freud's attempt to write the history of culture in these terms is to be found in *Totem and Taboo* (1953b), where he organizes the evolution of human consciousness and its unconscious latent base in three periods: animism, religion, and science, with psychoanalytic theory, finally, standing as interpreter of the preceding stages. In this we can see parallels to Hegel's discriminations of the history of art into the Symbolic, the Classical, and the Romantic, concluding with Hegel's own philosophy, which stands over all the artistic phases as their interpreter. Consequently, we find that in both theories there is a radical reformulation of the relationship between modernity and the past. Hegel said art was at an end, and he believed that the art of the past could be unlocked, interpreted to reveal its inner spiritual meaning through his philosophical method, which was simply his philosophy. Freud claimed art was now revealed to exhibit a psychological inner meaning that was repressed, put out of consciousness because it was painful and threatening. Freud saw himself as the discoverer of the method of interpretation whereby the latent repressed content could be brought into consciousness. Therefore we see in the thought of Hegel and Freud the belief that modernity is privileged as a scientifically insightful and in some sense "liberated" moment. Both thought that through their theories a new freedom and a more adequate understanding of both past and present would be gained.

When we think of Freud's evolutionary stage theory, however, we generally think of it in the individual sense more than we think of it as a theory of history. That is, to put it most simply, Freud's stage theory of oral, anal, phallic, genital often occurs to us as his more central concern and we usually put in the background his thoughts on animism, religion, and science. But they go together and they mirror one another so that in this sense also Freud is Hegelian. The triadic structures are disposed not only in time but constitute also, as it were, metaphorically a cross section in space. And that which unfolds in history also can be seen unfolding in the life history of the individual. Phylogeny recapitulates ontogony, in the psychoanalytic sense as well as in the embryological sense.

We might ask, then, looking at the parallels and similarities between Hegel's thoughts about the history of culture, and Freud's thoughts about both the history of culture and the history of developmental stages in the individual, how this is reflected in our situation today as posthistorical thinkers; what is meant by the phrase we hear so often today: the end of art; the end of history?

To regard the postmodern condition historically: the disconcerting awareness that history must be at least written differently, if not given up altogether, comes from art historians who look back to the way art history was written by, for example, Vasari, and later Hegel. The underlying assumption was that the story of art had a beginning, a middle, and an end. And that if we try to tell the story of art in modernity according to that model, it will no longer work. The art of today appears to be fragmented, stylistically ununified, and enclosing within itself elements of past modes of making that are neither a condition of decadence, nor a condition of original breakthrough toward a new unified style. In short, the art world of today presents a chaotic front. In the face of that confusion, the art historian poses a question: may it be that art history as a discipline structured as it has been in the past can no longer be supported and justified by the evidence? Perhaps art history as we know it is at an end. And further, may it be the case that this fragmentation suggests the truth of the thesis Hegel put forward: that art itself is at an end? Or at least, though it goes on in some ways, that art no longer satisfies and serves the spiritual needs it once did serve and gratify? And by further extension, we might be tempted to argue—some have been—that history itself is at an end and we live in a posthistorical world. What could that mean? In essence, it suggests that we cannot write history as we once did—not that events no longer occur, or that we cannot chronicle our own time and place, but that the unfolding of events does not exhibit an evolutionary pattern.

Now let us shift for a moment to the contemporary condition of psychoanalytic theory. There has been, I believe, an analogous attack upon traditional ways of conceptualizing the person and the culture that characterized early psychoanalytic writings. If it is true that Freud lived in a Hegelian universe and absorbed a way of conceptualizing the person and culture in stages in a kind of dialectical evolution as Hegel did, then we might see the attack on early psychoanalytic stage theory (psycho-morphology), as a part of a larger intellectual dissatisfaction and ferment of which I have just spoken. That is, we might pose a parallel question: is psychoanalytic history of the person now to be reconceptualized in and by means of a post-stage theory? One may note the questioning, reformulations, and rejection of drive theory in object relations theory, and in significant reformulations within recent classical writing (Schafer, 1976, 1983), as well as the revision of the concept of stages following upon sophisticated critical examination of development in infant observation (Stern, 1985). The profound influence of Winnicott's writing, at once original and category defying, is well known (Winnicott, 1971). Paralleling these theoretical reformulations is the description of the symptomatology of our time in terms of alienation, fragmentation, and identity diffusion; concepts so different from the neater, clearly delineated categories of the past.

Another way to put it is this: evolutionary theories of history and of the person grew up together in the late eighteenth and early nineteenth centuries, and we now look back to those theories with a critical eye. For the historian, this means we must write and conceive of history differently (just how is part of the posthistorical intellectual argumentation of this time we live in); and for the theorist of the person and psychic life in general, it means we must develop clinical and cultural theory of the person in new and more adequate terms.

However, though we are in a posthistorical frame of reference this does not mean that we derogate the models of evolutionary development postulated by Hegel and by Freud. Hegel, for his part, really established art history as a discipline; and among his philosophical contributions we recognize the creative insight that led to the assertion that cultural products and events have a history. And for his part, Freud developed a model of growing up that challenged the whole tradition of western biology and medicine. When I say that we are witnessing a renovation of Freud's evolutionary-developmental theory parallel to the renovation of Hegel's postulations about art history, I do not mean to suggest that these original and profound contributions have been or ought to be overthrown. Rather, the revisions of cultural theory that have occurred in the historical disciplines like art history suggest ways of gaining a more adequate theory of culture by looking from psychoanalytic theory to the challenges that have taken the form of questioning the possibility of history in our time.

Let us think then of the postmodern era as suffering from that which Freud called *Entfremdungsgefühl*. We are alienated from our feelings in a way that makes us feel dead, and turns us into confirmed skeptics. We say, "I see, but I do not believe," as Freud said to himself, standing on the Acropolis in Athens, "By the evidence of my senses I am now standing on the Acropolis, but I cannot believe it" (Freud, 1953c, p. 243). And Freud notes: "These phenomena are to be observed in two forms: the subject feels either that a piece of reality or that a piece of his own self is strange to him. In the latter case we speak of "depersonalizations"; derealizations and depersonalizations are intimately connected." The contemporary postmodern pathology may be seen as a form of Entfremdungsgefühl, but while Freud described the condition in terms of inner conflict, generated by a private developmental sequence, we today suffer from a feeling of cultural disconnectedness, of being distant from the past and from cultural objects. This state is reflected in those theories we refer to as "post" whatever—postmodern, postdeconstruction, postanalytic—by which we mean that we experience today a crisis of meaning so that we say history is at an end, objects have no constant content, meaning is only a function of the self.

I propose that one of the symptoms of cultural alienation is the mania for collecting and buying works of art, which one might see both as a symptom and as an attempt at self-healing. The museum has become a cultural warehouse crammed to the rafters with more than we can ever internalize and know. To own is to be; I own, therefore I am: this is the way we define our existence today. Our Cartesianism expresses itself not in thinking but in collecting. We are avid for justifications so that we can give purpose to an activity that has frequently become ludicrously aimless, empty, and witless.

I believe that a revivification of purpose and a sense of our own place in history can only be established if we attend more closely to a small selection of objects and the ways they function for us. Hegel's and Freud's closed systems no longer provide an adequate model. Today we replace the closed model by an open systems model, a model I shall sketch out, and so I would like to say a few words about the need to conceptualize a third space; the cultural space. I have found Winnicott's concept of the transitional object to be a significant contribution to the examination of this problem.

In postulating a third area, I believe that Winnicott is developing in his own way the epistemological model of modernity. Winnicott thought of his model as a revision of the traditional scientific-empiricistic model, which placed external reality on one side and subjective experience on the other. Winnicott imported into that model Freud's model, which added the unconscious to the side of subjectivity. However, Freud on the whole accepted without further revision the remainder of the scientific-empiricistic model. Freud's conceptualization of the unconscious made the model symmetrical by balancing the inferences that the natural sciences made to the external world with the inferences the psychological sciences (i.e., psychoanalysis) made to the internal world of the unconscious and primary process thought. However, in Winnicott's words, "A statement of human nature in terms of interpersonal relationships is not good enough even when the imaginative elaboration of function and the whole of fantasy, both conscious and unconscious, including the repressed unconscious, are allowed for." In elaborating that intermediate area of experiencing, the transitional space, Winnicott wrote, "I am here staking a claim for an intermediate state between a baby's inability and his growing ability to recognize and accept reality. I am therefore studying the substance of illusion, that which is allowed to the infant and which in adult life is inherent in art and religion, and yet becomes the hallmark of madness when an adult puts too powerful a claim on the credulity of others." In his discussion he notes further, "At this point my subject widens out into that of play, and of artistic creativity, and appreciation and of religious feeling and of dreaming," along with the pathological developments which also have their roots in this area of experience. So just as Winnicott said there is no such thing as a baby, but only a baby and a mother (1971), so we may say there is no such thing as a work of art, but only a work of art and an artist and a viewer at a point in time.

In adding a third space—the play-culture space—between external physical reality as dealt with by the natural sciences, and the internal physical reality dealt with by psychoanalysis, Winnicott did not elaborate an interpretative method to be used in tracing the development of and in analyzing the mature adult experience of the third space. A method appropriate to that space requires the integration of the psychoanalytic with the cultural sciences of philosophy and history.

Further, to require that the model have a historical dimension is to add to Winnicott's model a time component. Winnicott's focus was on the spatial component: the "third area" exists between internal psychic reality and external natural world. What is in the developed third realm? I will call the events "enactments," which would include works of art, the self of the artist, the history of art and culture. The self of the artist is a real presence in the third realm. I shall say a word about enactments.

Let us define culture as a tradition of enactments. And let us characterize enactments by means of the properties which the word itself represents. Enactments are complex objects with four dominant properties: 1) they are events whose presence declares an intention; 2) they are performances requiring space and time; 3) they are effectively charged objects (highly "cathected"; *Besetzung*); 4) they are representations that refer to other objects and events, both internal, external, and historical.

To grow up in culture is to experience and to know the objects that fill the third area or space. Some of those "objects" are theories that refer to external reality (physics, bio-chemistry, engineering) and some are theories that refer to internal reality (psychoanalysis, psychiatry). The diagram that I have envisioned represents psychoanalytic theory as I have repositioned it, a theory that mediates between nature (external reality), and culture (the intermediate space) on the one hand, and between culture and the internal realities of the mind on the other. There are three areas in which the psychoanalytic method of interpretation gives access to a dynamic interplay at a boundary: 1) the boundary between conscious and unconscious; 2) the boundary between nature and culture as dealt with in the cultural sciences; 3) the boundary between experience and external orders of nature and society. Those theories concerned with the study of cultural objects are the theories of the cultural sciences, *Geisteswissenschaften;* and those theories concerned with external nature are the theories of the natural sciences, *Naturwissenschaften.* A theory that has the power to analyze and explicate the middle ground, as I propose that psychoanalysis does, is a kind of critical theory as meant by the Frankfurt School. Psychoanalytic theory as I conceive it both explains a set of events—I would refer to them as "transitional events"—and provides understanding of the observing self, the person who comes to know those events as part of a cultural tradition. Psychoanalysis, so conceived, is a higher-order theory of the Geisteswissenchaften that stands above the theories of the so-called "social sciences," for it talks about their interpretations as well as offering its own interpretations. Such a theory encompasses aspects of both Hegelian and Freudian conceptualizations; that is, it is concerned with objects such as works of art, and with names, such as the names of artists. And this higher-order theory has a further requirement: to place or locate the user of the theory as a self within the field of study. Psychoanalytic theory of art and culture, as I am redrawing its boundaries here, embraces observer as well as observed; it has a sensitivity to the artist as well as to the work of art, to those who use the theory as well as to the events interpreted by the theory.

I shall turn now to two paired examples whose historical location and context determine part of the meaning they generate for us in the present.

Boccaccio and Buffalmacco (1313–1375; c. 1350)

The *Decameron*, a Renaissance *Gesamtkunstwerk*, takes as its cognomen *Principe Galeotto;* the Prince Galeot, the Pimp. By this we are to understand both an allusion and a method of reading the book. The allusion is to Dante's *Inferno* (Canto v) where Paolo and Francesca indict the book that made them lovers (the story of Lancelot and Guinivere) as a pander. The line in Canto v is, "Galeotto fu 'l libro e chi lo scrisse"; "A Galeotto was the book and he that wrote it." Once we have recognized the source of the cognomen, the implications for the *Decameron* become also a directive for reading. That is, in this case allusion looks backwards and forwards, and is itself, in a condensed way, historical. This book, the *Decameron,* is a pimp. What does that mean? There is a long tradition going back to Plato that conceives of the creative person, the artist, and even the philosopher, as like a pimp and a midwife. In the *Theaetetus* Socrates says: "There is an unscientific way of bringing men and women together, which is called pandering, and midwives, since they are women of dignity and worth, avoid matchmaking, through fear of falling under the charge of pandering. And yet the true midwife is the only proper matchmaker."

Socrates goes on to make the ironic point that he himself is merely a midwife, and by implication a pander; and indeed elsewhere he refers to himself as a pimp (*mastropos*). For his only power is to help others to give birth, and to examine the health of the newborn. Though infertile, he sees himself as possessing the power to bring fertile couples together to produce offspring. This he does through exciting them to a sexual frenzy. The philosopher-pimp uses the lure of sex to lead the seduced youth to intellectual mastery. The Socratic method is "soul-doctoring"; replacing the body object with the mind object. And with that miraculous foresight of genius, Socrates in the *Phaedrus* describes himself as a psychotherapist (soul doctor).

In adumbrating the meaning of the cognomen of the *Decameron,* and by metaphoric extrapolation, I can now understand how to read the book. It is a Principe Galeotto, a pimp and a pander, that uses sex on behalf of a higher, philosophic goal. But it does not stand alone in this endeavor; it draws upon all the arts to this end. The art closest to its content and method is that of the painter, Buffalmacco, who is the most frequently encountered real character in the *Decameron,* appearing in several of the stories in Days VIII and IX, and whose grand fresco, "The Triumph of Death," was displayed in the Campo Santo in Pisa during Boccaccio's lifetime.

Looking at the panorama of this Trecento artistic fantasy several interconnections to the *Decameron* become evident. Boccaccio and Buffalmacco have created transitional objects through whose agency we are joined to the complex historical reality of the Italian Trecento. Within "The Triumph of Death" we see not only the ravages of the plague that drove the Brigata (the ladies and gentlemen of the *Decameron*) out of Florence; we see also the garden where the three youths and seven maidens rescue themselves with song and story. It is my contention that this scene establishes an intimate link between the work of the two artists, and I believe that they exercise toward one another a kind of cultural power of inter-inanimation, by which I mean they give life to each other. The cultural power expressed by these enactments establishes relationships which, borrowing the terms of psychoanalysis, I would term a kind of transference and countertransference among enactments. By extending the use of these psychoanalytic concepts from persons to objects, I intend to establish a psychodynamic interpretation of tradition. Culture, I have said, is a tradition of objects. Now I would add: objects are not inert, not out there to be given whatever meaning we arbitrarily impose upon them; but they are experienced out there in their inter-inanimation, nurturing, as it were, their presences like persons who are in constant conscious and unconscious "conversation."

Looking again at the emptiness and relativism of the postmodern alienation of feeling, Entfremdungsgefühl, I believe that the psychoanalytic concept of transference can help us to understand our experience of the loss, and how we seek to repair that loss through a way of being with objects. There is a way of being with objects that lets them work in and through their inter-inanimations so that we see them not only in their confluence of contemporaneous meanings, but also in their historical settings.

The close interdependence of image and story has always been recognized. Here, in the amazing breakthrough of 1300 in Italy, when the new discoveries in material art, particularly fresco painting, pushed the development of art to a new visual accomplishment, new ways in which objects become psychodynamically interpreted are established. That is, through what I call a transference and countertransference relationship, narrative in language and narrative in images exchange powers. The *Decameron* contains painting within itself; it has internalized a material art, as it has also internalized a tonal art in its songs and dances.[1] The *Decameron*, then, is a historical transitional object that carries us back to Trecento, Italy. It exemplifies a fundamental unity in the arts in its own content, for it uses each art in a way that transfers its special, individual force to the other arts, and they in their interrelationship then create the aesthetic transitional object that allows us to move through the tradition of objects, to be at home in culture. And that being-at-home is what we feel has been lost in the postmodern period. But art object as transitional object has the potential to overcome our bereavement.

Psychological interpretations at this point must surrender to the demands of history. It is not enough to explore Boccaccio and Buffalmacco as makers of entertainments, linguistic and material. Their world is that of the Trecento—when the idea of "the end of art" was totally absent—but we can enter into that world of explosive inventiveness here and now, as a way of achieving a purpose in living that is an expression of Eros, of love. And that is the task of the artist-pimp, the Principe Galeotto, who joins couples as we are joined to objects with a definite purpose: new life.

Three hundred years later (and from the time of the Trecento, each period of three hundred years realized a dramatic change in the arts of visual representations) the conditions we meet and must interpret are those which mark the beginning of modernity.

Watteau and Kant (1684–1721; 1724–1804)

My two examples here encompass painting and philosophy. Philosophy and art in the modern period develop a new relationship that repeats, but carries to a new level of self-consciousness, the interdependence of the Athenian philosophers and artists, especially the writers of tragedy. The Enlightenment painter and the Enlightenment philosopher create between them a theory of cultural objects: one concerned with the fate of art itself (painting in the case of Watteau's work "Gersaint's Shopsign") and the other concerned with the fate of human beings, whose encounters with nature generate a deep conflict. First, the painting.

Watteau's painting is itself about painting, as befits a painting that serves as a shop sign. As we look into the shop (as if we were looking into a box) we have the voyeuristic pleasure of watching the art of painting, through its sensuous examples, stimulate erotic attractions and postures. Painting is a Principe Galeotto. Not only are the well-dressed bourgeoisie sticking their rumps out at us; they attend the noble thighs and posterior of a painted goddess, who elicits amorous advances. Her counterparts in the room (of course they too, for us, are painted), the beautiful women, gaze into mirrors to admire themselves and to solicit our admiration. Every glance is at once narcissistic and envious. The rich assemble here in this room—as we, the museum onlookers, assemble in our room that looks into the painted room—to be carried into the land of fantasy that the painter through his representation can create and sustain. It is a scene that we enter into through the agency of the object, our pimp, who promises adventures in erotic pleasures. However, we, like the painted folk, must hurry, for time presses and we shall not endure, as the clocks warn us. But with that reminder of life's shortness we cannot help but see the painting itself as timeless and enduring.

Not only is time a coercive force in the shop where art reigns; space too asserts its intuitional necessity. We live in space as well as time, and in this painting space beckons us: there is another space behind the space, a blue atmosphere that may be simply emptiness, or may be a space behind the space of the painting into which we might move to escape the harsh realities of painting, history, and the fate of matter; a fate that the painting itself as a material object must eventually suffer, though it saves itself as art.

As a material thing, "Shopsign" has had a weird career. It itself represents the world of art's commercialization, for now no longer are artists in the permanent employ of the monarch; the monarch must compete in the marketplace for his paintings alongside everyone else, just as the agent for Frederick the Great bought this painting in Paris, from Gersaint. It was sent to the Charlottenberg Palace in Berlin where it was cut in half, and two parts hung in the music room (some say the dining hall). And thus began the passion of the simple shop sign. In the process a bit of the top was cut off to give it a rounded edge; and in 1760 a marauding Russian soldier put a sword through it. Relief from its divided and slashed state came only in 1930, when it was stitched together and given once more its wholeness as art.

Relating the beribboned busts and satiny laps to our blue-jeaned stance in the Metropolitan Museum of Art is the peasant or worker standing at the edge of the shop, and the dog intent on biting a flea. The figure of the lower classes looks downwards and into himself; the dog looks at us but without seeing. Only we, the viewers, view with our eyes as painting is meant to be taken in, yet as we look, we suffer the curse of modernity: the marvelous world of art, here collected for us in our business and our social competition, is yet incomplete. What is it we lack? Painting—as is true with all the arts—cannot exist as art simply through being collected. The painting shows us the object-ness of art, but not its aesthetic essence. For that we need something of a reflective theory. And that was attempted, for modernity, in the thought of the philosopher, Kant.

The reality of art was far more complex, and aesthetic theory far more troubled than Kant's speculations present to us. In one sense Kant is retrogressive, in another he is radically ahead of other thinkers when he turns to the arts. I pair his thought (*The Critique of Aesthetic Judgment*) with the painting of Watteau because painter and philospher share a deep insight into the nature of art, and they illustrate the role of pimp and midwife as I metaphorically rely upon those terms to describe the creators' contributions to tradition. It might have seemed blunt and insensitive to the philosopher Kant to be placed in such low company, but his writing on art had a profound influence on the transitional phenomena of art, and the transitional behavior of artists and critics. The Third Critique, as it came to be known, was widely read, and through immediate translation affected both French and English thought. His arguments—in some instances better referred to as fantasies—provide a didactic complement to Watteau's vision in "Gersaint's Shopsign."

The basic search in both cases, that of philosopher and painter, is for an aesthetic domain in which we may find ourselves at home in contrast to the alienation and experience of Entfremdungsgefühl that we experience in nature before it is transformed and interpreted through the arts. Psychoanalytic contributions to an understanding of this condition begin with Freud's penetrating essay "The Uncanny" (1955). And I find one way to "read" both Watteau and Kant is with the help of Freud's essay. I shall not do that here, but simply offer my reading of the central argument of Kant's amazing study.

Kant says some of the things Watteau expresses, although much of Kant's argument is repressed, as if it too were part of a painting in which we are given figures and a "scene" but no written explanation. Kant's deepest insight is this: experience in nature confronts human beings with a double and often conflicted response to objects. One strand is that of the beautiful, the other that of the sublime; the two strands are not coordinate or even coherent, but the source of, on the one hand, satisfaction and pleasure; and on the other hand, fear, dread, and anxiety, although accompanied by an overwhelming—sometimes almost suffocating—excitement. In this conception, we see that Kant, in his defended and repressed way, suffered the turbulence of Romanticism in his philosophy.

The determinism of nature is met with and countered by the compulsion to repeat: laws of nature are rigid and deterministic; compulsion-repetition is rigid and repetitive, like the determinism of nature. But artistic compulsive repetition makes each object anew, in structures that are the work of genius; that is, lawlike, but not predictable. The artist faces off against nature; the puck is cast down; the two antagonists fight for the symbol; if nature wins, the artist dies; if the artist wins, nature is transformed into the comfortable garden-place of nature before the Fall. And the artist achieves the only immortality human beings can have: the only resurrection we can realize is the resurrection of art. In Kant's philosophic fantasy, the artist figures as a kind of hero, one who redeems humankind through his agency as maker-genius. Our lot in this natural order is made more auspicious, and even perhaps given some grounds for expectation of ease. For though we die, through the arts we live in an Edenic order in which at last we feel at home.

Historically considered, art searches for its right intention. Odd as that sounds, it is both a historical and a psychological claim. It is a claim that psychoanalytic theory can investigate and perhaps throw light on. For intention expresses itself in enactments and is one of the purposes they exhibit in history; enactments, however, are always individual products of individual psychic structures that organize the objects (enactments) in primary-process and secondary-process orders of thought. We have to determine whether or not primary-process thought is historically determined. I believe it is, but that requires much further study. It may be the case that the symbolic materials utilized in primary-process thought derive from the historical reality within which the artist works. There is no doubt that secondary-process thought expresses the presuppositions of an era, a people, a circle, a school.

If my comments have any claim to truth, then I conjecture that our interpretative strategies must be developed beyond our current methods, or rather, our current methods ought to look again at the views that twentieth-century positivism attempted to discredit, especially that mode of inquiry referred to as *verstehen,* in which the past is conjured up as if lived. Here psychoanalytic understanding can be helpful, for it seeks interpretative means through psychological reality, that is, through conscious and unconscious representations. It is the unconscious representations of art that provide the means to "live in" the past with something approaching full understanding of a point of view (a *Weltanschauung*) that differs dramatically from our own. But, as Mannheim pointed out, we shall never grasp fully our own unconscious assumptions; psychoanalysis when applied to the past can expose the unconscious assumptions of a distant time, yet always in terms of our own way of seeing. That is a constant relativism, one built into the human condition. So although I believe that the psychoanalytic can open up the enactments of the past to a deeper understanding than heretofore, the psychoanalytic method, like all methods in the cultural sciences, has built-in limitations.

So, beginning with the raising of the theoretical speculation upon the end of art, the end of the history of art, and the sense we have today of being alienated from the past, I have tried to give a somewhat psychological interpretation of the condition I called part of postmodernity, that condition Freud referred to as suffering from *Entfremdungsgefühl.* This feeling of alienation, which is endemic to our era, has led intellectuals who make theory to assert that we are in a post-post time beyond the past, which is to say we can no longer feel connected to a tradition, but must either cut free from any sense of tradition or join ourselves to all traditions. Well, that is part of our trouble, the need to encompass all while feeling at home in none. The psychoanalytic way with art and culture can diagnose and interpret, but it cannot mend or cure. The present therefore remains in some deep sense a time of alienation except that we can see how that alienation came to be and perhaps use that understanding in a new sublimation that will hoist us out of the slough of despond into which we have fallen and which we try to purify and clarify by means of minimalist theories of culture; theories for the post-post era in which we live. Let us use the availability of the tradition of cultural objects to project a more fruitful beginning. Yes, instead of bewailing the ending, let us begin afresh, . . . but here is the rub: we cannot know if that which we do and project is in fact a new beginning until it too has its ending.

As we study the examples I have presented along the way, we can see that they metaphorize living and leaving. And that is the task of transitional objects—to let us live in the world, and to help us when the time comes to leave the world. Joining couples that they may love is the pimp's work; bringing their offspring into the world is the midwife's job. From a cultural point of view, the artist and the work of art perform as pimp and midwife—and occasionally the philosopher has the stamina and imaginative creativity to do that too.

Notes

This paper was presented as part of the William Alanson White Institute's series "Psychoanalysis and Contemporary Culture," April 8, 1991.
1. See the thorough investigation of the power of inter-inanimation from painting to linguistic art and back again in Hans Belting, *Malerei und Stadtkultur in der Dantezeit* (Munich: Hirmer Verlag, 1989).

References

Eissler, K. (1961). *Leonardo da Vinci: Psychoanalytic Notes on The Enigma.* New York: International Universities Press.

Freud, S. (1953a). Interpretation of Dreams. *Standard Edition*, vol. 4, pp. 264–65. London: Hogarth.

———. (1953b). Totem and Taboo. *Standard Edition*, vol. 13.

———. (1953c). Disturbance of Memory on the Acropolis. *Standard Edition*, vol. 22, p. 243.

———. (1955). The Uncanny. *Standard Edition*, vol. 17, p. 217ff.

———. (1964). *New Introduction Lectures,* Lecture 35; "The Question of a *Weltanschauung,*" *Standard Edition*, vol. 22, p. 158.

Guess, R. (1981). *The Idea of A Critical Theory: Habermas and the Frankfurt School.* Cambridge: Cambridge University Press.

Hegel, G. W. F. (1975). *Aesthetics: Lectures on Fine Art.* Translated by T. M. Knox. Oxford: Clarendon.

Schafer, R. (1976). *A New Language for Psychoanalysis.* New Haven: Yale University Press.

———. (1983). *The Analytic Attitude.* New York: Basic.

Schapiro, M. (1941). Leonardo and Freud: An Art Historical Study. *Theory and Philosophy of Art: Style, Artist and Society.* New York: George Braziller, pp. 153–92.

Stern, D. (1985). *The Interpersonal World of the Infant.* New York: Basic.

Winnicott, D. W. (1971). *Playing and Reality.* London: Tavistock.

5

Psychoanalysis and Culture

Materialism, Humanism, and Psychoanalysis

CHARLES HANLY

Materialism, or naturalism, is the dominant ontology of our century. Materialism, in this sense, should not be confused with materialism as the pursuit of creature comfort and wealth. There is nothing wrong with these aims in themselves, but someone who espouses naturalism is not committed to their pursuit as the only or necessarily the most important aims of life. Naturalism, which is opposed to philosophical idealism, consists of at least these five tenets: matter is the substance of things and the ultimate source of their activity; there is no transcendental, unifying "ultimate reality" beneath or beyond the material furniture of the world; there is no teleology in nature; ideals should be judged according to the benefits they bring to people; the only way we have of discovering what is real is by means of scientific knowledge and pragmatic common sense, deepened by the insights into human nature expressed in art, literature, and philosophy. Naturalism is compatible with altruism; it only states that the expectation of a reward for it in an afterlife is not compatible with the best available information about what to expect.

Scientific discoveries continue to turn up facts about man and the world that support these tenets. To these facts, Freud had already made a contribution before he embarked on the investigations that led him to create psychoanalysis. In the late 1880s Freud, while a medical student, demonstrated features of the structure of the nerve cells of a primitive fish species that indicated their continuity with human nerve cells (Jones, 1953;

Gay, 1988). Freud's finding is an epitome of the direction of scientific discovery generally, insofar as it tends to confirm man's origin and destiny in nature and disconfirm the belief, still held at the time, that man's special creation would be vouchsafed by unique neurological features. It was not without reason that Freud proudly classified psychoanalysis, Copernican cosmology, and Darwinian biology in disturbing "the peace of this world" (1917, p. 285) because like them, psychoanalysis offends "the *naive* self-love of men" (p. 284).

Psychoanalysis implies a materialist ontology. Psychic life owes its existence to the brain, the organ of the mind. Those who would impute a mind-body dualism to psychoanalysis fail to appreciate that Freud's (1900) assumption that psychological processes could be investigated in their own right was methodological rather than ontological. It did not have the Cartesian or Platonic implication that the psychical could exist in its own right. Drives, which play such an important role in Freudian psychology, originate in physical needs, which very early become elaborated and experienced as wishes that motivate behavior. These wishes soon undergo transformations as a result of the action of defenses. And the defenses, while they can be studied psychologically, do not exist as purely psychic processes. Their actions are sustained by neurological activities about which we are still in the dark. And although sublimation, for example, changes the nature and quality of motives, behavior, and experience so that the result is no longer the same as the originally wished-for experience, the modified wish owes its existence to its more primitive original. Yet not a few humanists within and without psychoanalysis have found these ideas unacceptable. They have wanted to discard them along with the rest of Freud's metapsychology as being, like the *Project for a Scientific Psychology,* a vestige of nineteenth-century mechanics. It is claimed that Freud's working psychological premises, which are not those of the metapsychology, are to be found in his case histories and in his work on applied psychoanalysis.

But I think that it is a mistake to cleave Freud's case histories and his humanistic studies from his metapsychology. To be sure, the case histories are populated by convincingly drawn lives of complete personalities, as Freud ruefully acknowledged when he likened his case histories to short stories. But his patients are convincing because they are not disembodied; they are physical persons rooted in their bodies, in nature, in their families and society. In the metapsychological papers the ego, id, and superego are psychic processes with differentiated organizations, functions, and interrelations. They refer to the activities of thought and perception, desires and aversions and conscience in people. They are not structures of a separate psychic entity. The fundamental part Freud's theory assigns to sexuality in the formation of individual identity, character, and psychic functioning generally is only consistent with the idea that man is an evolved, rational animal. To claim that, because psychoanalysis is an exclusively psychological therapy, the psyche must be some sort of separate entity is mistaken. What happens in the brain is influenced by the nature of the excitations to which it is submitted. Psychoanalysis is a sufficiently powerful psychological process that it can bring about whatever organic changes are involved in the amelioration of such debilitating physical symptoms as impotence or frigidity. The discoveries which form the bedrock of Freud's psychology—infantile sexuality, dream psychology, symptom formation, processes of defense, the dynamic unconscious of drives and ego—as well as the theory in which he couched them support naturalism in just the way that the discoveries of Copernicus and Darwin do. This has posed a serious problem for those humanists who find humanism and philosophical materialism to be incompatible.

Psychoanalysis is not a philosophy (Freud, 1933) but a science that has important philosophical implications. In modern philosophy, Freud's contribution to the definition of human reality remains somewhat more of a challenge than an achievement. This is so despite the fact that the positivism of three great nineteenth-century predecessors of Freud—Comte, Mill, and Eliot—combined humanism with materialism and causal determinism. But since Freud, phenomenology (Sartre, 1943; Merleau-Ponty, 1945), which has been a major force in European philosophy, has reasserted the primacy of consciousness and rejected psychic determinism. Merleau-Ponty protests, "I am not the outcome or the meeting-point of numerous causal agencies which determine my bodily or psychological make-up" (p. viii). Wittgenstein, who first formulated the verification theory of meaning, concluded the *Tractatus Logico-Philosophicus* (1918) with the oracular statement, "That whereof we cannot speak, that thereof we must remain silent." The verification theory of meaning became the cornerstone of logical positivism and was used as a weapon to beat down idealist metaphysics. And although Wittgenstein did not in the *Tractatus* or later in *Philosophical Investigations* (1958) provide a basis for the meaningfulness of metaphysical assertions, there remains the ambiguity of the *Tractatus*'s conclusion. It could mean that there is nothing beyond nature about which to speak. Or it could mean that there is something beyond nature that has to remain a mystery because we cannot describe it. If the latter interpretation is correct, Wittgenstein's utterance provides an implicit defense of religious intuitions and mystical experiences about man, nature, and deity by protecting them from rational examination. Wittgenstein's early interest in psychoanalysis (one of his sisters was acquainted with Freud) gave way later in his life to his warning his students against it (1966). Ordinary language philosophy, which was inspired by Wittgenstein's later work but of which he approved no more than he did logical positivism, shared, initially at least, the animus of logical positivism against idealist metaphysics. But ordinary language philosophy proved to be a method sufficiently supple to accommodate science and religion. Each has its own vocabulary and provides its own contexts for giving meaning to it. Ordinary language can be used to defend psychic determinism or to reject it. By applying Ryle's account of mental concepts, MacIntyre (1958) was able to make the unconscious disappear into behavior. The hermeneutic school (Habermas, 1971; Ricoeur, 1970) has embraced psychoanalysis but in doing so has drawn its serpents' teeth; its narcissistically wounding theories of psychic determinism and the causal dependence of mental processes on physical ones. The hermeneutic school denies to psychoanalysis the place in natural science to which Freud assigned it. In this, the hermeneuticists are in agreement with the philosophers of science (Nagel, 1959; Popper, 1963; Grunbaum, 1984) who deny that psychoanalysis is a body of scientific knowledge. The philosophers of science add that in order to be taken seriously, psychoanalysis would have to be a successful empirical science. With this requirement Freud would have been in agreement.

This account is incomplete. But so far as it goes, it is a tale of the difficulty some of the most influential philosophers of our age have had in accepting psychoanalysis and working out its implications for philosophy. This is not surprising. Not a few psychoanalysts have had similar difficulties in accepting psychoanalysis. Some have used ideas borrowed from philosophy to modify psychoanalytic theory in order to make it approximate more to human nature, out of a disbelief that scientific postulates can comprehend humanity. Binswanger (1942) created existential psychoanalysis by carrying out a Heideggerean revision of psychoanalysis. Hermeneutic philosophy as well as ordinary language philosophy have been used by psychoanalysts to dispense with metapsychology. Even though this picture is one-sided, insofar as it does not include reference to the work of philosophers such as Hampshire, Hospers, Feuer, Lazerowitz, Wisdom, and Wollheim—who have, in various ways, exploited the resources of psychoanalysis to pursue philosophical inquires—none of these philosophers has influenced twentieth-century philosophical thought as much as those referred to directly or indirectly above. For the most part, philosophers have greeted psychoanalysis with indifference, they have criticized it, or they have made it over into something that Freud had not intended it to be.

But perhaps the assumption that psychoanalysis has something to contribute to philosophy is mistaken. Ryle (1949), after referring to Freud as "psychology's one man of genius" (p. 324), goes on to declare, "Let the psychologist tell us why we are deceived; but we can tell ourselves and him why we are not deceived" (p. 326). This cautionary division of labor would limit psychoanalysis to being a psychology of the neurosis, which of course it is, and leave to philosophy the description of healthy mental functioning. Psychoanalysis can safely be left to rummage about in the dark basement of the mind, but the mind's sunlit upper stories, where reason and morality reside, are the residences of philosophy. Ryle acknowledges that he himself, like others, does not know why he dreams or is sometimes tongue-tied in the company of certain people. He acknowledges that these goings-on raise psychological questions about their causation that require psychological answers. But so do some actions that he considers to have no psychological determinants at all. For example, Ryle says, "We know quite well why John Doe scowled and slammed the door. He was insulted." But there are other ways in which John Doe might have acted. He could have insulted back. He could have demanded an explanation from his insulter. Questions do arise. Why did John Doe take flight? Did he resentfully believe that there was some truth in the insult? If so, why? I do not wish to take more time speculating about the hidden motives and character traits of the anonymous John Doe except to suggest that there are theoretical reasons for wondering whether or not Ryle's John Doe is an anonymous expression of a group of repressed memories of his own. If this were the case, then there might be a psychological explanation for Ryle's need to philosophically shut the door on psychoanalytic enquiry. And if this were the case, then the reasons that philosophers have for the ideas they hold—including the philosophical ideas espoused in this presentation—may also be open to psychological explanation. Perhaps the upper stories of the mind are more connected with the basement than we like to think on the basis of a psychology informed only by conscious introspection and the more or less empathic observation of others. To this theoretical question, psychoanalysis does not have an a priori answer any more than there is deductive proof of my speculations about Ryle's unconscious reasons for insulating a large group of behaviors from psychoanalytic enquiry. The existence and nature of these connections have to be established empirically.

Let us explore one of several such connections that has a direct bearing upon philosophy. Morality is one of the characteristics (others are consciousness, freedom, rationality) that has been considered to be uniquely human and to warrant for man a special status in nature. It is true that human beings are able to know that something that they want to do is wrong and to refrain from doing it. There are things that we ought to do because they are right and we do them whether or not we want to do them. We are subject to categorical imperatives which dictate moral duties to us: what we ought to be, what we ought to do, and what we ought not to do. They exercise a powerful influence upon our lives both in what we do and how we feel about ourselves. Failure to live up to their demands can cause loss of self-esteem and depression. The repudiation of their injunctions can cause debilitating guilt. The introspective experience of moral conflict can leave the impression of the very dualism between physical desires and morality that led Plato and Kant to believe that moral reason has an origin and destiny beyond nature.

Freud has shown that moral ideals and categorical imperatives have a natural origin in the psychological development of the individual. To vastly oversimplify, they arise out of the identifications children form with the parents of the same sex, which form the core of the processes involved in the resolution of the Oedipus complex. This identification becomes the nucleus of the child's capacity to autonomously evaluate himself and his motives, and to regulate his actions. The prohibitions and permissions that once were imposed on her, the girl is now able to impose on herself and, with further ego and drive development, to test for herself.

Freud left this process of identification incompletely described, giving rise to a problem. Why is it that the identification involved in the resolution of the Oedipus complex is with the parent of the same sex when it is the parent of the opposite sex who has to be abandoned? The process of identification described in *Mourning and Melancholia* (1917) would suggest that the identification should be with the parent of the opposite sex. In the case of the oedipal identification, the object of the incestuous feelings is relinquished in favor of a strengthened identification with the rival object, because the sexual wish can only be satisfied by becoming like the rivaled object, even if this requires a delay and a detour. Thus the choice of identification is caused, on the side of the drive, by the tenacity of the libidinal wish and, on the side of the ego, by the humiliating realization that the sexual ambition greatly exceeds the capacity to do anything about it. This realization combines with the fear of punishment to oppose the drive demand. The strengthened identification with the parent of the same sex is the best compromise available. Thus five factors reinforce the image of the parent as an ideal: the need for libidinal gratification, the need to avoid punishment, the need to avoid narcissistic injury, the overestimation of the parent, who enjoys the forbidden pleasure, and the continuing need to preserve the affectionate, anaclitic tie to the parent. Also of great importance is the measure of realism that informs these factors; the tolerance for deferral and delay and differentiation between the ego as it is and as it would be. The resolution of the Oedipus complex and the groundwork for further development toward a mature moral conscience is consolidated by the repression and sublimations guided by the parental identification.

In this all too inadequate exposition, pre-oedipal preparations for the development of the superego and the contribution of identification with the parent of the opposite sex have not been mentioned. But rather than attempt to repair this fault, I would like, in this context, to focus upon another aspect of Freud's work about which humanists who have a legitimately high regard for critical thinking may wish to be reassured. One cannot read Freud's scientific work without forming a vivid impression of the high value he attached to reasoned criticism, which he regularly practiced on his own theories. It would be a failure to respect this value if one were to simply pass over in silence aspects of Freud's theory of the psychogenesis of the capacity for morality in human beings that remain or have become doubtful. Freud's hypothesis of the genetic inheritance of the Oedipus complex and the superego prohibitions was and remains inconsistent with what is known about the biochemistry of genetic inheritance. Freud's theory does not require the hypothesis. All that Freud's theory requires is that children be genetically predisposed to undergo a precocious phallic/clitoral sexual development during the period when they remain dependent for their survival on their parents or their substitutes. Freud's hypothesis of the acquisition of morality by women through cross-inheritance is not required by his theory either. This idea was needed to supplement the hypothesis of archaic residues, which was in turn linked by Freud to his speculation that humanity originated in an oedipal enactment. Freud's (1913) scientific myth of this enactment, unlike the Hesiodic myth, for example, casts women in an entirely passive role, uninvolved with the fateful events, merely awaiting the outcome, and profiting only secondarily and derivatively from the physical and mental travail undergone by the men. Finally, Freud drew upon the death instinct to account for the severity of the superego. Freud's psychological explanation of the genesis of adult morality in the resolution of the Oedipus complex does not require these special phylogenetic hypotheses. Identification as the mechanism of cultural inheritance, under the psychological conditions of the Oedipus complex, can account for an involuntary acquisition of values en masse, as it were, and the motives to enforce them without reliance upon a phylogenetic inheritance or a death instinct. The girl's fear of maternal punishment, and the pain of hating and wanting to destroy the very person who had been for so long and so recently the recipient of her anaclitic love, need be no less effective in repressing her Oedipus complex than castration anxiety in the oedipal boy. Childhood amnesia is no less common and no less extensive in women than in men. These qualifications of Freud's account of the genesis of morality in human beings only serve to render it consistent with what is now known about genetics and "the dark continent." The essential core remains intact. Freud's theory describes a fundamental truth about the human condition. It can provide to philosophy a key element in its search for a reality-bound understanding of human nature.

It explains why, according to nature, human beings should experience themselves as being subject to moral imperatives that have the character of divine ordinances or natural laws, without having the least idea as to how this has come about.

However, the direct influence of psychoanalysis on twentieth-century philosophy should not be exaggerated. For although it has made a number of crucial contributions to the construction of the edifice of modern positivism and humanism, these contributions still go largely unrecognized and unused by philosophers and humanists. Nagel, who has been one of the best exponents of naturalism in contemporary philosophy (1954), has also been one of the severest critics of psychoanalysis (1959). Naturalism in philosophy does not depend upon psychoanalysis. The tendency of scientific discovery and of evolving daily individual experience of reality provide sufficient evidence for the tenets of naturalism without psychoanalysis. Nevertheless, psychoanalysis has a unique contribution to make to the creation of a reality-bound humanism whether or not philosophers exploit these resources.

There are other limitations as well. The psychoanalytic account of individual psychological development and functioning presupposes that psychical processes are activities of the brain and central nervous system. It is based on the premise that an empirically accurate psychological explanation of character, psychical defenses, drive fixation, regression and maturation, psychic structure, and so forth will be consistent with their neurological and biochemical explanations when these explanations are found. But the psychoanalytic method does not enable psychoanalysis to reach beyond the psychological to the organic substrate.

Similarly, although psychoanalysis can give an account of the origins of morality, it is not itself an ethic any more than it is a political ideology or a religion. But psychoanalysis does bring morality down from the Olympian heights of religion and metaphysics to render it more serviceable to the needs of life. Psychoanalysis encourages a constant evaluation of moral beliefs and practices not so much according to the sacrifices they impose but according to the benefits they will bring. Freud (1930) explored the extent and inevitability of instinctual dissatisfaction. But Freud considered resignation to be a necessity to which one must submit rather than an achievement that authorizes the self-righteous determination to impose further sacrifices upon oneself or others. Freud identified the conflict that lies at the heart of human nature. In order to survive childhood and prepare for maturation, one must repress spontaneously occurring sexual and aggressive wishes; in order to reach maturity one must relinquish these wishes and repressions as much as possible. By clearly and realistically describing the consequences of unnecessary sexual repression, Freud set in motion a reevalution of sexual morality and a search by individuals for a more integrated and gratifying personal life that goes far beyond philosophy. From the perspective of generations who, hopefully, will be able to enjoy its benefits without suffering its excesses and failures, this process in our culture will probably be seen to have had many false starts and bizarre turnings. At its best, it will have brought about as much reconciliation as nature will allow with what, besides birth and death, is most representative of nature in man—the sexual and aggressive drives. Freud's observations led him to the view that the most effective means of controlling the drives is through their gratification; this self-mastery is best when it is achieved through the gratification of sexual love between a man and woman and through the gratification of aggression in work. In this view there is a certain element of stoicism, as well as the more obvious hedonism of the pleasure principle. It is a stoicism not of resignation, but of submission to the demands of our own instinct life. The ego is, as it were, called upon to give up its narcissistic, omnipotent, illusory mastery of the drives for the less ambitious and more realistic task of finding fitting objects and actions for their satisfaction.

Freud's account of the genesis of morality has the advantage of being able to help us understand how and why morality, values, and ideals can go wrong. By explaining their genesis and the nature of their power, psychoanalysis teaches us not to idealize ideals and offers the potential for an improvement in moral education (potential that is very far from being realized). This century has witnessed appalling spectacles of violence and devastation for the sake of ideals. The ideals that rationalized the recent German conquest of other nations and the Holocaust were experienced by multitudes and their leaders as ennobling, higher purposes of such worth as to justify any sacrifice. (Freud admired German militarism in the early phases of the First World War until he became aware of the senseless cruelty of the war and the component of envious hostility in his pride and anxiety concerning his soldier sons.) It has been claimed that the violence that has occurred in our century has been facilitated by a scientific culture that, having undermined traditional faith, has left people vulnerable to the pursuit of strange gods. The bizarre claim has been made that psychoanalysis helped to create the cultural conditions that fostered Nazism. Psychoanalysis is a godless doctrine just as any other natural science is, but unlike others it can help us understand why men need to submit themselves to gods of destruction, and, despite Freud's pessimism about it, perhaps learn how to find better alternatives. As a therapy, I have never observed psychoanalysis to have any other than a civilizing influence upon aggression.

If the considerable opportunities for direct contributions of psychoanalysis to philosophy are still largely ignored by philosophers, an indirect influence has been exerted through what one might call vernacular psychology. Of course, many academics still wish to ignore psychoanalysis and to ridicule those who take it seriously. And this attitude is preferable to that of those who would cleanse psychoanalysis of "the stench of mortality" and dress it in fine academic robes. That Freud never appreciated such efforts is evident from his reply to Einstein, who expressed his long-standing admiration for the beauty of the logical structure and literary expression of Freud's ideas, but who reported that he had only recently come upon some evidence that had convinced him of the correctness of the repression hypothesis. Freud replied, "Of course, I always knew that you admired me only out of politeness and believed very little of any of my doctrines, although I have often asked myself what indeed there is to be admired in them if they are not true, i.e. if they do not contain a large measure of truth" (Jones, 1957, p. 203). Yet every humanist, whether philosopher, historian, or literary scholar, must frequently rely on a background of psychological ideas in his or her work, and these ideas not occasionally form premises of arguments. As Freud himself said, his ideas concerning infantile sexuality, the Oedipus complex, the primacy of sexuality in life were already part of a vernacular psychology before he gave them scientific formulation and made them available to systematic observational testing, building the foundation for a new therapy. It was a vernacular psychology upon which the poets (in the generic sense) relied and to which they contributed—a psychology of character, motives, and relationships. The poets, on the whole, have been better at this underground work than theologians. They have been obliged to enlighten by entertaining and thus, while they have not abandoned morality, they have had to be curious about sin, whereas the theologians could only contemplate it by chastising it, an attitude of mind that interferes with its observation, let alone its just appreciation. Philosophers have existed uneasily somewhere between the poets and the theologians—too intent on being rational to be either pious or profane. Freud recognized the intuitive, sometimes only implicit, grasp of the concepts of repression, the dynamic unconscious, and the Oedipus complex in, for example, Plato, Diderot, Schopenhauer, and Nietzsche. Psychoanalysis has had a great impact upon the general culture as a result of its influence on literature and the arts, but also upon the healing and educating professions.

Among the strengths of the secular twentieth-century spirit has been the iconoclastic pursuit of realism and efforts to ameliorate the human condition. This spirit has not dominated modernity but it has been present. There can be no question that this is the spirit that Freud gave to psychoanalysis. It is to be found everywhere in his work: in his early studies of hysteria, which exposed the inadequacies of both the poorly sublimated humanistic moral attitude toward the illness and the fatalistic organic-genetic understanding of it; in his psychology of dreams, which at once removed dreams from the realms of mysticism and superstition and physiological disorder. Many more examples could be enumerated.

Two characteristics of Freud's work are especially important in defining the spirit of his thought. His iconoclasm was inadvertent. It was a by-product of his search for the facts of human nature and the theoretical formulation of their significance. It was a by-product of his demand for self-honesty and realism. The psychology that he created from this search is not psychologizing—that is to say, it gives the organic its due, as any scientific psychology must. If one were to summarize all of this one might say that Freud's work represents what is best in the scientific and the humanistic spirit of our age.

It is not surprising that psychoanalysis has, without trying to, come to have an indirect influence on philosophy. At the very least, it establishes limits. Reason, to which philosophers are especially committed, can no longer be regarded as the sovereign, autonomous, even self-sufficient function that it had previously been conceived to be. Arguments such as Descartes's and Locke's argument that the idea of an unconscious thought is self-contradictory are no longer as convincing as they once were. Psychoanalysis has raised doubts about the veridicality of consciousness even when it confines itself to its own contents. Introspective knowledge has been toppled from its throne. But one must be careful not to exaggerate or to allow enthusiasm to push one beyond the limits of realism. Sartre (1943) not so long ago "refuted" the hypothesis of an instinctual unconscious using an edition of Locke's (1689) argument. However, it is also true that existentialism is as dead as ordinary language philosophy. Perhaps part of the reason for the demise of existentialism is the sense of incredulity that is aroused by a theory of motivation that has to assert, as a consequence of the denial of a dynamic unconscious, that a pedophile is a pedophile because he chooses to take pleasure in sexual relations with children and that he could choose to be a mature heterosexual by choosing to take pleasure in sexual intercourse with women were it not for his putting this equiprobable alternative out of play by, in bad faith, attributing his sexual preference to childhood trauma. This kind of mind control can now be more easily recognized for the illusion that it is. And perhaps this incredulity is, in part at least, a consequence of the preconscious influence of a vernacular psychology that has been influenced by Freud's discoveries, even on those who would not identify themselves as Freudians.

I dare conclude by asking why psychoanalysis has been greeted with so little enthusiasm by philosophers because the same question can be raised about psychoanalysts as well. From psychoanalysis's earliest days some of them have shown a remarkable zeal for reforming Freud's findings by reinterpreting them, on the basis of conceptual innovation rather than on the basis of new facts. I believe that part of the reason for this more or less universal reaction to psychoanalysis is alluded to by Freud in his comment to Einstein. Just about anyone would prefer to find the facts of human nature and the human condition to be different than Freud found them to be. The degree of disquiet these ideas arouse in anyone is directly proportional to the extent to which the memories that might confirm them are subject to repression. Philosophers have rightly objected to this line of argument when it has been used in an ad hominem way to reject counterarguments and their evidence. Freud would have agreed with the objection. He pointed out (1927) that to trace the belief in God to the wish for a God does not by itself falsify the belief. However, the probability that the belief in God is only a wishful idea is greatly increased by the failure of every attempt by philosophers to construct sound arguments to prove its truth. To state it paradoxically, people believe in God because the world is not such a place as an omnipotent creator who had the best interests of people at heart would have created. Nature is not always very user-friendly as far as we humans are concerned. A realistic awareness of the world causes in us irremedial feelings of helplessness that tend to motivate a belief in a being sufficiently powerful and beneficent to bend the course of nature to our needs. What we believe is not always what we choose to believe, any more than what we do is what we choose to do.

If philosophers, like some psychoanalysts, have wanted to repudiate or dilute psychoanalysis, it is in part, I believe, because they have thought it not to be a humanity. And there is a still-pervasive received definition of humanity that makes this perception true. This definition, which was originally religious, has been retained in thoroughly secular and even atheist schools of thought. The essential idea of this definition is that man is not altogether part of nature. The details differ but the idea informs Sartre's distinction between *pour soi* and *en soi,* as it does the unspoken meaning beyond meaning in Wittgenstein's thought. It is an idea that requires the assertion, in some way, of the uniqueness of consciousness, the differentiation of motives from causes, the repudiation of psychic determinism and the drives, and the autonomy of moral values, judgments, and actions. This idea has always been a necessary part of Judeo-Christian religious belief. Our ancient religious ancestors demonstrated their ingenuity and fitness for survival when they managed to protect their still-uncertain grasp on reality—and their belief in God that helped to secure that grasp—with the guilty illusion that they were themselves responsible for all those things in life and the world that caused them so much pain and helplessness. In this illusion, there is implicit the narcissistic, omnipotent thought, "what a being is he whose misdeed has brought about such a transformation of nature." This narcissistic compensation contributed to shaping Judeo-Christian cosmology by imposing on it the teleological axiom that man is the meaning and purpose of nature. Modern secular philosophers have accepted and integrated the findings of science that have destroyed the traditional cosmology, but some (certainly not all, for many philosophers belong to the naturalist school) have retained, as it were, a window of narcissistic opportunity that allows some degree of retention of the old pride of place for man in nature.

Although the humanism inherent in psychoanalysis deprives man of the status of cosmic sinner or fallen god, it provides an understanding of how and why such beliefs about man persist. This understanding is at the same time a caution against exaggerating the resources of psychoanalysis. Accidents, disease, natural catastrophes, and death may be subjectively associated with castration. But overcome our castration anxiety as we may, we will not thereby have altered our vulnerability to them in the least. Human beings, who are obliged by nature to value their own existence and to strive to protect their own persons, cannot help but be somewhat narcissistically offended by the hazardousness and, at best, indifference of nature. Anxieties that cannot be reduced by realistic action cause illusions. While such illusions are contrary to reality-bound reason, they are evidently not contrary to nature. The remarkable thing is not that people cling to illusions, but that they have managed to give them up to the extent that they have. The psychology that Freud founded has contributed greatly to whatever education to reality our century has been able to achieve. Freud's contribution to the development of a modern culture that continues to struggle to replace traditional religious values and beliefs about man and his place in nature with scientific knowledge are unique and fundamental. Freud's psychology is at once a science of the human psyche, a therapy for its disorders, and a humanity that illuminates the comedy and tragedy of human existence.

References

Binswanger, L. (1942), *Grundformen und Erekenntnis des menschlichen Daseins*, 2, Aufl. Zurich: Niehans, 1953.

Freud, S. (1900), The interpretation of dreams. *Standard Edition*, 5.

Freud, S. (1913), Totem and taboo. *Standard Edition*, 13: 1–161.

Freud, S. (1917a), Introductory lectures on psycho-analysis. *Standard Edition*, 16: 284–285.

Freud, S. (1917b), Mourning and melancholia. *Standard Edition*, 14: 237–258.

Freud, S. (1933), New introductory lectures on psychoanalysis. *Standard Edition*, 22: 1–182.

Gay, P. (1988), *Freud: A Life for Our Time.* London: J. M. Dent & Sons.

Grunbaum, A. (1984), *The Foundations of Psychoanalysis.* Berkeley: University of California Press.

Habermas, J. (1971), *Knowledge and Human Interests*, trans. J. J. Shapiro. Boston: Beacon.

Jones, E. (1953), *The Life and Work of Sigmund Freud*, vol. 1, p. 48. New York: Basic Books.

Locke, J. (1689), *An Essay Concerning Human Understanding*, ed. Peter H. Nidditch. Oxford: Clarendon, 1975.

MacIntyre, A. C. (1958), *The Unconscious*. London: Routledge & Kegan Paul.

Merleau-Ponty, M. (1945), *Phenomenology of Perception*, trans. C. Smith. London: Routledge & Kegan Paul.

Nagel, E. (1954), Naturalism reconsidered. In *In Quest of Value*, ed. F. C. Domineyer. San Francisco: Chandler, 1963, pp. 71–84.

Nagel, E. (1959), Methodological issues in psychoanalytic theory. In *Psychoanalysis, Scientific Method and Philosophy*, ed. S. Hook. New York: Grine, pp. 38–56.

Popper, K. R. (1963), *Conjectures and Refutations: The Growth of Scientific Knowledge*. London: Routledge & Kegan Paul.

Ricoeur, P. (1970), *Freud and Philosophy*. New Haven: Yale University Press.

Sartre, J. P. (1943), *Being and Nothingness*, trans. H. E. Barnes. New York: Philosophical Library, 1956.

Wittgenstein, L. (1918), *Tructatus Logico-Philisophicus*, trans. C. K. Ogden. London: Routledge & Kegan Paul, 1922.

Wittgenstein, L. (1953), *Philosophical Investigations*. New York: Macmillan.

Wittgenstein, L. (1966), *Lectures and Conversations*, ed. C. Barrett. Oxford: Oxford University Press.

Devil's Religions

SOME REFLECTIONS ON THE HISTORICAL

AND SOCIAL MEANINGS OF

THE PERVERSIONS

JANINE CHASSEGUET-SMIRGEL

I'gin to be aweary of the sun
And wish the estate o' the world were now undone.
—Shakespeare, *Macbeth*

Freud's initial ideas on the subject of the perversions are to be found in a letter he wrote to Fliess on January 24, 1897, from which I shall quote a few extracts:

> The idea of bringing in the witches is gaining strength and I think it hits the mark. . . . Their secret gatherings, with dancing and other amusements, can be seen any day in the streets where children play. I read one day that the gold which the Devil gives his victims regularly turns into faeces; and the next day Herr E., who describes his old nurse's money deliria to me, suddenly (by a round about path via Cagliostro—the alchemist—*Dukatenscheisser*) said that Louise's money was always faeces. So in the witch stories it is merely being transformed back into the substance from which it arose. . . . I have ordered a copy of *Malleus Malificarum* . . . I shall study it diligently. The Story of the Devil, the vocabulary of popular swear-words, the song and habits of the nursery—all these are now gaining significance for me. . . .

I have an idea shaping in my mind that in the perversions, of which hysteria is the negative, we may have before us a residue of a primeval sexual cult which, in the Semitic East (Moloch, Astarte), was once, perhaps still is, a religion. . . .

Perverse actions, moreover, are always the same, with a meaning and made on some patterns which it will be possible to understand. I dream, therefore, of a primeval Devil religion, whose rites are carried on secretly, and I understand the severe therapy of the witch's judges. The connecting links teem. (p. 242–43)

Freud did not subsequently return to the ideas expressed in this text, but the striking fact is that he had no misgivings about juxtaposing phenomena as seemingly different as "deviant" forms of sexuality, popular beliefs, and witchcraft. The basic idea is that perversions are equivalent to "Devil religions." Freud's contribution to social anthropology, like his method, can be questioned but that is not my intention. I only want to point out that Freud clearly says there is a link between the internal and external worlds: the nuclear complex of the human psyche, i.e. the Oedipus complex, acts as an (unconscious) organizer of social space. It is at the root of ethics, religion, and the structuring of society. This, as we know, is a central theme of *Totem and Taboo* (1912–13) but already in *The Interpretation of Dreams* (1900) the theme is tentatively outlined when Freud attributes the origin of monarchy to feelings of veneration for the father.

Then, in "Obsessive Actions and Religious Practices" (1907) he establishes connections between obsessional and religious ceremonials, comparing obsessional neurosis to a *private religion* and highlighting the unconscious meaning of obsessional rituals and the hidden motives leading to the formation of religions: the two originate, in part at least, in guilt feelings. I intend to go back to Freud's initial intuitive view of the perversions as "Devil religions" and to try to give just a brief glimpse of the historical and social meanings attached to sexual deviations, since I cannot hope to deal at any length with so vast a subject in this essay. I shall in fact enlarge on ideas advanced in my work on the perversions and I apologize for any repetitions this will entail.

In viewing perversion as a Devil religion, we find two concepts of the Devil, the one relating to anality and the other to the "Luciferian" idea of the Devil, the "bearer of light" who snatched a spark of God's fire; the fallen angel who rebelled against the Creator. As regards this megalomanic aspect of the Devil, we find that the Vulgate names Lucifer in the prophecy of Isaiah (Chapter 14, verses 12–14):

> 12. How art thou fallen from heaven, O Lucifer, son of the morning! . . .
> 13. For thou hast said in thine heart, I will ascend into heaven. I will exalt my throne above the stars of God, . . .
> 14. I will ascend above the heights of the clouds; I will be like the most high.

Note that the original Hebrew Bible contains no mention of Lucifer.

Lucifer became henceforth part of the different Gnostic heresies or mystical theories, such as those of Jacob Boehme (Koyre, 1929). For those who rebel against the Creator, Lucifer represents the master and the model.

Whereas only Satan, the Adversary, the Accuser, the Slanderer (cf. Etudes Carmelitainis, 1948; de Urtubey, 1980) appears in the Old Testament, the idea of revolt against God, of the inordinate arrogance of appropriating the Creator's power, is nevertheless present from the start—with man's fall—and reappears, with the building of the Tower of Babel in particular.

As for the New Testament, Lucifer is prefigured in The Revelation of Saint John the Divine (the Apocalypse). The beast to which the dragon has bequeathed its power is a representation of Satan. ("And the great dragon was cast out, the old serpent called the Devil, and Satan, which deceiveth the whole world." [Chapter 12, verse 9]) It is endowed with truly "Luciferian" powers: "And there was given unto him a mouth speaking great things and blasphemies. . . . And he opened his mouth in blasphemy against God, to blasphemize his name and his tabernacle, and them that dwell in heaven" (Chapter 13, verses 5–6). Arrogance is the principal characteristic of Lucifer.

The "gentleman's" conception of the anal phase needs to be enlarged to gain a better understanding of the links Freud refers to in his letter to Fliess and in a few other later texts (in particular 1908). It is notable that we find that the Devil (Baal-Zebub, the stinking "Lord of the Flies") with his gift for fecalizing everything, including things of value, is capable of eradicating the genital order in favor of the anal universe.

In previous studies I have tried to show that whatever their content, perversions always unfold against an identical background of anal-sadistic regression. Their aim is to *destroy reality*, composed of differences, and in its place to establish the reign of anality where all differences have been abolished. Among other things, I have pointed to the well-known equation "feces = child = penis" (1917). A literal "interpretation" of the equation is central to the perversions. As a matter of fact, feces, unlike penises and babies, are a possession that is shared by adult and child, man and woman alike. A genital, impregnating penis implies male adulthood. Giving birth to a baby is the mark of a pubescent woman. On the other hand, the anal universe of feces, the anus, and buttocks is undifferentiated, a universe where differences of sex and generation have either ceased or do not as yet exist. At the same time it escapes the dimension of time since it ignores the necessity of growing up, or developing in order to acquire adult genital capacities. Additionally, because feces are constantly renewable, castration does not involve a definitive loss, in opposition to the next development phase, the genital one. Infantile helplessness has been banished, in fact. This is a world of magic, a fabulous sunken Atlantis to which one accedes through regression—to the detriment, it is true, of the sexual truth—and by denying the human condition, including the fact that the child can never be an adequate sexual object for the adult.

In previous works I have quoted many passages from the writings of Sade to supplement the clinical examples supporting my propositions. The Divine Marquis has nothing but contempt and repugnance for the vagina, "the shameful slit," and without exception his heroes loudly proclaim their preference for "that other temple," meaning the anus. I find it hard to consider that this is only an effect of castration anxiety related to the woman's lack of a penis. This is disparagement of the feminine attributes that distinguish the mother from father and son, and is aimed at effacing infantile insufficiency; in other words, the small boy's feelings of inadequacy, unable as he is to fill the maternal vagina and to give the mother a child. (As you will have gathered, I am speaking of the boy, because perversion is mainly a male disease, in the same way that hysteria or anorexia are mainly female.)

I would like to suggest that our understanding of the masculine castration complex should therefore be extended to include the young boy's painful feelings of inadequacy and the steps he takes to palliate these. Whole chunks of psychic life are involved here, the possibility being, in the case of perversion, a subsequent refusal of genitality with concomitant *idealization* of pregenitality, anality in fact.

It is important to understand the dual nature of Satan (symbolized as the Devil in relation to anality and as Lucifer in representation of man's arrogance in rebelling against God) because it brings a better understanding of the opposition between law and perversion and the relationship perversion bears to hubris, arrogance, and immoderation.

THE FORBIDDEN MIXTURE: HUBRIS AND HYBRID

To start with, I should like to call to mind some well-known passages from the Bible. Let us take the famous commandment: "Thou shalt not seethe a kid in his mother's milk." The commandment is repeated several times in the Torah (Exodus 23:19, Exodus 34:26, Deuteronomy 14:21). Psychoanalysts usually read into this a formulation of the law against incest (the mother and the child being united by the same substance: milk). But an article by Woolf (1945) goes a step further than this first approximation and puts forth hypotheses that are more convincing. Woolf disagrees with the interpretation of the commandment as symbolizing the law against incest, judging it to be insufficient. He bases his argument on a book by H. Bialik (1916) that points out that seething the kid in his mother's milk formed part of the worship of Astarte (Freud, we remember, compared perversion to the cult of Moloch and Astarte before defining it as a Devil religion in the letter to Fliess from which I have just quoted). Astarte is the goddess of love and fertility: "seething the kid in his mother's milk means placing the child back in its mother's belly, giving it into the full and undivided possession of the mother. The son belongs to the mother." Woolf's thesis is that the biblical commandment represents an attempt to destroy the matriarchal law. The child does not belong to the mother (Astarte, goddess of fertility and harvests). Consequently, the quality of *isolation* that characterizes ritual Jewish eating habits is the result of the struggle of Jewish monotheism against the paganism all around it, an intrapsychic struggle just as much as an external one. In essence, this commandment reflects the conflict between the matriarchal and patriarchal forms of society.

This very interesting hypothesis confronts us with the fact that "mixtures" (milk and meat in our case) imply *the father's exclusion* in favor of the mother-child fusion. In Leviticus, Chapter 19, verse 19, the Almighty says: "Ye shall keep my statutes. Thou shalt not let thy cattle gender with a diverse kind; thou shalt not sow thy field with mingled seed; neither shall a garment mingled of linen and wool come upon thee."

In the preceding chapter (Leviticus, Chapter 18, verses 6–17) the Almighty lists the commandments more closely connected with incest. However, I should like to point out that the aim of these commandments is to prevent the breaking down of the barriers set up to preserve the *essential nature* of things:

6. None of you shall approach anyone that is near of kin to him to uncover their nakedness: I am the Lord.
7. The nakedness of thy father, or the nakedness of thy mother, shalt thou not uncover: she is thy mother; thou shalt not uncover her nakedness.
8. The nakedness of thy father's wife shalt thou not uncover: it is thy father's nakedness.
9. The nakedness of thy sister, the daughter of thy father, or daughter of thy mother, whether she be born at home, or born abroad, even their nakedness thou shalt not uncover.

10. The nakedness of thy son's daughter, or of thy daughter's daughter, even their nakedness thou shalt not uncover: for theirs is thine own nakedness.

Verses 20–23 forbid adultery, the sacrifice of children to Moloch, homosexuality, and intercourse of a man or woman with an animal. Note that these biblical prohibitions are based on the principle of division and separation. In pathology this quality appears as an *isolation* mechanism at the root of obsessional neurosis. We know that in neurosis of this type anal-sadistic regression has replaced genitality, but that anal drives are subject to intense defense techniques. Freud (1926) associates isolation with the taboo of touching and bodily contact, whether it be aggressive or tender, with the object.

I have advanced that isolation in obsessional neurosis is a more generalized mechanism that tries to fight off the anal-sadistic desire for muddle and confusion. In this sense it would take the form of a reaction formation against the typically perverse ideas of indivisibility and amalgam (the reduction of objects to feces).

"The woman shall not wear that which pertaineth unto a man, neither shall a man put on a woman's garment." I quote from Deuteronomy, Chapter 22, verse 5. If we now turn to Genesis, we see that it is entirely based on the principles of distinction, separation, and differentiation: "In the beginning God created the Heaven and the Earth. And the Earth was without form and void." God brings order into this original chaos, the *tohu vabohu,* and divides it up:

> And God divided the Light from the Darkness. . . .
> God said: Let there be a firmament in the midst
> of the waters and let it divide the waters from the
> waters. And God made the firmament and divided

the waters which were under the firmament from the waters which were above the firmament. . . . And God said: Let the earth bring forth grass, the herb yielding seed and the fruit tree yielding fruit after his kind, whose seed is in itself, upon the earth: and it was so. And the earth brought forth grass and herb yielding seed after his kind, and the tree yielding fruit, whose seed was in itself, after his kind."

Verses 14 to 20 deal with the separation into night and day:

"And God made two great lights; the greater light to rule the day, and the lesser light to rule the night: he made the stars also. And God set them in the firmament of the heaven to give light upon the earth. And to rule over the day and over the night, and to divide the light from the darkness."

Verses 20 to 26 deal with the creation of animals:

"And God said, Let the waters bring forth abundantly the moving creature that hath life, and fowl that may fly above the earth in the open firmament of heaven. And God created great whales, and every living creature that moveth, which the waters brought forth abundantly, after their kind, and every winged fowl after his kind, . . . And God said, Let the earth bring forth the living creature after his kind, cattle, and creeping thing, and beast of the earth after his kind, and it was so. And God made the beast of the earth, after his kind, and cattle after their kind, and every thing that creepeth upon the earth after his kind: and God saw that it was good."

In this passage, the adverbial phrase "after their kind" is repeated like a leitmotiv. Now in this differentiation between the species we see no intermingling, or more precisely, an absence of hybridization. The commandment not "to sow thy field with mingled seed" is also translated as "hybrid seed." The man who does not respect the law of differentiation challenges God. He creates new combinations of new shapes and new kinds. He takes the place of the Creator and becomes a demiurge. Notice that the word "hybrid" comes from the Greek *hubris,* which means violence, excess, extremeness, outrageousness. Hubris is for the Greeks, we know, the greatest sin.

To me it seems that the biblical commandment prohibiting hybridization of seeds, materials, and animals in the name of the principles of separation and division, and the connection between this and the barrier against incest and perversion aimed at an amalgam, the return to undifferentiated matter, follows from what Mircea Eliade writes in this passage from his book *Blacksmiths and Alchemists* (1977):

> Maimonides explains that the Jews were forbidden to use lemons from trees that had been grafted, by a need to prevent the orgiastic practices that went on when neighboring peoples carried out grafting. Ibn Washya — and he is by no means the only oriental author to have let himself be carried away by such images — even speaks of grafts of various species of vegetable that were fantastic and "against nature" (saying, for example, that by grafting a branch from a lemon tree onto a laurel or an olive tree, lemons no larger than an olive could be obtained). But he specifies that the graft will only take when performed ritually at a certain conjunction of the moon and the sun. He explains the ritual as follows: "A

very beautiful young girl must hold the branch to be grafted in her hand, while a man has *shameful and against nature sexual intercourse* with her. During coitus, the young girl grafts the branch onto the tree." The meaning is clear: to guarantee the success of a union which ran counter to nature in the plant world, there had to be an against nature sexual union. (p. 28)

It seems clear that hubris, pride, immoderation, the wish to seize God's power, *hybridization*, are expressed in the mixture, in the wish to return to primal chaos from which a new reality will emerge, and that such an undertaking is consubstantial with perversion.

In Greek, the original meaning of *nomos,* the law, is "that which is divided up into parts." Thus we find that the principle of separation is the foundation of the law. A further meaning of nomos is "division of land" "province," "region," "pasture," "grazing land"—that is, direct applications of the principle of separation (Bailly Dictionary, 1894–1950).

Anomie implies confusion and undifferentiated values. For Kierkegaard, this is evil of the highest degree.

The noun has much in common with the law, considered as separation, division. It is a part of speech which names a person, place, or thing, which takes it out of chaos and confusion and gives it a definition. In fact the book of Genesis relates the story of creation not merely as a process of division and separation, but—and this comes to the same thing—as one of naming. In verse 5, it says: "God called the light Day and the darkness he called Night." When He made the firmament (verse 7), "God called the firmament Heaven" (verse 8). In verse 10, it says: "God called the dry land Earth and the gathering together of the waters called he Seas." So we begin to understand the fundamental reasons which oppose law and perversion and which likewise oppose the paternal quality of order to anal-sadistic confusion, the return to undifferentiated matter, to primal chaos.

Like Woolf, I read into the Jewish prohibition against seething the kid in its mother's milk a formulation to prevent the child's return to the maternal bosom by introduction of the paternal principal, *the paternal law.* We can add here the total isolation of the Shabbat from all other days of the week— the Havdalah—and the fact that on entering the Shabbat one reaches quite another dimension of life, a dimension which ends when the Shabbat is over.

As I have stressed previously, perversion is equivalent to a reading of the Bible in reverse. I have also stressed the idea that all laws based on separation are paternal in nature. Obviously this is no new idea but it brings out the opposition between paternal law on the one hand and, on the other, perversion, based on amalgamation. Sade, and perverts in general, make a point of turning law and ethics to ridicule, caricaturing and inverting them, at times consciously, at others unconsciously. In this way, teachers charged with "bringing up" children will be the means of their initiation into debauchery. This fantasy is far from rare: in common fantasies the child is subjected to erotic brutalization on the part of the male or female teacher (Freud, 1919) or has been ordered to take part in all manner of sexual games organized by the teacher. True, this is displacement of the father's, the mother's, or even the parental image onto the male or female teacher, but the essential question is the use to which the teaching or legislative function is put: not to contain drives by the enforcement of laws and the fear of punishment, but rather to *subvert* it. This function is no longer directed at the child's betterment (via castration anxiety). It has entered into the service of pleasure and its enjoyment.

Thus law is held up to ridicule. Such mockery of the law is present throughout Sade's work. Priests are dissolute, monks debauched, boarding school teachers depraved, right down to the pope himself. But debasement of the role of educator is at its height in Sade's *Philosophy in the Boudoir*, to which the subtitle "Or Teachers of Immorality—Dialogues for the Education of Young Ladies" was added in 1805. "Any mother will make her daughter read this," the epigraph announces. As we know, the book is about a young virgin's erotic initiation into incest, blasphemy, and crime, and it extols atheism. The fifth dialogue contains the exhortation: "Frenchman, a little more effort," from which it appears that this is not just the education of the young woman, Eugenie, but the education of a whole people (we are in the year 1795).

In the first "dialogue," Madame de Saint-Ange tells her brother, the Knight of Mirvel, of the plans she has for Eugenie, this with the complicity of Eugenie's father.

> Madame de Saint-Ange:—It's a matter of education.... The Knight:—Oh you rogue, how you'll enjoy the pleasure of educating the young thing! What delights await you in corrupting her, in stifling in her young heart all the seeds of virtue and religion sown there by her teachers....
>
> Madame de Saint-Ange:—Quite certainly I shall spare no effort in perverting her, in debasing, *toppling over backside* all the false principles of morality which may already have turned her head....

On reaching the boudoir, Dolmance says, so this is "the school where classes are to be held." Eugenie becomes "our schoolgirl," "our pupil," and she receives "lessons," the object being to "train her." In the full swing of debauchery, Madame de Saint-Ange mumbles: "Let us continue the lesson." Eugenie exclaims: "Oh, my divine teachers!" and addresses Dolmance as "my dear, adorable teacher."

In short, this is a parody of teaching, the aim of which is to "elevate," whereas here the aim has been reversed to leading the subject, "the pupil," back into the universe of amalgamation: the world of group lovemaking, sodomy, homosexual and heterosexual incest. The law, comprised of limits and separation, as we have seen, is debased for the purpose of establishing the reign of amalgamation.

Any situation destined to bring about a metamorphosis—from a lower to a higher level—is liable to undergo a reversal and to become perverted, especially if it takes place within a fixed framework and is ritualized. The psychoanalytic session itself can also succumb to such a temptation.

After a session of debauchery where incest and sodomy are practiced, Verneuil says to his partners:

> My friends, . . . we consulted fate on our pleasures not long ago; I now feel we should consult the Almighty on the same subject. . . . You, Gernande, will be the first to question God.
>
> Gernande: — Despicable image of the most ludicrous nonentity, you who are only at home in a bawdy house and *useless, except for regulating the pleasures of the ass,* what must I do to have another erection? Tell me; I shall execute your commandment.

This episode is very like a Black Mass, to which, when viewed in a certain perspective, many Sadian scenes can be compared.

When there is subversion of the law (as in *The 120 Days . . .*) and a parody of religion devoted to the worship of God, when sham gods, each yet another figure of Satan, are substituted for

God or the Trinity (as in the Apocalypse), then the passage leading from amalgamation to separation and demarcation can be followed in the reverse direction. Here we are very close to the worshippers of Satan and the religions of the Devil. Because in every instance we are dealing with metanoia, a reversal of values aimed at a return to primal chaos. Stating that law has been turned "head down" is not enough, for it is imperative to understand the intention behind this reversal. It is not simply the reversal of a system of values. A code, when reversed, remains a code. It appears that this reversal of a system of values is only the first stage in an operation whose end is the destruction of all values. This is a magical process. First law is reversed; this is the initial step in the return to chaos, like a film being rewound at top speed to get to the beginning. The flower's petals refold and it becomes a seed again. Perverse ritual aims at reconstituting chaos, from which a new kind of reality will be brought forth. Absence of law is consubstantial with chaos, an affirmation found in one "Midrash Rabbah": Without Torah, the whole world would become "shapeless" and "empty" again, in other words, would turn into the *tohu vabohu* it was before.

It follows that the creation of monsters or chimera is something one finds frequently in perversion, as is a fascination with hybrid creatures, with "living organisms whose conformation is other than the natural one of their species or sex" (Quillet-Flammarion Dictionary, 1957), and a fascination for inverting the use to which the body's organs are put. The objective is precisely to escape the divine order, the paternal dimension, to set oneself up as the creator or to envisage such an eventuality. Two examples come to mind, amongst others, one being the way a perverse patient enthused over the switch of a bedside lamp a friend had made from the testicles of a squirrel (at least so he said). The other example is the work of the photographer Joel-Peter Witkin. Here, masculine and feminine organs are intermingled, an animal's beak is superimposed on a human face, a monkey is dressed up in clothes and given the name "Manuel Osorio," and there are portraits of a female dwarf, Siamese twin sisters, and any number of physical handicaps and mutilations (in *Joel-Peter Witkin* [1989] for example). The photographer in fact defines himself as "perverse."

"DEVIL'S RELIGIONS"

Here I shall do no more than place a few markers. Before discussing "Luciferian" sects, I want to say that *alchemy* and the transmutation of reality it pursues do not seem to be irrelevant to our subject as regards certain of their aspects.

In the first place, alchemy is linked to the Aristotelian idea of a primordial matter from which every other kind of matter is created. The different metals are composed of a unique substance which differs only in its various stages of "maturity." Discovering the way to artificially hasten this maturity would make it possible to transmute one metal into another and, finally, to turn any metal into gold. Here we have a concept from which the principle of division has disappeared totally.

The alchemist's conception of the world is then one which enables him to split essences, or rather to deny their existence (and so, in the words of Genesis, to deny the existence of "kinds"). To find existence again from primordial matter (*materia prima, materia confusa:* Eliade, 1956, p. 101) is equivalent to the idea that it may be possible to return to the state of homogenous, undifferentiated matter from which a new reality, new forms, can be created (Eliade even speaks of a return to a "chaotic" state; p. 101). It is evident that in some respects the alchemist's ideology, Gnostic doctrines, even various mystical theories and practices, as well as Luciferian cults, are all related. In a brief essay on "Mephistopheles and the Androgyne, or the

Mystery of Totality," Mircea Eliade presents a certain number of rites, myths, and traditional theories "implying the union of opposites and the mystery of totality" (1962, p. 98). These can be detected, he says, in "the cosmogonies which explain the Creation by fragmentation of a primordial Unity, in the orgiastic rituals seeking the reversal of human conduct and the confusion of values, in the mystical techniques for the union of opposites, in the hermaphrodite myths and rites of androgynisation, etc." (p. 100).

The Gospel of Thomas, which was popular among the first Gnostics, quotes Jesus as saying: "When you make two human beings into one, and when you make the inside as the outside, and the outside as the inside and the top as the bottom! And if you make the male and the female into one so that the male is no longer male and the female no longer female, then you will enter into the Kingdom." It would seem, from this quotation, that male-female amalgamation is aimed at a fundamental and absolute undifferentiability.

The witches in the opening scene of *Macbeth* echo the Gospel of Thomas:

> Fair is foul, and foul is fair.
> Hover through the fog and filthy air.

In passing, it is worth noting the atmosphere of filth and of shapelessness which pervades this scene, in other words the anal chaos in which this fiendish reversal of values takes place, prelude to the abolition of all values, where nothing is clearcut, where things merge one with the other like the vile mixture brewing in the witches' cauldron:

> Double, double toil and trouble;
> Fire burn and cauldron bubble. . . .
> Make the gruel thick and slab (act 4, sc. 1)

From my point of view, *Macbeth* can be considered as a gradual building up into a Black Mass, which is reversed at the end and the natural order of things restored. The words "hell" and "devil" are repeated more than any others, second to which comes the word "night." When Macbeth falls prey to the shades of darkness, almost the same words as those used by the "weird sisters" spring to his lips: "So foul and fair a day I have not seen" (act 1, sc. 3). "Unnatural" things, events which go "against nature" (as does perversion) are observed; nature itself seems to be contaminated:

> by th' clock 'tis day,
> And yet dark night strangles the travelling lamp:
> Is't night's predominance, or the day's shame,
> That darkness does the face of earth entomb,
> When living light should kiss it?
> 'Tis unnatural,
> Even like the deed that's done. (act. 2, sc. 4)

Nothing is missing, not even the *infanticide* that is the central element of a Black Mass. The important fact about this reversal of the natural order of things, true for both Macbeth and the Black Mass, is that its aim is to acquire power, in Macbeth's case political power. My hypothesis is that perversion represents a similar magical process aimed at a return to the state of indistinctness, a manifestation of hubris, of man's desire to discredit the power of the Father-Creator, and to shape a new reality from chaos (which is anal). On the subject of ritual androgynisation, Mircea Eliade remarks:

> Since sexual conduct is exactly the opposite of what it normally should be, this amounts to suspension of laws and customs. The total confusion of values implicit in the reversal of behaviour is typi-

cal of all orgiastic rituals. Morphologically, intersexual transvestism and symbolic hermaphroditism are characteristic of ceremonial orgies. Ritual "totalisation," reintegration of opposites, regression to primordial indistinctness are present in each case. *In short, the goal is the symbolic reinstatement of "chaos," the state of unity without differentiation that preceded the Creation. This return to confusion manifests itself in a supreme act of regeneration* and an enormous increase in power.

In the famous passage in which Lady Macbeth calls on the spirits of darkness "to unsex me here," to "come to my woman's breasts, and take my milk for gall," is it not true that besides ridding herself of the "milk of human kindness" she is also seeking to become completely possessed by the weird sisters, to become, as they, neither man nor woman but both man and woman? "You should be women and yet your beards forbid me to interpret that you are so," Banquo says when he meets the witches on the heath (act 1, sc. 3). The witch's imago is ambiguous and far from clear-cut: anal and maternal simultaneously, like that of the Erinyes and chthonic divinities in general, like that of the Night that Lady Macbeth invokes ("Come, thick Night, and pall thee in the dunnest smoke of Hell"). A regressive mother is one who implies not the reciprocal complementarity of father and mother but elimination of the paternal dimension.

In his book *The Societies of Evil or the Devil in the Past and Today* Jean-Claude Frere (1972) reviews "Luciferian" societies from the Middle Ages up to the present time. He underlines "the importance of the role of sex in the often disorderly expression of erotic passions when magic rites take place. . . . Sabbaths, black masses and many Luciferian initiations . . .

must be accompanied by magic rites of a sexual nature in order to be perfect and to acquire complete meaning" (p. 20). In one of the first Luciferian societies, which met in Orleans around the year 1000, "magic sexual rites with the union of son and mother, brother and sister, father and daughter, especially when she was a consecrated nun, were practiced at the secret gatherings" (p. 26). Frere shows that the Luciferian refuses to submit to universal nature governed by divine harmony, that he has declared an interminable war on God's creation.

We are wrong, I believe, to consider sexual orgies (and particularly incest) as an end unto themselves in these ceremonies. They are the means, even if the end can be lost from sight, for subverting the divine order of things, based on separation, for the purpose of transmuting reality, as in the witch's cauldron. Etymologically, perversion means "reversal" or "deviation." Reading the sacred tetragrammaton in the reverse order often forms part of the Luciferian ceremony, just as, aside from sexual aspects, Black Masses consist of reading Mass backwards. In addition, the Eucharist is black, as well as the candles, Satan is called "the Very-Low," etc.

If, as Freud tried to show, moral standards of behavior, religion, and social organization are the consequence of projection into external space of the Oedipus complex and the paternal relationship in which monotheism is rooted, perversion, on the other hand, is linked to eradication of the father from the internal psychic universe and from the structure of society. On the religious level, there is a tendency to regress to paganism, to reinstate the cult of goddess-mothers like Astarte.

It is evident that in simply referring to alchemy and its ideology, the myth of the hermaphrodite, certain orgiastic rituals catalogued by Mircea Eliade, and some of the permanent features of Luciferian ceremonies, I have explored only the surface of a vast subject. My main objective has been to emphasize that *perversion represents a permanent temptation for the human mind.* It seems that throughout time and space man has never been free of the temptation to elude paternal law and the paternal universe, and has employed a great variety of means to bring about their eradication. On a certain level, this struggle and the struggle against reality merge.

As I have noted elsewhere, periods of great historic upheaval are preceded and for a time accompanied by an outcrop of behavior which can be called "perverse." The Enlightenment of the eighteenth century, which engendered the French Revolution, produced works of art and literature in which transvestism is particularly prominent (it is present in both *Cosi Fan Tutte* and the works of Marivaux). The works and life of the Marquis of Sade were closely knit in with various episodes of the French Revolution. It is not so easy to find such prodromes for the October Revolution. However, Dostoyevski's book *The Devils* (1870) describes the Netchaiev Group (nihilism being one stage leading up to the Revolution). Stavroguine, a member of this group, rapes the young girl Matriocha. The rape of a young girl, an act which abolishes the difference of generations, is a recurrent theme in Dostoyevski's work, written during this period of violent political upheaval. (At the same time the name Matriocha suggests the mother.) The same theme was taken up in Visconti's film "The Damned" (1969), which retraces the rise of Nazism. The hero, Helmut Berger, commits incest with his mother, rapes a young girl, and dresses up as Marlene Dietrich. By so doing he abolishes sexual and generational differences and destroys reality itself. It has become commonplace to associate the multiplication of transvestite cabarets in Berlin with the advent of Nazism. Two films at least — Bob Fosse's "Cabaret" (1972) and Ingmar Bergman's "The Serpent's Egg" (1977) — set out to show how perversions and Nazism developed in parallel. Also, in Losey's "Mr. Klein" there is a scene with a transvestite.

Can it not be said that multiplication of perversions on the eve of a violent historic upheaval represents the unconscious collective action of "miming" a new reality through the perverse act in order to bring it into existence magically? Just as the unnatural sexual intercourse Mircea Eliade describes was destined to magically ensure the success of grafts that also ran counter to the laws of nature. But it is equally true that there is a parallel tendency to uphold law and paternal values. The human mind is the permanent battlefield where these two tendencies vie one against the other.

The practices of Abbot Boullan, the founder of a new religious order, give a clear and condensed picture of a Luciferian sect. He used to heal sick nuns by rubbing them with a mixture of consecrated hosts and excrement. Mass was celebrated in a chapel where nuns stood naked and the abbot had sexual intercourse on the altar with the order's cofounder, a woman. He ended up by sacrificing a newborn baby. The sacrifice of a fetus or a newborn baby is a widespread practice in sects, from certain Gnostic sects dating back to the early days of Christianity up to the Manson affair and the murder of the pregnant Sharon Tate. It is perhaps possible to connect this with the cult of Moloch.

As I have pointed out in "The Archaic Matrix of the Oedipus Complex" (1984–86), besides representing a content of the mother's body and proof of the father's superiority over the young boy, who is incapable of fathering a child, the fetus and the baby both represent whatever develops, evolves, and is situated in time; they represent both life and reality and the inescapable necessity of growing and maturing.

This rapid panorama of doctrines as different as alchemy and gnosis and the rituals of Luciferian sects does not claim absolute historic exactitude (I have consulted only a limited number of books) and above all it does not claim to be exhaustive. To lend weight to my proposition I have tried to point to some of the encounters between man's need to free himself of the bonds of law, and the need which seems to transcend space and time, with man's pride presumptuously and perversely assuming the Creator's power. Over and above the sexual gratification that perversion affords, I believe that it is basically a religious ritual, or rather the parody of a religious ritual, destined to bring a neo-reality into existence from the very ruins of the paternal universe. My aim here has been only to try to resurrect one of Freud's initial ideas according to which the perversions can be considered as Devil religions, for the purpose of showing how this idea may provide us with some insight into those moments in history when "the estate of the world is undone."

Whereas Freud showed that social, political, and religious organization is rooted in the Oedipus complex, perversion tends to subvert the established order—in MacDuff's words, "measure, time and place" (act 5, sc. 9)—and to eradicate the Oedipus complex. However, I believe it would be inexact to qualify "Oedipians" as conservatives and perverts as progressives. In fact the former, as I have had occasion to note in my clinical practice, can turn out to be marvelous discoverers and creators who integrate models (parental substitutes) and then are able to surpass them. Perverts, if left to themselves, would almost certainly lead the world to its ruin. They hate reality to too great an extent not to seek its destruction. For mankind to progress without becoming mad in the process, a conviviality between "Oedipians" and "perverts" may be necessary.

References

Bialik, H. (1916), *Halachah and Aggadah*, English trans. Sir L. Simon, London: Zionist Federation, 1944.
Bible (1944), *King James' Bible*, Cambridge: Cambridge University Press.

Centre National De Photographie, Paris (1989), *Joel Peter Witkin*, catalogue prepared for the exhibition of his work organized by the Spanish Ministry of Culture.

Chasseguet-Smirgel, J. (1984), *Creativity and Perversion*, New York: Norton; London: Free Association Books.

—— (1984–86), The Archaix Matrix of the Oedipus Complex, in *Sexuality and Mind*, New York: New York University Press.

Dictionnaire Bailly (1894–1950)

Dictionnaire Quillet-Flammarion (1957)

Dostoyevski, F. (1873), *Les demons*, Paris: Fernand Hazan, 1963.

Eliade, M. (1956), *Forgerons et alchimistes*, Paris: Flammarion, 1977.

—— (1962), *Mephistopheles et l'Androgyne*, Paris: Gallimard.

Etudes Carmelitaines (1948), *Satan*, Paris, Brussels: Desclee de Brouwer.

Fackenheim, E. (1980), *La presence de Dieu dans l'histoire: Affirmations juives et reflexions philosophiques apres Auschwitz*, Paris: Verdier.

Frere, J. C. (1972), *Les societes du mal ou le diable hier et aujourd'hui*, Paris: Grasset.

Freud, S. (1892–1899), 'Extracts from the Fliess Papers' in *Standard Edition*, 1.

—— (1900), *The Interpretation of Dreams*, S.E., 4/5.

—— (1907), Obsessive Actions and Religious Practices, in *S.E.*, 9.

—— (1908), Character and Anal Eroticism, in *S.E.*, 9.

—— (1912–13), *Totem and Taboo*, S.E., 13.

—— (1917), On Transformations of Instinct as Exemplified in Anal Eroticism, *S.E.*, 17.

—— (1919), A Child is Being Beaten: A Contribution to the Study of the Origin of Sexual Perversions, in *S.E.*, 17.

—— (1926), *Inhibitions, Symptoms and Anxiety*, S.E., 20.

Koyre, A. (1929), *La philosophie de Jacob Boehme*, Paris: Vrin, 1979.

Sade, D. A. F. (1967), *Marquis de Sade: Oeuvres completes*, Paris: Cercle du Livre Precieux.

—— (1966), *The 120 Days of Sodom and Other Writings*, New York: Random House.

Shakespeare, W. *Macbeth*, Collection bilingue, trans. Pierre Leyris, Paris: Aubier Montaigne, 1977.

Urtubey, L. de (1980), *Le diable dans la psychanalyse*. Unpublished dissertation.

Woolf, M. (1945), Prohibitions against Simultaneous Consumption of Milk and Flesh in Orthodox Jewish Law, *Int. J. Psycho-anal.*, 26: 169–76.

Some Reflections on the Failure
to Develop an Adequate
Psychoanalytic Sociology

COMMENT ON HANLY AND

CHASSEGUET-SMIRGEL

ELI SAGAN

Although I have spent the past twenty years trying to understand the relationship of the development of the psyche to the evolution of culture and society, both of these papers made me consider certain connections I had not confronted before. My work has been based on two assumptions. The first is that the development of the psyche is the paradigm for the evolution of culture and society and the second is that in order to understand social and cultural evolution, we must take a psychoanalytic approach to analyzing psychic development.

One could take a nonpsychoanalytic developmental model and apply it to society as Jürgen Habermas has done, basing his theoretical approach on the work of Lawrence Kohlberg, who in turn elaborated the findings of Piaget. Habermas takes Kohlberg's pattern of psychic moral development from preconventional to conventional to postconventional morality and finds that the historical evolution of society replicates that exact paradigm. The problem with all this, as in the work of Piaget, is that no room is found in the theory for contradictions, paradoxes, repression, ambivalence—precisely those conflicts that psychoanalysis has made us so aware of. In a word, the problem with the Piaget-Kohlberg-Habermas project is that it has eliminated conflict from the equation. And just as Brenner has underlined for us the fact that we cannot understand the psyche without seeing it as fundamentally in conflict with itself, so is it important to understand that we can never comprehend society without perceiving that it is in conflict with itself. In fact, these conflicts, contradictions, ambivalences, and their resolution or nonresolution through compromise, are exactly what society is about.

What I bring to the task of respondent is training in sociology and history. I am not a clinician. I cannot, for instance, really make a judgment on Chasseguet-Smirgel's conception that all perversions are primarily, if not overwhelmingly, anal-sadistic. Many readers, I imagine, have their own clinical experiences involving patients struggling with addictions to perversion, and are therefore in a much better position to make a judgment as to what degree the anal-sadistic drives play in perverse activity.

I can, however, discuss intellectual history since Freud's death. It is interesting to think about what psychoanalysis was in 1939 and what it is today. What progress have we made in understanding the world? Hanly reminds us that at the time of Freud's death psychoanalysis was a theory of the psyche and a therapy intended to promote psychic health. I would like to suggest that for Freud psychoanalysis was, equally importantly, a theory of society. It may seem strange at first to hear this, but if we take the full corpus of Freud's work on society, including *Totem and Taboo, Group Psychology, The Future of an Illusion, Civilization and Its Discontents, Why War?, Moses and Monotheism,* and many short works, it seems safe to say that Freud wrote more about society than any other subject, except possibly dreams.

Even *The Ego and the Id*, considered a seminal work of strictly psychic theory, takes on an entirely different aspect when we consider Talcott Parsons' notion that the concept of the superego is the great meeting place of psychoanalysis and sociology. It answers, among other things, the question of how the system of values, a crucially important concept for twentieth-century sociology, is passed from one generation to the next—how, in effect, society reproduces itself. We will return later to the question of whether or not the superego represents the moral system, as well as the system of values, within the psyche.

Freud himself set great value on the application of psychoanalysis to an understanding of society. "I have always been of the opinion," he wrote in 1925, "that the extramedical applications of psychoanalysis are as significant as the medical ones; indeed, that the former might perhaps have a greater influence on the mental orientation of humanity." And near the end of *Civilization and Its Discontents* he set out a significant challenge that has yet to be taken up: "One day someone will venture to embark upon a pathology of cultural communities."

It seems not unreasonable to state that since Freud's death, remarkable progress has been made in psychoanalysis both in the theory of the psyche and in therapeutic technique. It seems equally clear that in the realm of a theory of society, the creation of a psychoanalytic sociology, there has been practically no progress. We remain, essentially, where Freud left us in 1939. Some valuable work has been done in the fields of literature, art, mythology, and religion, but a grand historical understanding of social change eludes us.

The question immediately suggests itself as to what factors may have contributed to this outcome. There seem to be four significant elements. First, of fundamental importance, is the failure both within and outside the psychoanalytic community to face up to the full importance of aggression in social life. Though we would all answer that, yes, aggression is important in human existence and agree that it is one of the two fundamental drives, still some mode of repression is operative that makes us reluctant to look at this Medusa except when its full impact is reduced by being reflected in a defensive shield. Freud himself, who only came to a full confrontation with aggression late in his life, queried: "Why have we ourselves needed such a long time before we decided to recognize an aggressive drive?" He reflected on his reluctance to accept the notion and commented on "how long it took before I became receptive to it." We all know the story of the intense resistance that met Freud's ideas of the overwhelming importance of sexuality, and especially infantile sexuality. But in historical terms, it took a remarkably short time to overcome much of that particular resistance. By the 1920s the sexual revolution of the twentieth century had begun, and by the 1940s the world was clearly one of Freudianism and sexuality.

But the resistance to facing the full import of aggression, especially outside the psychoanalytic world, remains enormous. Just recently I had the disturbing experience of having one of the most important historians of the genocide of the Jews tell me that he did not think the Holocaust was about hatred. In many aspects, in regard to aggression, we are still back where Freud was with sexuality in 1905.

Even within psychoanalysis a significant reluctance remains. One of the great values of both papers is that they confront the problem of aggression directly. Certainly Chasseguet-Smirgel's emphasis on the anal-sadistic has broad implications for an understanding of the destructive elements in social life. And Hanly's addressing the question of why so many twentieth-century philosophers have rejected the findings of psychoanalysis is related primarily, in my view, not to matters sexual, but to matters of aggression. When he says that "the upper stories of the mind are more connected with the basement than we like to think," that basement is full of uncontrolled hatred and rage. And if philosophy is intent on defining people as "not altogether part of nature," which requires "the repudiation of psychic determinism and the drives," it may be of value to suggest that what disturbed the thought of Sartre and Wittgenstein was not human beings' sexual nature, but their destructive nature. It is psychoanalysis's insistence on the instinctive, and therefore universal, nature of aggression that makes it so unpalatable for so many.

The problem for sociology is that we will never begin to understand society without paying full attention to the aggressive drives. Hanly reminds us of the "appalling spectacle of violence and devastation" of this century, but it is not only this terrible century that we must think about. The history of society is a story of cannibalism, head-hunting, human sacrifice, slavery, warfare, and genocide. Freud summed it up in one sentence: "The history of the world . . . is essentially a series of murders of peoples." That is, of course, only half the truth, but a very important half.

The problem for psychoanalysis is that very little has been done to explain how these aggressive drives operate through history and social evolution. We cannot go beyond Freud by merely repeating, in various ways, that *homo homini lupus*. Are these aggressive drives capable of sublimation and transformation? And if so, what are the *social* circumstances that make those transformations possible? Without thorough and complex answer to these questions, there can be no psychoanalytic theory of society.

A second consideration, probably of equal importance, is our deep reluctance to be critical of Freud; our tendency to transform theory into dogma. Several years ago, Robert Wallerstein wrote a profound article in which he hypothesized that we have not yet learned how to mourn Freud properly and that a strong indication of that is our inability to subject received Freudian theory to the same kind of critical review that would be given to any theoretical enterprise. We are thereby, he suggested, doing a disservice to ourselves and to Freud.

One example of this, wherein we can use some theoretical insight taken from sociology, may be helpful. Sociological theory differentiates between a value system and a system of morals. The value system of a society consists of all those attitudes toward reality which the society considers good, proper, orderly, and legitimate, or disorderly and illegitimate. However, there are always certain values considered legitimate within society that are, in actuality, immoral. Slavery is one obvious example. It is an extraordinary experience to read Aristotle, one of the greatest moral minds ever, on the subject of slavery. He asserts that some are slaves by nature (*physis*) and that, therefore, slavery is just and legitimate. The value system of the society in this regard had been so completely internalized by Aristotle, through the operation of his superego, that he was powerless to see the immorality in the institution of slavery.

Slavery is just one example of this conflict between values and morals. In a racist or anti-Semitic society, the value system legitimates prejudice. In a sexist society, the system of values legitimates sexism. Anti-Semitism, racism, and sexism are clearly immoral. And these conflicts between values and morals are some of the most important examples of the conflictual and ambivalent nature of culture and society.

In all discussion of the nature of the superego from Freud onward, however, no distinction has been made between values and morals. Values and morals have been treated as if they were identical, with the superego representing the psychic structure by means of which world-views are internalized into the individual psyche. It is true that many, if not most, of the values that are internalized by the superego have a moral dimension. But many do not, as primitive patriotism, racism, and Aristotle's commitment to the inherent justice of slavery demonstrate. In essence, the superego does not represent the moral system within the psyche, but only the system of values, and it is moral or immoral only insofar as the values internalized are such.

Nothing illustrates this with greater power than the history of the genocide of the Jews and the value system that the perpetrators brought to their task. One cannot read Robert Jay Lifton's book on the Nazi doctors without becoming fully aware that without the superego—true, a Nazi superego, but no less a superego for that—the Holocaust would have been impossible. He demonstrates that the Nazis used all the trappings of the superego to promote genocide: purifying, healing, curing, oath, community, the *Volk*, social usefulness, ideal society; sacrifice and dedication, ideology, idealism, and morality. I quote: "My honour is my loyalty . . . to have stuck it out and, apart from exceptions caused by human weakness, to have remained decent, that is what has made us hard. This is a page of glory in our history." These words resonate with superego imperatives. They were delivered, nevertheless, by Heinrich Himmler.

It does not answer the theoretical question to respond that what I have been emphasizing is a corrupt superego, for the notion that the superego can be wholesome or corrupt implies a value by which a particular superego can be judged. That value cannot, then, be given by the superego itself and must be external to it. This is not to deny that there are corrupt and wholesome superegos and all matter of combinations in between, but to say that implies a capacity for moral judgment within the psyche independent of the superego. What exactly that capacity might be is too large a question to be addressed here, but it does seem that it is not helpful to assume that Freud has answered the question of morality within the psyche. The question of values, yes. Morality is a much more complicated issue.

The superego cannot, in itself, tell us *why* slavery is immoral. I assume that is what Hanly means when he says that psychoanalysis is not an ethic. But we cannot stop there because we have come to a potentially treacherous place. Where, then, are the grounds of our morality? If psychoanalysis is not an ethic, and God is dead, and reason occupies only the upper story of the mind, by what right do we say that slavery, or anything else such as racism or genocide, is immoral? Even if psychoanalysis is not itself an ethic, it has a scientific obligation to answer that question.

One answer, of course, is the nihilist one: the psyche has no capacity to make moral judgments. It can only tell us how the superego transmits the values of parents and society from one generation to the next. In a word, there are no morals, only values.

That is not my view. In disagreement with Hanly, I believe that psychoanalysis is an ethic. Unable to address at length that complicated issue here, to put it quickly and as simply as possible: those advances which the philosopher or the sociologist calls moral, like the abandonment of slavery, for instance, are all movements in the direction of psychic evolution, that is, psychic health. Slavery means the ownership of one human being by another. To use the insight Chasseguet-Smirgel has given us, such ownership, anatomically speaking, takes place in the behind. Slavery represents a primitive, anal mode of trying to dominate the world. Capitalism, which emphasizes the accumulation of money and not the accumulation of other people, or "souls" as the Russian nobility liked to refer to their serfs, represents a fundamental sublimation of anal instincts, which makes possible psychic development. The abandonment of slavery is, simultaneously, moral *and* psychic progress. That all of this has enormous implications for a theory of culture and society seems unarguable.

The third consideration has to do with the fact that theoretical problems of society and history take, under the present conditions of scholarship, a huge amount of time. One continues to wonder how Freud, an avaricious reader, ever found time to read all that he did. When he decided to attempt the problem of totemism, he managed to read almost everything available on the subject. Not content merely to digest Frazer's important article in the Encyclopedia Britannica, he waded into the four massive volumes of *Totemism and Exogamy* and even rendered complaint about how large was the amount of reading he had undertaken. Were he to set himself the same research task today, he would have to foreswear making a living for his family and devote his twelve to fourteen hours a day to absorbing the material from perhaps two to three hundred different cultures.

It is one thing to set oneself the task of writing a article, let us say, on the homosexual dimensions of the relationship between Iago and Othello. That involves reading the play, doing some work on the psychoanalytic theory of male homosexuality, extracting valuable insights from one's clinical experience, and then using the sharpest intuitive insight one can muster. Such an effort is manageable and can, and does, produce important articles.

It is a far different thing, however, to approach the enormously difficult and fascinating problem, let us say, of why the early Christian Church was so oppressive of sexuality, why it insisted on creating a society in which the holiest people, those with the most prestige and power, were supposed to be living completely repressed sexual lives. What did all that mean? What implications did it have for the development of the psyche and for the evolution of culture and society? Something very complex and ambiguous was going on, something both good and bad for human beings. And no quick generalizations will serve. Such a problem would take three or four years of reading—just reading, no patients, no classes, no conferences, maybe a two-week vacation in the Caribbean where one could sit under a beach umbrella while reading Origen—three or four years merely to decide what one's position was on the crucial questions. It would then take an additional two or three years to assemble the material necessary to convince others that one was right. Who among us has that kind of time, or even inclination?

The problem is that among historians, who do do that kind of work, with very few exceptions, psychoanalytic theory is not in favor. Psychoanalysis, for instance, has made practically no contribution toward understanding the Holocaust, because those who have done or are doing the massive research work are uninterested in its findings; people like Raul Hilberg, who is indifferent, or Hannah Arendt, who was openly hostile.

This is why, on the basis of my admittedly limited historical knowledge, I cannot accept Chasseguet-Smirgel's notion that "periods of historic upheaval are preceded by an outcrop of behavior which can only be called perverse." It appears to be, even if true for certain circumstances, too global a conclusion. Does such hold true for the American Revolution? The world of Washington, Madison, and Jefferson does not give the impression of being overcast by the polymorphous perverse. And what of the great English Revolution of 1640, the first proto-democratic revolution in modern history and the very first in which the *demos* executed the king? Whatever the Puritans were, anal-sadistic and incestuous does not seem to fit.

And what do we make of the fact that the early years of the Roman Empire did see an efflorescence of perverse sexual behavior, including the exhibitionistic escapades of Augustus's daughter, which resulted in the banishment of the poet Ovid, the anal-sadistic behavior of the emperor Caligula, and the reputed activities of Nero, which included recurring incest with his mother? Instead of a period of great social upheaval, what followed, starting with the emperor Vespasian in 69 A.D. and ending with the death of Marcus Aurelius, was a period of over one hundred years of the most stable, glorious time of Roman Empire, an era that Gibbon described as one of the happiest ever in which to be alive.

This particular critique of Chasseguet-Smirgel depends upon the reading of some ten or fifteen books on the Roman Empire, and it is, naturally, subject to even greater critique by someone who has spent much of his or her life doing the necessary work. It may seem a hard conclusion to draw, but if we are not going to do the historian's work, we may not make much contribution to historiography.

The fourth, and last, concern that has contributed to the failure to develop a psychoanalytic theory of society is our almost total neglect of the history of child rearing. This seems a singularly remarkable thing. Enormous changes have occurred in the mode of child rearing over the last four hundred years, changes that have vast implications for the development of the psyche and the evolution of society. One would think that such a course of development would be of crucial interest to psychoanalysts and psychoanalysis, but this has not been the case. The central work on the history of child rearing has been done by those outside the psychoanalytic community, some of the most important being Philip Aries in France, Lawrence Stone of Princeton University, and Lloyd de Mause. The only work of importance known to me that came from within the psychoanalytic community was Spitz's work on the history of the repression of masturbation in children. What Spitz elaborated was that, starting at an almost unbelievably low, inhumane point, around the middle of the nineteenth century, the response to the child's need to masturbate became less and less oppressive and more and more understanding of the nature of instinctual life. Even with what we now know, it is still startling to read Freud's case of Little Hans. In the first few pages he tells us that Hans's parents were followers of his, progressive people attempting to raise their child in the most intelligent manner possible; and on the very next page he has Hans's mother threatening that if he touches his penis again, she will call the doctor to come and cut it off. We can only imagine what the nonprogressive parents were saying to their children at that time.

Now, whatever else has happened since the nineteenth century, whatever disabilities our present society suffers from over-permissiveness or the breakdown of the stable-neurotic family, the fact is that progressive, humane parents do not threaten their children today in that manner. And the implications of this revolution in child rearing reach far beyond the family. It is my view that no stable democratic society is possible without what can only be described as a nonauthoritarian child rearing.

Stone and others have elaborated the revolution in child rearing that began in Europe about 1600. Previous to that, all children were swaddled; those who could afford it gave their children out to wet nurses; no child had a room of his or her own; the main stated aim of child rearing was to beat the spirit out of the child, either physically or psychologically. Around 1600 all this began to change, and we can observe a steady development of a more sympathetic mode of nurturing since then, except for a remarkably violent, regressive period in the nineteenth century, which has yet to be explained (a regression, nevertheless, which was overcome in the twentieth century).

Significantly, this revolution occurred first in England and North America and then in France, exactly those countries that were destined to lead the world into modernity, a stage of society embracing the first stable democratic societies on Earth since Athens, and the very first to include women in the polity. Some European societies came very, very late to this modern mode of child nurturing. Included among these latecomers are the societies that gave us the two totalitarian catastrophes of this century.

Can we really, then, understand the anal-sadistic, the polymorphous perverse, without paying attention to the mode of child rearing? There must be a thousand different ways to toilet train a child and at least a hundred significantly different modes exhibited in the various countries of Europe over the last two hundred years, with great changes from one thirty-year period to the next. One has only to read the advice given to mothers by pediatricians and others from 1800 to the present to see what variety is possible. Can this mode of anal training have no effect on the anality of adults who have been subjected to it in childhood? Everything in psychoanalytic theory insists that it must have a significant effect. What we can observe is that even something as seemingly basic to the psyche as toilet training is *historically* determined, a fact of history. It is not enough, as an example, to say the words "sphincter-morality," without perceiving that even the control of the sphincter is dependent upon history, that is, upon social change and evolution.

What is suggested by all this is that, when Chasseguet-Smirgel detects a particular relationship to anal-sadistic perversity in twentieth-century German culture, she may be quite accurate in her intuition. To fully understand it, however, one may have to look at the child's first encounter with anality and the crucial response of the parents to that experience. Alan Dundes's work on anality and the Germans, for instance, seeks to examine the whole range of that encounter, from childhood to adulthood. In summary, the history of child rearing may prove to be the royal road to the social unconscious.

I would also like to address a few more specific matters raised by the papers. It may be that Hanly, in the quest for a scientific psychoanalysis, leaves no room for what can be described as necessary illusions. There are certain stances toward reality, which in our rational mind we know to have no validity, but which we really cannot live without. There is a marvelous story of Isaac Bashevis Singer, who was interviewed after he won the Nobel Prize and was asked whether he believed in free will or not. "Of course I believe in free will," he responded, "do I have a choice?" It is reminiscent of V. S. Pritchett's notion that if courage is an illusion, it is one illusion worth having.

The same ambiguity, the same need for what Keats called "negative capability," surrounds the question of whether life has a meaning or not. The rational part of the mind knows that, of course, life has no meaning, that there is no such thing as a soul, that human beings occupy no privileged place in nature. But, can one really live with the perception that life is meaningless? Macbeth's great cry of despair that "Life's but a walking shadow. . . . a tale told by an idiot, full of sound and fury, signifying nothing" is the lament of a man who is depressively ill. Freud said we must either fall in love or grow ill. Similarly, if we abandon the "illusion" that our will is free or that courage is possible or that life is full of meaning, we are facing an inevitable pathology. There are limits to our scientific rationality.

Related to this, it seems important to distinguish between ideals, idealization, and ideology. Ideals and idealization are essential for social and psychic health. Without ideals, there can be no love of country, no society, and certainly no democratic society. That all men are created equal and are endowed by their creator with certain inalienable rights is clearly not a statement about political reality, but is a necessary ideal toward which a democratic society must strive. On the personal level, without idealization no one would fall in love, get married, conceive children, or pursue a career. Further than this, idealization is essential for the sublimation of primitive narcissism, and may be the very first step in that sublimative process.

What Hanly finds has brought such destruction to this century is not ideals but ideology. Ideology is the perversion of idealization. The pursuit of ideology is not a sublimative experience, but a de-sublimative one. And in this process of de-sublimation a good measure of primitive aggression is unleashed. Violence and devastation are not merely side effects of the institutionalization of ideology, they are a necessary goal. Some psychoanalytic writing confuses idealization with overidealization and sounds like idealization is something we could and should dispense with. When Hanly cautions not to idealize ideals, I assume that it is overidealization that he has in mind.

Finally, to return to Chasseguet-Smirgel's paper on analsadistic perversion, there seems to be a very important theoretical question implied that is not quite spelled out, a question that I hope she will give us an answer to someday. There seem to be two different kinds of people engaging in two different forms of this perverse activity. There are people who perform anal-sadistic acts in private on a recurring, probably compulsive and addictive basis. But they exhibit no desire or inclination to make a religion out of their preferences. They need their analsadistic satisfactions but they exhibit no need to perform these acts under a social — that is, superego — ritual umbrella.

There are others, however, who are not content merely to perform perverse acts. They wish to make them part of a satanic ritual performance, to turn them into a caricature of a religion; to make them a part of "beliefs and practices," as Durkheim said of true religion, "which unite into one single moral community called a church, all those who adhere to them." Their intent is not only to attain anal-sadistic satisfaction but, at the same time, to abolish the moral universe. Their intent is to debase and corrupt, and, if you will, shit on the superego.

Why should these two different modes of behavior exist? Why this social, communal, anti-superego dimension? If we could fully understand what is going on in all these variations on the Black Mass, we might learn an enormous amount about the nature of the superego and its perversion into ideology.

The last point I wish to address is very complicated, hard to deal with in a short time, but important enough to pay some attention to. Chasseguet-Smirgel's discussion demonstrates that on the symbolic level of ritual, religion, or social action, regression is not the same thing as merely returning to a formerly achieved stable position. Regression from Jehovah's ordered, oedipal, patriarchal universe does not mean return to an orderly, pre-oedipal, pre-genital, anal world. It involves reversion to a place where chaos and destruction abide. Similarly, on a social level, fascism was not merely a regression from the modern, democratic, freedom-infused world back to an orderly, authoritarian, patriarchal monarchy. It too was a reversion to a place where chaos and destruction abide.

Once an advanced psychological position has been even partially achieved, it is abandoned only at great cost. Always, this de-sublimative experience involves an explosion of aggression. Regression to an anal-sadistic world creates a much more violent world than that of the original anal-sadistic state. Regression to authoritarianism, under fascist impetus, creates a much more destructive world than monarchy ever made possible. De Tocqueville saw in the 1830s that, in the future, there would be no more return to a patriarchal monarchy. Either democracy would prevail or unlimited power would be concentrated in the hands of one man and this power would "take a new form and display features unknown to our fathers." There can be no orderly return to a former position, once it has been transcended. The explosion that dismembers the superego is almost uncontrollable.

6
EPILOGUE

Freud and Culture in Our Fin de Siècle Revisited

ROBERT S. WALLERSTEIN, M.D.

Freud's psychoanalysis was born in one fin de siècle and is revisited in this volume in another, at its first century mark, and under the particular impetus of the 1989 commemoration of the fiftieth anniversary of Freud's death marked by an American tour of selected antiquities from Freud's personal collection. The appearance of this exhibition at Stanford University in early 1991 was the occasion for the weekend conference entitled "Psychoanalysis and Culture: The Contributions of Sigmund Freud," upon which this present volume is based. The happenstance of the two fin de siècles and the differing world cultures that they reflect, as well as Freud's own death very close to the midpoint of this hundred-year history, provides context for consideration of the two framing points for psychoanalysis. The first is reflection on what psychoanalysis was a century ago, as Freud single-handedly brought it into being, and on the world view within which he lived and with which he (mostly) identified. This then needs be juxtaposed against what psychoanalysis now is—as well as any distinguished current group of psychoanalytic practitioners and psychoanalytic scholars can represent it—and where it may today be going, and what, of its current posture in its relation to its contemporary cultural surround, we can feel was at all prefigured by Freud. In developing these themes I will circumscribe my task, in this summarizing chapter, by staying close to the issues and the ideas articulated in the texts of the various chapters, rather than trying to more broadly encompass all that could be implied in the remarks just stated of a full intellectual comparison of the differing cultures of the two fin de siècles and the changing position of psychoanalysis as it has evolved within whatever degree of shift in prevailing world culture. That would be subject for a book of its own, by a cultural historian who is at the same time intimately familiar with psychoanalysis.

Stated for our purposes here, the fin de siècle in which Freud matured reflected the fullest flowering of what has been called the modern world or modernism. It was the era of the wide dispersion through the culture of the Darwinian evolutionary concept with its placement of humankind into a scientifically understandable position within the natural order of our planet; of Marxian economics with its heady promise of a rationally ordered (and inevitable) progression of the conditions of material well-being for the earth's population; and of the explosive transformations of our intelligence of the natural universe triggered by Einstein's relativity theory and progressing via successive fundamental discoveries through the elaborations of quantum mechanics, with all the fateful consequences that was to have for our bewildering advances in science and technology, including ultimately the awesomeness of nuclear power.

The unifying theme of the modern world-view encompassed by these advances was of the orderly progression of knowledge of an ultimately knowable universe and a controllable material and social world. Knowledge accretion was automatically equated with progress, and science and its spectacular growth was the exemplar—even in the realm of human affairs and the social order, the Marxian economic claim was of the 'scientific' nature of socialist economics and of its historical inevitability. The hallmarks of this scientific perspective were the conceptions of objectivity, rationality, the neutral dispassionate observer, empiricism and pragmatism, and what in philosophy was called positivism, materialism, naturalism. The prevailing commitment was to a reality-bound understanding of nature (and within that, of human nature) and, philosophically, to a correspondence theory of truth. The early decades of the twentieth century saw the rise of the Vienna Circle, of logical positivism, and of the verification theory of meaning.

No culture as complex and diverse as our Western world is as monolithically one-sided as I have just sketched, but this was the generally prevailing zeitgeist within which Freud, the medical scientist and neuroanatomist trained within the so-called Helmholtz School of Medicine, created psychoanalysis in an effort at a biologically anchored, natural science of the mind, a presumed general theory of mental functioning, at first of psychopathology and abnormal functioning but ineluctably to be expanded into a comprehensive theory of the functioning of the mind, in both its abnormal and normal states. Freud's aborted effort to ground this neurophysiologically, essayed in the Project for a Scientific Psychology (1895), is well known, and when reluctantly given up, was simply transmuted into a psychologically confined general science of the mind, the Freudian metapsychology in which various astute observers have seen the persisting structure of the natural science model, with all its ontological anchorings.

Additionally, Freud lived and worked within the patriarchal society of turn-of-the-century Central Europe and the particular imprint of Victorian bourgeois Vienna, and again, numerous observers, both sympathetic and critical, have pointed to the marked coloring this gave to the universalist and assumed normalist assumptions, embedded in psychoanalytic conceptions of gender and sexual development, of the nodal position of the oedipal drama in character formation and in illness predilection, and of gender-linked superego formation and its central role in linking individual psychic development to the requirements, constraints, and values of the cultural surround.

Further to make this case, Freud made strenuous efforts throughout his lifetime—and for the greater part of it, reasonably successfully—to define the parameters of his new science of the mind, and to hold it together as a unified enterprise, against both destructive or diluting pressures or seductions from without and also against fractious human divisiveness from within. The story of Freud's endeavors in this direction, including the formal creation of the International Psychoanalytical Association (IPA) in Nuremberg in 1910, the later creation of the secret committee of the seven ring holders, etc., and the ultimate breaking of the unitary theoretical structure of the IPA, first with the rise of the Kleinian movement as a new theoretical direction within organized psychoanalysis, even while claiming a more direct descent from and closer adherence to the declared original mind of Freud than the Viennese followers with whom he was more identified, and the subsequent proliferation of theoretical psychoanalytic positions (metapsychologies); the story of all that I have told in considerable detail elsewhere (Wallerstein, 1988). The overall point is that Freud created psychoanalysis within a natural-science, biologically-underpinned, and universalist framework, drenched with the values of a patriarchal morality and world view, and he succeeded, more than the originator of any other discipline or school of thought, in impressing that framework and that cast upon the whole fabric of the discipline for a period extending far beyond his lifetime, and enduring in substantial ways even until today.

And yet, at the same time, this was never the whole of psychoanalysis even in Freud's day, and even in Freud. Much has been written about the tensions between science and humanism, or between science and art, in the Freudian corpus, between the experience-distant metapsychological edifice, the general theory, and the experience-near clinical theory, linked closely to the observational data and to the experiences of the consulting room; tensions between, in other words, the universal generalizations of the (metapsychological) psychoanalytic effort at an encompassing theory of the operations of the mind, and the particularities of the unique life history and development and psychic formation collaboratively (re)constructed in the ongoing psychoanalytic encounter. Indeed it has become fashionable of late to talk of this as telling a (life) story or creating a narrative with all the resonances (if not the imaginative skills) of the poets, the playwrights, and the novelists, the Shakespeares and the Dostoyevskis. The point is that this tension between the theoretical (seeking universal truths about the human condition) and the clinical (seeking to understand and to meliorate the sufferings of the unique individual), to state it at its simplest, also always existed in Freud's psychoanalysis, even in its earliest days, though it was usually minimized in the public face of psychoanalysis, whose practitioners sought acceptance and respectability within the modernist world, fueled by the power and promise of science and its drive for unfolding truth and progress. Yet, though Freud never achieved Nobel Prize recognition for scientific achievement, he was awarded the German government's Goethe Prize for literary accomplishment.

To now, again in oversimplified fashion, span the sociocultural changes in the century between the two fin de siècles that frame the history of psychoanalysis, the modern world has given way, at least in significant quarters, and in the perspectives of significant cultural spokesmen, to what has come to be called the postmodernist stance toward theory, culture, and knowledge, strongly rooted in contemporary literary criticism and in major segments of contemporary philosophy. The cataclysmic events of our century have shattered naive beliefs in the inevitability of progress and in the beneficence, and even the truth claims, of science. Presumably scientifically anchored universal truths about human functioning and the human condition, outside of history and outside of context, have given way to a concern with historicization and contextualization, in effect, of the particularities of unique conditions and confluences of intersecting and interacting influences, akin, that is, to that facet of psychoanalysis first revealed in Freud's classical case histories and reflected now in the varieties of relational, interactional, interpersonal, intersubjective, and social-constructivist conceptualizations that constitute what is called the major paradigm shift taking place in contemporary psychoanalysis. In its extreme, the ultimate logic of the postmodern or deconstructionist claim is that rather than the written text (read, for psychoanalysis, the patient's life) containing specific meanings put there by the author (read, by the patient's life experience) in a form that can be communicated to and retrieved by the reader (the conception of veridical interpretation), the text is ultimately but an arrangement of words on paper, which different readers with different subjectivities, and at different points in geographic space and historic time, will respond to differently, so that the 'reality' of the text, what it "means," will be constructed anew with each reader. My parenthetical insertions indicate clearly enough the very direct analogues to this philosophic literary posture in the contemporary psychoanalytic writings, for example, of Schafer (1992) on analysis as a succession of narrative acts, a telling of life stories, and of Hoffman (1991) whose "social-constructivist" perspective shifts the task of analysis from a concern with interpreting reality to a focus on the interactive process by which therapist and patient create and shape, out of their mutual impact on each other, their uniquely constructed reality.

And, of course, in keeping with this shifting zeitgeist over the past century of psychoanalysis just described has been the decentering of the patriarchal social and family structure within which Freud lived, marked by the rise of feminism and the women's movement, the now open avowal of the gay and lesbian orientation as an alternative lifestyle, and also the divorce revolution, with the altering family structures brought about by all of these influences—the so-called companionate or two-career marriage, the single-parent household, the growth of stepparenting and of combined families, etc.—and all of this in the context of the greater acceptance and celebration of ethnic diversity and multiculturalism, with emphasis now on the contingent roles played by differing cultural traditions and their differing modal family structures. And, finally, specifically within psychoanalysis, the final fragmenting of Freud's vision, that of maintaining a unified theoretical structure to which all organizationally affiliated psychoanalysts would adhere, all this giving way to the full acceptance today of the diversity—or pluralism as we call it—of defining psychoanalytic theoretical frameworks, the (American) ego-psychological, or now post ego-psychological, the Kleinian, the object-relational (as developed by the British Independent group), the self-psychological, the interpersonal (originally, Sullivanian), the Lacanian, the Bionian, etc. These now all have their staunch adherents in the marketplace of psychoanalytic ideas, and are in healthy contest for the allegiances of practicing psychoanalysts. There are of course efforts at theoretical amalgamation across perspectives (like Kernberg's efforts at an amalgamated ego structural/object relational framework, where units of self- and object-representations linked by affectively charged valences form the building blocks of the gradually evolving tripartite psychic structure), and, contrapuntally, arguments advanced so cogently in Greenberg and Mitchell's groundbreaking book, *Object Relations in Psychoanalytic Theory* (1983), of the utter incompatibility of what they counterpose as the drive/structural and the object-relational models of psychic functioning. The compounding of diversity within diversity!

How then can we place the themes and the contents of this book, as they reflect the evolving psychoanalysis of Freud, within the boundaries of the two fin de siècles whose major defining attributes I have sketched out in such broad brush strokes? Paul Robinson, a historian of culture *and* of psychoanalysis, has tried in his introductory chapter to tease out central problematics that persist within psychoanalysis as reflections of the tugs between what psychoanalysis was in its beginnings, and what it is fitfully evolving into today. In the search for these unifying themes, or rather thematic statements, he has drawn heavily on the not quite explicit critiques of Carl Schorske, an eminent historian of psychoanalysis, in his keynote address to the Stanford conference, and on the discussion by John Toews, another eminent historian concerned with psychoanalysis, who offered a detailed critical discussion of two other of the psychoanalytically grounded accounts in the book—Peter Loewenberg's historical account of the problems and consequences of modern-day nationalism, and Marcelo Suárez-Orozco's anthropological account of the (violent) ambience of soccer and its fans in one of the nations of strongest soccer fanaticism, Argentina.

The point that Robinson states that Schorske makes by inference, and Toews very explicitly, is that so much, not just of psychoanalytic praxis, where it is less mischievous, but of psychoanalytic comprehensions of culture in all its aspects— history, anthropology, literature and art, philosophy, etc.—is still grounded in the now outmoded modernist, universalist, and preferentially masculinist world view that automatically privileges universalism and normalization over particularism and historicization, men over women, heterosexuality over homosexuality, and mainly sameness over difference. The cry is to overcome the tension between a psychoanalytic theory freighted with its modernist inheritances and predilections— the declared legacy and still powerful imprint of Freud—and the postmodernist concern with difference and heterogeneity, with historicization and contextualization. As an aside here, one can say ironically that this declared contemporary thrust toward difference, toward context, toward the particulars of historic time and geographic space threatens (in this view) to become a new universalism of its own.

And, as another aside, in posing the so-called modernist-drenched psychoanalysis of Freud in opposition to the so-called more liberated, relational, constructionist, and pluralistic post-modernist psychoanalysis toward which we should be moving inexorably today, we do a major disservice to Freud, who, as I have already briefly indicated, in his own tugs between science and humanism, or between the universals of a general theory of the mind and the particulars of the individual (re)construction of a unique life history, was himself much closer to the central psychoanalytic issues and dynamics of today than some of his critics and detractors (like Sulloway and Masson and Green-baum—a trio about whom Paul Robinson has written a book [1993] devoted to this very theme) have given him credit for.

The faulty understanding here, and there is a faulty under-standing, actually lies more with those psychoanalysts who were trying to immutably preserve and distill the legacy of Freud, whether clinically—like Kurt Eissler, who in his famous 1953 paper on parameters defined a rigorously austere and unneces-sarily rigid psychoanalysis as the so-called classical technique bequeathed to us by Freud—or theoretically, like Heinz Hart-mann and his collaborators, who architected the (American) ego-psychological metapsychology paradigm (systematized to the fullest extent possible by David Rapaport) in an effort to create a biologically based general science of the mind in the natural science mold.

But these clinical and theoretical models which prevailed— at least in America—in the 1950s and 1960s have given way clinically to the focus on the nature of the dyadic interpersonal relationship within the transference-countertransference interplay, which emerged into prominence through the writings of Hans Loewald, signalled particularly in his landmark 1960 paper "On the Therapeutic Action of Psychoanalysis," and Leo Stone, propounded most fully in his 1961 monograph "The Psychoanalytic Situation." It is a trend undermining Eissler's austere vision, and one given further impetus by Samuel Lipton's incisive 1977 paper comparing Freud's actual technique with Eissler's so-called classical technique, which Lipton demonstrated to be a misreading of Freud and a crystallization of analytic technique in a spirit antithetical to that of Freud.

And theoretically, the once hegemonic position of Hartmann's natural-science ego-psychology paradigm has given way to a widespread retreat from that drive- and structure-based, biologically grounded model to a current focus on the relational, the interactional, the interpersonal, the subjectivistic, and the constructivist perspective in psychoanalytic praxis and theory, alongside the previous, more unitary focus on the interpretive process alone, leading, via repetitive working through, to insight and change. That is, there has been a turn from the primacy of the objective, natural-science model of veridical interpretation of defense and underlying impulse, embedded in the so-called "one body psychology" of the ego/structural paradigm, to the growing concomitant appreciation of the tenets of a "two body psychology," within which relational and interactional perspectives have assumed conceptually an enlarging, and ultimately a co-equal importance in the processes both of understanding (the theory) and of change (the praxis).

Lastly, I should point to another dilemma or question that Robinson raises without proposing a response. In commenting on Richard Almond's psychoanalytic account of Charlotte Brontë's *Jane Eyre,* Paul Schwaber's psychoanalytic account of Leopold Bloom in James Joyce's *Ulysses,* and Jerome Winer's discussion of the two, he raises the question of the propriety of ascribing a particular kind of past and a particular constellation of motivations and impulses (all psychoanalytically constructed and understood) to fictional characters who cannot be psychoanalytically interrogated in depth as can real and living patients, with whom a plausible and accountable past and motivational set can be jointly (re)created and consensually agreed. This question raised by Robinson is not even posed by any of the three authors referred to nor is it a special theme of the book. As an aside, I only want to raise the contrapuntal question: Does not the genius of the Shakespeares and the Dostoyevskis of the world reside in their very capacity to create characters of such convincing authenticity and verisimilitude that if we went to a dinner party and sat next to Hamlet, for example, and could talk with him, that we could come home and say, "Guess what? I met Hamlet tonight." Where does our conviction about the recognizable coherence and particular personhood of a major Shakespearian or Dostoyevskian character come from anyway? Or, what is the reach, as well as the limitation, of the application of the psychoanalytic method and psychoanalytic understanding to fictional characters? This question I think *is* implicit in both the Almond and the Schwaber presentations.

But my own main intent in this concluding chapter, differing from Paul Robinson's in his introductory chapter but meant to be complementary to his effort, is to look not for unifying themes and central problematics that would focus the book thematically, but rather, oppositely, to highlight the variety of directions and underlying assumptions that have enriched and diversified psychoanalytic interactions with the multiple aspects of contemporary culture. These have brought psychoanalysis solidly beyond the legacy of a single creative genius, with all the directions that he opened up or presaged, unto today, when psychoanalysis has become the combined responsibility of its diverse worldwide collectivity in interaction with a thoroughly psychoanalytically infused world culture. For, in W. H. Auden's (1940) inimitable words in his moving elegy upon Freud's death, "To us he is no more a person, / Now but a whole climate of opinion," and today intellectual discourse can scarcely exist without recourse to psychoanalytic concepts and meanings, like rationalization and ambivalence and repression and defenses, used, quite unself-consciously, even by those who still stoutly deny the unconscious and psychic determinism.

Within, then, this intent to mark out the diverse themes and contents of this book, I can simply indicate sequentially the range of preoccupations and questions posed by the contributors to this volume. The first several contributions were historical (temporally) and anthropological (geographically); Carl Schorske in his essay did indeed sound the comparative note of the juxtaposition of what he described as Freud's two Egyptian digs, the first grounding the Leonardo fantasy (Freud, 1910) on the vulture-headed Egyptian mother-goddess, Mut, extrapolated into the world of the bisexual, the polymorphous, the preoedipal, and the maternally sensuous; and the second, some three decades later (and therefore presumably more definitive?), in the Moses and Akhenaton (Amenhotep IV) story (Freud, 1939), reasserting the stern and moralistic patriarchy, the father principle adjuring the growing child away from the gratification of infantile symbiosis into the creation of the Puritanical world of moral principle and adult achievement. But I read this differently both from Schorske's identifying this juxtaposition of masculine/feminine or heterosexual/homosexual-bisexual as the central problematic of psychoanalysis at the hundred-year mark, or Robinson's assumption that it reflects Freud's final opting for the patriarchically hierarchical and Puritanical world of his surrounding Vienna and Central European culture. To me this juxtaposition posed by Schorske, as well as the other he stated of masculine England vis-à-vis feminine Paris and bisexual, anxiety-laden Rome, is rather an expression of the eternal dialectical two-sidedness of Freud containing within himself both the thrusts of the objective modern world of general and universal sciences as well as of the harbingers of what has come to be called the postmodern subjective world of contingency, context, and difference. Freud, to me, both is a creature of his time and transcends it.

And this is exactly where John Toews takes both Loewenberg and Suárez-Orozco so severely to task, declaring both to be exponents of a psychoanalytical imperialism based on the presumed primacy of psychoanalysis over other disciplines, and thereby clearly being the dominant window upon an otherwise obscure world. Toews charges that neither addresses Freudian theory as a specific historical/cultural discourse, but rather that both move in the opposite direction of asserting the universal psychic structure and processes of a male-centered psychology as the hidden wellsprings of meaning in our culture (thus conjoining the charge of a universalizing psychology and a privileged masculinism). To Toews that is the problem of psychohistory, that by remaining rigidly loyal to a psychoanalytic theory of a universal unconscious desire in its oedipal, object-related dimension, it cannot connect psychic processes to the specificities of history and of culture, and therefore fails to offer more than banal generalities to the complex cultural issues it takes under consideration.

I have already made clear my own position that these sharp disjunctions and dichotomies constitute an oversimplistic rendering of the subtle flexibility and adaptability of a psychoanalytic perspective. Witness for example the distinction that French analysts make between the pragmatism, meliorism, and quest for the objective and the veridical that they feel color what they call anglophone analysis, and their own francophone incorporation of semiotic and linguistic conceptions of culture into psychoanalytic discourse about the nature of psychic reality (and this is as true of the French who are opposed to the tenets of Lacan as it is of his followers). It is this encompassing of such diversity within contemporary psychoanalysis that makes possible a psychoanalytic theory that encompasses both the understanding of the mind in general and the specifics of differing history-bound and culture-bound individual, subjectively lived experience in particular.

But my own central concerns with Peter Loewenberg—and with Marcelo Suárez-Orozco—are other, centering on what to me is the major problem posed at least implicitly by Loewenberg, and inherent in both papers, but not really addressed at all by either of them. Loewenberg, in his psychoanalytically framed portrayal of the perils of nationalism run amok, that has marked so much of the unparalleled horrors of our twentieth century, provides instances, albeit small ones, in the Italian-Austrian border disputes and in the cantonal organization of Switzerland, where somehow these nationalism-grounded ethnic, cultural, and linguistic oppositions have been peacefully transcended. What Loewenberg does not provide, it seems to me, is any effort to explain—psychoanalytically or otherwise—how these instances came about, when we are faced, as I write this, with the tragic failures of Bosnia and Rwanda and Somalia. Loewenberg has stated so clearly the saving Swiss notion that all human communities are equal before the bar of history, but he includes not a word about how the Swiss have succeeded in living by this tenet, and at what price, as compared with the citizens of former Yugoslavia (or just Bosnia), who have not.

And Marcelo Suárez-Orozco, in his quite parallel anthropological disquisition on the meaning of the conflicts unleashed by soccer and its fans in so many parts of the world, does not even pose the issue of how these can be transcended, so that soccer can be returned to its supposed raison d'être as just a sport. Yet if psychoanalysis is ever to exert a civilizing and mitigating effect upon the excesses of our "civilization," this would be for me the central issue for our psychoanalytically informed cultural historians and cultural anthropologists to address.

The next sequence of papers, on psychoanalysis and literature, by Richard Almond on *Jane Eyre* and Paul Schwaber on the character of Leopold Bloom in *Ulysses*, with discussion of both by Jerome Winer, seem to me to focus on a different range of issues, though Robinson does see in these, as well as in the historical and anthropological contributions, the continued privileging of the universalizing and normalizing in the uncovering of literary narratives grounded in masculinist and heterosexist constructions of human relations (within Freud's paradigmatic oedipal struggle and its resolutions). To me, a central issue posed by Almond is his focus on the maturing and transformative power of a relationship, in this case the unfolding love relationship between Rochester and Jane Eyre, developing ineluctably across the startling reversals of its tumultuous vicissitudes. Almond has tried, intriguingly, to draw parallels between the highly contrived change processes of the successful psychoanalytic and psychotherapeutic encounter and the more ubiquitous, natural, and also serendipitous change processes that account for the character maturations and transformations of the fully lived life, using here the prototypical instance of a powerful love relationship. Schwaber, with a more complex tale, essayed a less ambitious effort, merely to make sense, internally within Joyce's novel, and without any claimed lessons for real life outside, of the crises of Bloom's Jewish identity and how the events of his father's suicide and his infant son's death reverberated under particular circumstances to illuminate his Jewishness in all its vulnerability and social isolation in Catholic Ireland.

Winer in his discussion gently questions Almond's suggestion of the comparabilities of the change processes inside the therapeutic situation with those that life in all its vicissitudes (including love) brings. Clearly Rochester both needs love and falls in love in a way that no analyst should. Where Winer does see a parallel is in the fact that in both instances—the stylized events within the therapeutic situation and the natural events of life circumstance and happening—central unconscious organizing fantasies can be enduringly altered (transformed), though not at all necessarily via comparable mechanisms. And this Winer pursues as well in his discussion of Schwaber's portrayal of Leopold Bloom. Here he traces the transformation of what he sees as Bloom's central fantasy, organized around the regressively re-created primal scene with its dual roles and dual identification, to the more developmentally advanced fantasy of the dual identification with the strong father and the trusting, dependent son whom he protects and nurtures. It is indeed a transforming sequence of psychic experiences, salvaging not only Bloom's Jewishness, but also his manhood.

But Winer raises another concern as well, one that has been a thorny issue in the efforts at psychoanalytic research, but one that reflects critical concerns in the broader array of social science and cultural scholarship as well. In psychoanalytic investigation, it was dubbed in a critical review by Seitz (1966) the "consensus problem." It describes the common observation that different clinicians, confronted with the same clinical data from the consulting room, can arrive at quite different (though not necessarily antithetical) and equally plausible dynamic formulations, and that we have no consensually established canons of inference to enable accepted and reliable judgments as to which formulation yields a truer understanding of the development and nature of the patient's pathology. Consensus is too often bent in the direction of authority or seniority; hardly an acceptable basis for proper knowledge accrual and scientific advance. Here this issue is introduced by Winer's inquiry as to whether Almond (in *his* formulation) took sufficient account of Jane Eyre as an early parent-loss case, with common enough consequent implications of that status for later psychic conflict and functioning. This is another of the issues simply touched on in this volume but one of real consequence for psychoanalytic clinical work, psychoanalytic research, and, to the extent that there are parallel issues in the psychoanalytic understandings of literature (and art), in that realm as well.

In all of this though, in the pieces by Almond, by Schwaber, and by Winer, there are allusions, but which are never explicitly taken up and grappled with, to the issue I previously raised of the limitations of psychoanalytic literary criticism. For when we talk about Jane's or Bloom's motives and meanings, we are actually talking about what reader and author separately, and differently or similarly, fantasize about a fictional character. These are not real people (no matter how much patterned upon actual people) with real lives and real histories, and they are certainly not subject to the psychoanalytic inquiry out of which our convictions in real analyses arrive. This to me is certainly a major defining issue for works of this genre, and as with the other issues I have discussed in this essay, I do not feel that it has either a simple or clear-cut (i.e. one-sided) solution.

From literature, the book moves to art and art criticism, both the art of high culture and that of the popular and everyday child's picture book. Here the book offers no discussant to extract shared themes and to contrast and compare how they are dealt with. Lynn Gamwell's is a very particularistic vision indeed, of the art of our century being an art of silence, of withdrawal into muteness as the quintessential expression of the loss of meaning that she sees in our past century's culture. This Gamwell relates to so many well-known phenomena of our twentieth-century world—the decline in unifying religious world views, the surfeit of communication especially at the most common levels of the pop culture, the threat (only very partially receded now) of nuclear extermination, the degradation of our biosphere and the inexorable pressures of its ever-growing population. All in all what she sees is a secular world of science (and misplaced faith in it), of atheism, of annihilation (unto actual genocide); a world, that is, where words and cultural expressions have lost meaning and must be always distrusted, where art necessarily becomes as mute as the proverbial psychoanalyst.

That this is but a singular and particular vision, perhaps shared by some not-quantifiable cohort, is made clear in the implicit confrontation of Gamwell by Ellen Handler Spitz's vibrant exposition of the very positive formative role that the best children's books play in the maturational and developmental process of growing children. And *pari passu,* how the psychoanalytic understanding of the organizing fantasies that reverberate in these books can illuminate their appeal and their central meanings, and thus shed light on the interplay (the reciprocal illumination) between developmental theory and the lived and evoked life experience, and on the mediating role of this child-centered art form in establishing and conveying these

meanings and resolutions. Ultimately it is part of our understanding of both the creation and the transmission of culture.

Which brings me to the final section of the book, on philosophy and the culture at large, with presentations by Charles
Hanly, a philosopher turned psychoanalyst, and Janine Chasseguet-Smirgel, a psychoanalyst with philosophical interests.
Hanly's central topic is philosophy itself, and his essay com-
prises a spirited defense of the continuing position of a materialist, natural science, and evolutionary, biological ontology for
psychoanalysis, and with it, an adherence to a correspondence
theory of truth (rather than to a coherence theory of truth as
espoused by those wedded to a hermeneutic, phenomenological
and/or linguistically based conceptualization of the nature of
our field). Hanly's posture, with its defense of empiricism, of a
verification theory of meaning by way of established correspon-
dences to an existent external reality "out there," and its reality-
bound understanding of human nature, would of course be seen
as a regressive, inertial drag by those (like Toews most emphati-
cally) seeking to place psychoanalysis most firmly within the
tenets of the extremes of postmodernist subjectivity and contextualization. But from another perspective, Hanly's offering
can also be read as a reminder that in the ongoing dialectic between modernist and postmodernist world views, neither pole
should be (or can be) submerged by the other.

In distinction from Hanly's chapter, that by Janine Chasseguet-Smirgel can be seen as an effort at applied philosophy,
psychoanalytically framed of course. Her discourse roams over
devil religions (Satanic cults), perversions, the pervasiveness
of anal temptations and the tug of anal-sadistic regressions,
and the differing emphases and messages in the Luciferian
and Satanic representations of the anti-God. Her own unifying
theme in these various manifestations of organized human be-

havior is that of the deliberate and systematic destruction of reality, which is constituted by differentiation and composed of differences, with the intent to reduce all of reality to an undifferentiated and chaotic rubble. Within the perverse character this entails the wiping out of what the French call the double difference, the differences of gender and of generation, in favor of the anal sameness of meaning that characterizes the sexual perversions. This is a reversal of what Chasseguet-Smirgel defines as "the natural order of things"; a return to the medieval psychology of alchemy in which anything can be transmuted into anything else, and represents a permanent temptation to the human mind, explicitly enacted in the moral and sexual perversions. In its sweep this is a comprehensive and explicitly psychoanalytic rendering of a whole segment of our world and its culture, as well as of a whole cohort of deviant individuals within it, in both publicly organized and also privately materialized enactments; in both the culture and in individual psyches. Though it too can be read critically for its universalizings—of everything from cult religions to the Marquis de Sade's literary fantasies—it can also be read as an exemplar of one kind of cultural illumination that a committed and steadfast psychoanalytic perspective can bring.

It was Eli Sagan's task to encompass both Hanly's straight philosophy, seeking to establish the philosophical assumptions that underlie the psychoanalytic vision that Hanly finds congenial, and Chasseguet-Smirgel's applied philosophy, seeking to explain (but not explain away) a variety of cultural and individual psychic expressions under one particular psychoanalytic umbrella. Sagan's choice was to sidestep this specific task in favor of a more general underlying issue: the need for a psychoanalytic sociology on a par with the far more developed psychoanalytic psychology. Sagan reminds us that, despite our conventional perspective, psychoanalysis actually did not start that way with Freud. Though Freud is properly credited as the originator of psychoanalysis as both a theory of the (individual) mind and a treatment for the disorders of the mind; he also, if we take the full corpus of his work on society (including *Totem and Taboo, Group Psychology, The Future of an Illusion, Civilization and Its Discontents, Moses and Monotheism*, and many, many shorter works), can be said to have paid almost as much attention to the disorders of society as to the disorders of the psyche—with the need for comparable amelioration in both arenas. Sagan outlines his reasons, some more convincing than others, for the subsequent lag in the development of an articulated psychoanalytic sociology, with a few side references to some who have ventured into this still largely unformulated and unsystematized realm. For our purposes, it is another of the wide open vistas for scholarly intersection, between psychoanalysis and a neighboring discipline of human custom and behavior, that this volume holds forth for us.

Put altogether, what can we make of all this? In counterpoint to Robinson's endeavor to see the commonalities and the unities of perspective discernible through the various and varying chapters of the book, and to ground them within the framework of the century-long shift between the two fin de siècles, from the modernist to the postmodernist world view, with special focus on the evidences of psychoanalytic holding back from being quite up to date in our new world, I have tried rather to reflect the diversity of themes, of issues, of problems, essentially of areas of yet-to-be-explored scholarship that emerge in any such multidisciplinary effort to locate psychoanalysis in our culture today. Along with this intent, and of course related to it, is my thrust to place psychoanalysis into a reverberating and dialectical tension between modernism and postmodernism, not to be fully captured by either stance; a position that, as I have indicated, Freud himself was also party to, more than he is usually given credit for.

Such a theoretical preference as I have just stated demands, of course, its own justification, or statement of credo, which I offer, in closing this summarizing chapter, by way of extended quotation from an article I have written for a very different purpose:

> The "postmodern sensibility in psychoanalysis" . . . has indeed been a useful corrective to a number of problematic, and by now outmoded, aspects of analytic thinking, like the tendencies toward a misplaced scientism that inhere in a natural science ego psychological paradigm; or the seduction into an authoritarian stance by the analyst committed to the erstwhile modern ideal of the presumed objective observer who can always correctly assume the role of "arbiter of the patient's reality" (in a phrase from Gill) and declare accurately what is transference distortion and what is realistic perception; or the conception that there are no theoretical limits, other than in biology, to the uncovering of the past of a knowable mental life and development.
>
> Where, however, the postmodern perspective creates a problematic for my argument concerning psychoanalysis and the analytic therapies, is in its tacit discouragement, as misguided and ultimately fruitless, of any quest that aspires towards ever increasing clarity and knowable precision of consensually agreed conceptual distinctions; since in their essence our understandings are always historicized and contextualized, they are always no more than

social constructions, geared to what is considered satisfactory or unsatisfactory understanding within each particular sociohistorical zeitgeist. Yet, we need not be caught up in the extremes of a relativist and socially constructed model of the postmodern world anymore than in the fully objective, natural-science model of the earlier modern world. It is true that psychoanalytic treatments involve two inter-acting subjectivities and sensibilities, and depending on the experiences of the particular encounter over time, can result in a range of finally agreed-upon story lines. But it is also true that, although analyst and patient together socially construct an understanding of the patient's life experience, that life experience also exists independently of the analyst, and that therefore some story lines fit better than others, correspond better to the felt life experience, and that analyst and patient can reasonably openmindedly arrive at such judgments. There is still a real world, a reality, "out there" or else we could not have arrived at a science and a technology that works, and provides us the material world within which we live. (Wallerstein, 1999)

The above paragraphs were written in another context, of course, that of the impact of the diffusion of postmodern perspectives on our understandings of the nature and the mechanisms of the therapeutic process, rather than that of the perspectives of this book, those of locating psychoanalysis contextually within the cultural evolution of the past century, and of interrelating psychoanalysis with the many facets of our culture with which it imbricates. But my point is the same; that we, psychoanalysis, and our culture at large, are within a dialectic between modern and postmodern perspectives that can provide the best possible platform for our continuous advances into the next century, so long as we do not feel impelled into a one-sided adherence, with all the truncating of our possibilities that that would entail. This, in closing, brings me full circle to the effort at unifying perspectives presented by Paul Robinson in his introductory chapter.

References

Auden, W. H. (1940). In Memory of Sigmund Freud. In *Another Time.* London: Faber and Faber.

Eissler, Kurt R. (1933). The Effect of the Structure of the Ego on Psychoanalytic Technique. *J. Amer. Psychoanal. Assn.* 1:104–143.

Freud, Sigmund (1895). Project for a Scientific Psychology. *Standard Edition* 1:281–397, 1966.

———— (1910). Leonardo da Vinci and a Memory of his Childhood. *Standard Edition* 11:56–137, 1957.

———— (1939). Moses and Monotheism: Three Essays. *Standard Edition* 23:1–137, 1964.

Greenberg, Jay R., and Mitchell, Stephen A. (1983). *Object Relations in Psychoanalytic Theory.* Cambridge: Harvard Univ. Press, pp. 437.

Hoffman, Irwin Z. (1991). Discussion: Toward a Social-Constructivist View of the Psychoanalytic Situation. *Psychoanal. Dial.* 1:74–105.

Lipton, Samuel D. (1977). The Advantages of Freud's Technique as Shown in his Analysis of the Rat-Man. *Int. J. Psycho-Anal.* 58:255–273.

Loewald, Hans (1960). On the Therapeutic Action of Psycho-Analysis. *Int. J. Psycho-Anal.* 41:16–33.

Robinson, Paul (1993). *Freud and His Critics.* Berkeley: Univ. Calif. Press, pp. 281.

Schafer, Roy (1992). *Retelling a Life: Narration and Dialogue in Psychoanalysis.* New York: Basic, pp. 328.

Seitz, Philip F. D. (1966). The Consensus Problem in Psychoanalytic Research. In Louis A. Gottschalk and Arthur H. Auerbach, eds., *Methods of Research in Psychotherapy.* New York: Appleton-Century-Crofts, pp. 209–225.

Stone, Leo (1961). *The Psychoanalytic Situation: An Examination of Its Development and Essential Nature.* New York: Int. Univ. Press, pp. 160.

Wallerstein, Robert S. (1988). One Psychoanalysis or Many? *Int. J. Psycho-Anal.* 69:5–21.

——— (1999). Psychoanalysis and Psychotherapy: A Half-Century Perspective. In *Festschrift in Honor of Joseph Sandler,* March.

Index

evolutionary stage theory of, 239, 272-73, 275, 276-77; and France, 2, 14-17, 25, 30-32, 367; and gender differences, 14-19, 107-8; on group formation, 106; and Hegel, 270-75; and history, 108-13, 268, 269, 272-73; on homosexuality, 101; iconoclasm of, 307; on instinctual dissatisfaction, 304-5; on isolation, 320; on Jews and Jewishness, 11, 13, 17-20, 22, 24-26, 30, 107, 204; on Leonardo, 2, 4, 33n20, 33n22, 269; literary references in works of, 4, 117, 307; on love, 350; medical research by, 293-94; metapsychology of, 294-95, 357; and Michelangelo's Moses, 4, 19-20; on morality, 300-305, 332, 343; on narcissistic desire for identity, 105; on oedipus complex, 111, 112, 117, 300-303, 314, 335, 369; on "oral" phase of life, 51; on perversions, 313-15, 318, 335; on primal scene, 208, 212; on primary process, 179; and Project for Scientific Psychology, 357; on psychoanalysis as disturbing to peace of world, 294; on psychotherapeutic relief, 187, 212; reading and research by, 345; on religion, 221-22; reputation of, 1-2, 8; in Rome and Rome neurosis of, 17-20, 24, 30, 367; Ryle on, 298; on science, 221, 277, 358-59; self-analysis of, 18, 108; on society, 338-39, 375; on stability of self and reality, 6; on transference, 199; on unconscious, 224, 227, 277;
universalism of, 3-6, 111; verbal optimism of, 225; and vernacular psychology, 306-7; on Weltanschauung of psychoanalysis, 271; on World War I, 305
— works: "Antithetical Meaning of Primal Words," 23; "Child Is Being Beaten," 204, 324; *Civilization and Its Discontents,* 338, 339, 375; "Contributions to the Psychology of Love," 23; "Disturbance of Memory on the Acropolis," 19; *Ego and the Id,* 338-39; "Female Sexuality," 23; *Future of an Illusion,* 221, 338, 375; *Group Psychology and the Analysis of the Ego,* 101, 106, 338, 375; "Human Bisexuality," 19, 20; *Interpretation of Dreams,* 17, 269, 271-72, 314; *Moses and Monotheism,* 2, 12, 14, 20, 22, 23-32, 205, 225, 338, 375; *Mourning and Melancholia,* 300; "Obsessive Actions and Religious Practices," 314-15; "Recommendations to Physicians Practicing Psychoanalysis," 226; *Totem and Taboo,* 23, 272, 314, 338, 375; "Uncanny," 286; *Why War?* 338
Friedlander, K., 193
Fromm, E., 80, 81
Frustration-aggression hypothesis, 67

Gallina (chicken) motif, 86-87, 92n23
Gamwell, L., vii, 7, 219-238, 372
Gay, P., 1, 294
Geertz, C., 73-74, 97-99, 113n1
Geisteswissenschaften, 279